Access your Online Resources

Working with Children's Language is accompanied by a number of printable online materials, designed to ensure this resource best supports your professional needs.

Activate your online resources:

Go to www.routledge.com/cw/speechmark and click on the cover of this book.

Click the 'Sign in or Request Access' button and follow the instructions in order to access the resources.

Working with Children's Language

This revised and updated second edition of *Working with Children's Language* has been created to support practitioners who work with young children with delayed language acquisition.

Rooted in a developmental theory of language learning, it covers topics such as attention control and listening, the role of play, verbal comprehension and the acquisition of spoken expressive language. Each chapter offers a straightforward overview of current research relating to the specific language skill before introducing a wealth of targeted games and activities that can help support the development of those skills.

Key features include:

- A structured approach to language learning that can be followed as a programme or adapted for informal use by individual practitioners.
- Accessible activities, games and ideas suitable for small group or individual intervention, linked to specific aims based on developmental norms.
- Photocopiable and downloadable resources, including a record sheet to track progress in each skill against aims and outcomes for individual children.

Clearly linking theory and practice in an engaging and easy-to-follow format, this is an invaluable resource to support children in early years settings and Key Stage 1 whose language is delayed, but who are otherwise developing normally. It is a must-have book for early years practitioners, teachers, SEND professionals and speech and language therapists with varying levels of experience.

Diana Williams initially trained as a speech and language therapist before moving into higher education as a lecturer and then as an educational developer. She is the author of several publications that provide practical resources for therapists and practitioners working with children in the Early Years Foundation Stage. These include the practical manuals *Early Listening Skills* for use with children who have hearing loss and *Early Visual Skills* for use with children who have underdeveloped visual perceptual skills. She also created the popular board game 'Find the Link', designed for use by individuals and small groups to develop word finding and categorisation skills.

The *Working With* Series

The *Working With* series provides speech and language therapists with a range of 'go-to' resources, full of well-sourced, up-to-date information regarding specific disorders. Underpinned by robust theoretical foundations and supported by intervention options and exercises, every book ensures that the reader has access to the latest thinking regarding diagnosis, management and treatment options.

Written in a fully accessible style, each book bridges theory and practice and offers ready-to-use and well-rehearsed practical material, including guidance on interventions, management advice, and therapeutic resources for the client, parent or carer. The series is an invaluable resource for practitioners, whether speech and language therapy students, or more experienced clinicians.

Books in the series include:

Working with Children's Language, Second edition
Diana Williams
2022 / pb: 9780367467913

Working with Voice Disorders: Theory and Practice, 3rd edition
Stephanie Martin
2021 / pb: 9780863889462

Working with Children's Language

A Practical Resource for Early Years Professionals

Second Edition

Diana Williams

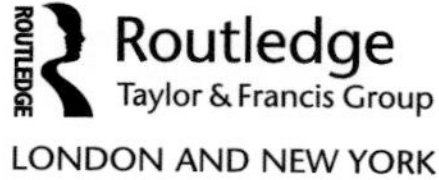

LONDON AND NEW YORK

Second edition published 2022
by Routledge
2 Park Square, Milton Park, Abingdon, Oxon, OX14 4RN

and by Routledge
605 Third Avenue, New York, NY 10158

Routledge is an imprint of the Taylor & Francis Group, an informa business

First edition published by Speechmark 1997

British Library Cataloguing-in-Publication Data
A catalogue record for this book is available from the British Library

Library of Congress Cataloging-in-Publication Data
A catalog record for this book has been requested

ISBN: 978-1-032-06382-9 (hbk)
ISBN: 978-0-367-46791-3 (pbk)
ISBN: 978-1-003-03110-9 (ebk)

DOI: 10.4324/9781003031109

Typeset in Interstate
by Apex CoVantage, LLC

Access the companion website: www.routledge.com/cw/speechmark

Contents

Acknowledgements

I would like to thank colleagues in health and education who contributed to the first edition of *Working with Children's Language*, which laid the foundation for this second edition. I am also indebted to the families and the children I have had the pleasure to work with and who helped frame the experience from which this book has grown. I would especially like to acknowledge the encouragement and generous support in making the decision to undertake this project from my co-author in the first edition, Jackie Cooke. Her input was very much missed this time round.

INTRODUCTION

Now in a revised and updated second edition, *Working with Children's Language* is a photocopiable resource to support language development in children within early years settings and Key Stage 1. This manual offers a broad range of accessible ideas and practical activities based on a developmental theory of language acquisition. It is designed primarily to support language development in children whose language is delayed but who are otherwise developing normally. These children develop language in a typical pattern but are delayed in their rate of acquisition. Many of them have difficulty learning language in an incidental fashion and may need specific intervention. This is reflected in the book's fairly structured approach to language teaching; however, the activities can easily be adapted for more informal use and are suitable for use by a range of early years practitioners, therapists and teachers.

How the book is organised

The five chapters examine different aspects of language skills and are divided into two parts: theory and activities. Chapter 1 describes the development of the infant's early communication skills from birth to the appearance of first words. Chapter 2 outlines the development of attention control and listening skills, examining their importance to language learning. Chapter 3 explains the role of different types of play in language development and stresses the importance of play to the development of social interaction skills. Chapter 4 looks at the comprehension of spoken language, beginning with the first verbal labels and early concepts through to longer, more complex, utterances and question forms. Chapter 5 describes the growth of expressive language, from the child's first words to complex utterances, taking into account the functions, meanings and form of language. The chapters are interrelated as the concept of separating the different areas of a child's development is only possible in theory; in practice we are faced with the whole child, developing along a number of parallel lines. For this reason, there is some cross-referencing between chapters, and certain skills have been included in more than one chapter.

DOI: 10.4324/9781003031109-1

How to use this book

Theory

Each chapter has a straightforward overview of theory relating to the key stages of language development with reference to current research and practice. It includes an outline of some of the most pertinent factors that might impact on the development of specific skill areas. This section serves to introduce the reader to the work of practitioners and researchers in the field of language acquisition and language impairment that readers can access using the bibliographic information.

Activities

Each chapter has a section outlining practical suggestions and activities to support language development subdivided into specific skill areas.

Chapter1 has activities that support early communication skills written specifically with parents and caregivers in mind. Practitioners may wish to use this photocopiable section to provide advice and guidance that encourages parents'/caregivers' communication with their child.

Chapters 2 to 5 have activities to support the development of specific language skills through a range of individual or group interventions. These sections are introduced with a set of *general guidelines* written in easy-to-read bullet points. They are subdivided according to the particular skill that they develop, for example, *Attention to people: Activities to encourage eye contact*. Each skill area has clear *aims*, *outcomes* and *strategies* with a list of *suggested materials and resources*. The reader can look up the goal that they are intending to achieve and find a range of accessible games, activities and ideas listed there. These activity sections can be photocopied and distributed to other practitioners who support the child's learning and development.

General guidelines

General guidelines provide advice and guidance on intervention relevant to the aspect of language addressed in the activities section. Guidelines in Chapter1 are written specifically with parents/caregivers in mind. Chapters 2 to 5 have guidelines highlighting relevant approaches to language teaching for use by practitioners, including advice on recording observations of the child's development.

Each skill area has:

Aims and outcomes

The *aim/s* provide a general statement about the overall goal for learning.

For example:

Aim: To recognise and understand familiar objects by name even when these objects are not in a familiar context or routine.

The *outcome/s* focus on the child and the result of their learning. They describe what the child will be able to say and do when they have made progress.

For example:

Outcome: Identifies familiar objects by name without contextual cues.

The aims and outcomes are suggestions that practitioners can adapt to create SMART targets for a specific child or group of children, if applicable.

Specific – This needs to be specific to the individual child. What is familiar to the child? What is the targeted vocabulary? In what ways will the child demonstrate knowledge and understanding? For example, the more general term 'identifies' might be specified as 'looks toward', 'points to', 'fetches', 'gestures' or 'names'.

Measurable – How can you see progress towards the outcome? This might be measured in terms of frequency or amount – How often? How many?

Achievable – What are the individual needs of the child? Is it age appropriate? What are the child's desired outcomes?

Realistic – Is it functional? How does it fit with the child's daily routine? What resources are available?

Time-bound – Set a time frame for achieving outcomes with a realistic date for review.

A SMART target might be 'Points to three everyday objects (cup, spoon, plate) 5/6 times on request by the adult during mealtimes' (Add review date).

Further guidance on how to write goals and set SMART targets are contained in the *Statutory Framework for the Early Years Foundation Stage* (2021); *Early years: Guide to the 0 to 25, SEND code of practice* (2014); and *Special Educational Needs and Disability (SEND) Code of Practice: 0–25 years* (2015).

A photocopiable record sheet is provided at the end of Chapters 2 through 5 to record progress against aims and outcomes for specific children.

Strategies

Specific advice is provided to support the planning of activities and the choice of teaching approaches in regard to that skill area. These should be used alongside the general guidelines for the chapter.

Suggested materials and resources

A list of suitable materials, toys and equipment is suggested for each skill area. These items have been selected as the most relevant for the activities in a particular section but may be adapted or substituted as necessary. Objects, toys and homemade items provide an opportunity to link activities with the cultural experience of the child. The list can also be used to stimulate ideas for adapting and extending activities and games. Using a variety of materials in this way will also help the child to generalise their skills.

Activities

The activities address key skills within each area of language development and are linked to specific aims based on developmental norms. Additional ideas are provided for older children with links to the curriculum where applicable.

Suggestions are made for both individual work with the child whilst other activities are more suitable for groups. It is useful to consider the benefits of both types of intervention.

Small group intervention:

- Provides a more natural communication situation.
- Provides more opportunity for learning social skills and conventions.
- Eases the pressure on individual children.
- Makes healthy use of children's competitive instincts.
- Allows a wider range of games and activities to be used.
- Helps the child to practise and generalise skills they have learnt in individual sessions.

Individual one-to-one intervention:

- Enables more time and concentration to be given to specific tasks.
- Provides the child with undivided attention.
- Reduces environmental distractions and allows the child to focus on the task.

General guidelines for learning and teaching

Teaching should be based on careful formative assessment that regularly reviews the child's progress (DfE, 2021). It is strongly advised that any child with a suspected speech, language or communication problem should be initially referred to a speech and language therapist for a comprehensive assessment.

Certain teaching and learning principles have been stressed throughout the book. It is important to remember these when designing an individual intervention programme for a child or a group of children. However, some factors are common to all language teaching, and these are highlighted here.

- Take account of all the variables that may affect the child's language competence, for example, his attention control, memory and dexterity.
- Plan activities that are developmentally appropriate for the child, taking into account their level of functioning in other areas, such as symbolic understanding, language development and performance skills.
- Choose materials and resources that acknowledge and build upon the child's interests; for example, a fascination with minibeasts can be incorporated into activities for learning prepositions.
- Provide materials and resources that are relevant to all the children's cultures and reflect diverse communities.
- When planning an activity, it is important to consider the child's level of symbolic understanding. For example, miniature toys require a greater degree of symbolisation than real objects and therefore increase the complexity of the activity for the child.
- The adult's language should be modified according to the child's level of comprehension.
- Ensure the child is physically comfortable and generally at ease with the situation.
- Allow children to play freely with new equipment before they are asked to perform specified activities with it.
- Teaching should normally proceed in small steps that support the consolidation and extension of learning and development.

- Children should proceed at their own pace – some may need carefully graded levels of activities, while others will not.
- Remember that children will not all progress at the same pace, so activities and approaches will need to be differentiated for individual children.
- Repetition and practice are essential for consolidation of learning.
- Generalisation activities, and carry-over into the home environment where possible, must be built into the child's language programme.
- Parents/caregivers and other significant people must be included wherever possible.

Teaching strategies

Some commonly used techniques are included below:

Role reversal: as the name suggests, the adult and child swap roles; for example, the adult models a word by naming a picture for the child to find, and then the child names a picture for the adult to find.

Forward-chaining: the child starts off an activity and the adult completes it. Gradually, children are expected to do more and more of the task by themselves.

Back-chaining: the adult shows the child an activity and leaves them to carry out the last step; for example, the adult builds up a sequence of red and blue beads and helps the child to place the final bead to complete the sequence. They repeat the activity, gradually leaving more and more for the child to do. This has the advantage of giving the child the satisfaction of completing a task.

Forward- and backward-chaining are techniques often applied to the teaching of multistep tasks. Both methods have been found to be effective, and choice is governed by the context, activity and preference of the adult and child (Slocum and Tiger, 2011).

Commentary:

Self-talk – adult commentary is focused on what the *adult* is seeing, hearing, touching or doing. The link between words and their referent must be clear so the child associates what they are hearing with the object, action or event. The adult can also vocalise about their thoughts, so the child is exposed to examples of critical thinking, for instance, making links, generating new ideas and problem solving. Questions can be posed and answered by the adult – What might happen next? What if I do this? Why did that happen?

Parallel talk – adult commentary is focused on what the *child* is seeing, hearing, touching or doing. This should be a real-time experience as things happen, so the link between words and their referent is made clear. The adult can also use this time to model critical thinking, so if a tower of bricks topples, the adult might comment: "What happened?" - pause - "it fell down", "too tall".

Such commentary can be conversational in nature with a back-and-forth element as the adult leaves pauses for the child to respond; however, there should be no requirement or prompts for children to copy words or make any sort of response.

Modelling: the adult gives many examples of the required language targets, which is useful for reinforcing and generalising learning. These differ from recasts (see next section, 'Responding to Errors') as the models are not dependent on what the child is saying.

Expansion: the adult expands on what the child has said by filling in missing words, for example, child instructs the adult "brush" as they point to a dolly, and the adult models back an expansion, "brush *dolly*". The original meaning and intention of the child's utterance is retained.

Extension: the adult extends what the child has said by adding in more descriptive words, for example, "the car is beeping" might be extended to "the red car is beeping" or "the big car is beeping". Again, the original meaning and intention of the child's utterance is retained, with the additional information being optional.

Both expansion and extension can also be used to provide an example of a specific language target.

Sentence Closure: the adult models a word or structure and then elicits it, by requiring the child to finish the sentence, for example, 'I'm drinking milk. Mary's drinking milk. You're drinking...'.

Responding to errors

It is best to decide beforehand upon a strategy for responding to the child's errors so that they can be dealt with swiftly and consistently by everyone involved with the child. Here are some suggestions for responding to errors:

- **Recasting** (Cleave et al., 2015) or **reformulating** (Clark, 2018) is a way to provide the correct example following an omission or error by the child in their speech or language. The words and meaning of the child's utterance are retained, but corrections are offered by the adult. If the child mispronounces a word, for example, "dups" for "cups" the adult models the word clearly in response - "Yes, I need *cups*". There should be no attempt to prompt imitations or repetitions from the child. Omissions and language errors can be responded to in the same way. For example, "I runned in park" might be recast as "You ran in the park" or "I want eat" might be recast as "I want to eat too". It is important that a reformulation is made within the next conversational turn by the adult, so feedback is given immediately to the child (Clark, 2018).

Until the child has fully consolidated a new skill, errors are to be expected. In the early stages of learning, every appropriate effort should be rewarded as you gradually shape the correct responses. Slowly reduce the rewards and reinforcement as the child becomes more proficient.

Glossary of terms for the most prevalent developmental conditions that impact on language development

Information on the language and communication difficulties associated with these conditions are highlighted within the 'Factors Affecting' section of each chapter.

Attention-Deficit Hyperactivity Disorder

Children with Attention-Deficit Hyperactivity Disorder (ADHD) typically present with shorter attention spans, impulsivity and hyperactivity (Barkley, 2006). It is a neurodevelopmental disorder that affects children and adolescents but often continues into adulthood. Approximately 60 to 100 per cent of children with ADHD will have one or more other conditions (Gnanavel et al., 2019) including poor pragmatic language skills (Green et al., 2014) and dyslexia.

Autism

Autism (also known as Autistic Spectrum Disorder (ASD)) is a developmental disability that affects how individuals perceive the world and interact with others, with 1 per cent of people on the autistic spectrum (National Autistic Society, 2021). It is a lifelong condition that affects individuals differently and to varying degrees, hence the term 'spectrum'. Autism affects many different areas of development but in particular social communication and interaction.

Developmental Language Disorder

Children with Developmental Language Disorder (DLD) present with a significant impairment in learning and using language, which is unlikely to resolve, particularly without specialist help, (RCSLT, 2020). There is significant variability between children, who may have difficulty with a range of skills including understanding and processing language, use of language, and social interaction. DLD is "not acquired or associated with a known biomedical cause"

(Bishop et al., 2017, p. 2), although it may occur alongside other conditions like ADHD, developmental dyslexia and speech sound disorders (RCSLT, 2020). (Readers should note that it may also be referred to in the literature under the previous terminology of 'Specific Language Impairment'.)

Research has shown that it affects two children in every class of 30 pupils (Norbury et al., 2016) and is likely to persist through childhood and into adulthood. Speech and language therapists provide management and targeted therapy for children and young people with Developmental Language Disorder, and a referral for assessment is essential if there are concerns about an individual child.

Hearing loss

There are two main types of hearing loss in children:

1 A permanent sensorineural deafness due to impairment in the inner ear (cochlear) or auditory pathways to the brain.
2 A conductive hearing loss affecting the outer ear, ear canal and middle ear often associated with otitis media with effusion (glue ear). The National Deaf Children's Society (2017) report that 8 out of 10 children will experience glue ear before the age of 10.

Children vary in the level or degree of hearing loss, which might be described as mild, moderate, severe or profound. Some hearing losses affect all frequencies equally (flat loss), while others may affect a specific range (for example, a high frequency loss). A bilateral loss affects both ears, and a unilateral loss affects one ear. Specialist support and advice is available from Teachers of the Deaf and Speech and Language Therapists.

Vision impairment

Vision impairment where a child is blind or partially sighted might arise from damage to or dysfunction of the eye, optic nerve or the brain. Children will vary in the amount and effects of a sight loss; for example, some may have difficulties seeing at a distance, others seeing close up, and some may have a narrow field of vision. Nearly 50 per cent of children with a vision impairment will have other conditions, including hearing loss and learning disabilities (RNIB, 2021). A specialist teacher of vision-impaired children will be able to offer support and advice.

1

EARLY COMMUNICATION SKILLS

DOI: 10.4324/9781003031109-2

Introduction

This chapter describes the development of early communication skills from birth to the emergence of the first spoken words by the child. The skills described are not just basic to early communication but are fundamental to the development of language, cognition and social interaction. It provides an introduction to the topics covered in other chapters, and it should be read in conjunction with these to give a wider view of the developing child. The early communication guidelines and activities are written specifically with parents and caregivers in mind. Practitioners may wish to use this photocopiable section to provide advice and guidance that encourages parents'/caregivers' communication with their child.

Factors affecting early communication skills

There are many factors that might affect the development of a child's early communication skills.

- **A sensory impairment:** A sensory impairment affecting hearing or vision is likely to impact on a child's early communication skills.
  Examples include:
  - *Hearing loss:*
    Hearing loss impacts on the quality and quantity of vocalisations produced by an infant with a significant hearing loss when compared with their hearing peers (Fagan, 2014). Infants vocalised less often (Fagan, 2014), and the production of canonical syllables occurred much later (Iyer and Oller, 2008).
  - *Vision impairment:*
    Studies have found that children with significant vision impairment show delayed exploratory play, with more repetitive, stereotyped behaviour towards objects (van den Broek et al., 2017). They also take more time to explore objects, as they see or touch only a small part of an object, and it was more difficult for them to discover switches and levers.
- **An underlying neurodevelopmental disorder:**
  - *Autism or Autistic Spectrum Disorder (ASD):* Reciprocal interactions between parents/caregivers and infants who have early onset ASD are disrupted with reduced motor activities and vocalisations by the child (Apicella et al., 2013).
- **Environmental influences:**
  - *Child-directed speech:* There have been many studies of parental language which have shown that parents modify their language when talking to the child. The

parents simplify their language and use shorter sentences (Snow, 1972; Broen, 1972; Elmlinger et al., 2019) in what is known as infant-directed speech. This reduction in complexity does not affect the meaning or reduce the information the parent wants to convey. The quality and quantity of this infant-directed speech is important in promoting infants' language acquisition (Rowe, 2008).

- *Socio-economic status:* Research suggests that children from lower socio-economic status families are more likely to have language difficulties. This seems to relate to the quantity and quality of input, with parents speaking less to children (Rowe, 2008), in a more directive manner, using a simpler and less diverse vocabulary (Hoff, 2013).

- **Biomedical conditions:** Babies born prematurely are at a higher risk of difficulties in the mother–infant relationship. For example, preterm babies have been found to look and smile less in face to face interactions with their mothers and are generally less responsive to her communicative initiations (Feldman and Eidelman, 2006).

Always seek professional advice where there are concerns regarding delayed or atypical development.

Early interactions

Although the child is communicating from the moment of their first cry, there is a fundamental difference between their behaviour before they are 6 months and after about 9 months. For the younger child, vocalising is not purposeful; it is a reflex action, reflecting feelings of hunger, discomfort and pleasure (Bloom and Lahey, 1978; Stark, 1980). The older child, however, does communicate with intention (Bates, 1976; Halliday, 1975), and vocalisations start to have meaning between 9 and 12 months. Intention develops as the child becomes aware that their behaviour has an effect on their environment and that movements and sounds can stand for feelings, needs and desires (Franklin, 2014). Both these realisations are helped by the parents'/caregivers' responsiveness to the baby's behaviour (Bloom, 1988).

Early actions and vocalisations are reflexive, but parent/caregivers give them meaning and respond to them (Oller, 2000; Cole, 1982). This is the beginning of a social interaction; for example, the child smiles, so the parent/caregiver smiles back and probably also talks and plays with the child, which leads to further smiling. The forms of these communicative episodes gradually change over time as the child matures and is able to take a more active part.

Attention to a common referent

The ability to jointly attend to a common referent is a necessary prerequisite to communication and language development (Houston-Price et al., 2006). Until 3 to 4 months of age the infant's focus of attention is mainly towards the parent/caregiver, with a preference for looking at faces (Adamson, 2019). In response, the parents/caregivers concentrate upon the child, playing with their toes, tickling their hands, imitating their mouth movements and facial expressions.

After 5 months the infant is less interested in this social interaction, as they become attracted to objects and events external to themselves (Gratier et al., 2015). By 6 months the infant can recognise and follow another person's line of regard, which means that the parents/caregivers can direct the child's attention to objects and events in the environment (Cole, 1982). At this stage, the child's focus is very much on the object, whether in exploratory play or as a passive observer of others.

By around 9 months infants are able to engage in a triadic interaction (Sharma and Cockerill, 2014), shifting attention between the adult and the object of mutual interest. At first the infant will look back and forth, and then later start showing or giving the object to the adult. Once mutual attention to the child's object of interest is established, the adult gains the infant's attention by using a high-pitched voice, exaggerated intonation, facial expression and eye contact, bringing the face close to the child's line of regard and smiling (Bruner, 1975; Stern, 1977).

By 12 months the child is able to initiate joint attention taking a more active role in directing the adult's attention with a point. There is a shared understanding of intentionality and a mutual desire to engage in collaborative communication.

Co-actions

Co-actions are activities that the child and adult engage in simultaneously. They begin at about 3 months and include mutual gaze, sustained eye contact, synchronised head movements, making faces, smiling and co-vocalisations, all incorporated into play routines (Nomikou et al., 2013; Stern, 1974). Either the parent or the child may initiate the activity, and the other joins in a reciprocal, synchronised interaction (Reyna and Pickler, 2009). At 3 months vocalisations will increase when an adult responds to the child, especially by talking, cooing or making other sounds (Weisburg, 1963). Mutual gaze and co-vocalisations are particularly common and provide experiences that can be shared by both parent and child. These behaviours are available to the baby almost immediately and are exploited by the parents, who adapt their own responses to the changing capacity of their infant (Rączaszek-Leonardi et al., 2013).

Alternate actions

Gradually, at about 4 to 6 months, co-actions give way to alternate exchanges reflecting the infant's emerging interest in object play and joint activity (Gratier et al., 2015). Initially the parent imitates the child; immediately, they cease an activity to encourage him to repeat it. The child repeats the activity, and an alternate exchange is established. If the infant doesn't respond, then the parent takes both turns, leaving a pause for the child's response until they do join in appropriately (Snow, 1977; Stern, 1977). Parents also hold two-way conversations with their children, taking both speaking parts but leaving appropriate pauses for the baby's coos and gurgles. Later, the parents initiate an exchange by imitating a sound or facial expression they know the child can do and encouraging the child to join in (Cole, 1982).

Co-vocalisations still take place and tend to predominate during times of high excitement and emotion while alternate exchanges occur at mid-levels of arousal (Stern, 1977). Stern believes that this pattern has a parallel in adulthood; for instance, people tend to wait their turn in a rational discussion but all shout together when angry or excited.

From 4 to 6 months parents can differentiate between the child's varied vocalisations and impute different intentions to them. If the parents consistently respond to the child's call, they will soon learn to expect a response. This is the beginning of their appreciation of cause and effect and of their intentional behaviour, as they learn that vocalising can bring about social interaction and the satisfaction of their needs (Franklin, 2014).

At 8 to 10 months infants show a significant increase in intentional behaviours, especially those oriented towards achieving goals. This marks the beginning of the means-end distinction (Cole, 1982). The child will repeat actions that evoke an interesting response from adults.

From 8 to 12 months infants begin to indulge in other kinds of alternate actions, such as 'give and take' games, when the child demands a toy, gives it back and demands it again, or puts it down and 'asks' for another one (Bruner, 1975). The child is learning many things during this game. They are taking turns, which is vital for later reciprocal exchanges, including conversation and games with rules.

Early concepts

Object permanence

This refers to the realisation that an object exists in time and space even though it can no longer be seen or acted upon. The very young child acts as though an object that is out of sight is also out of mind. At 6 months they will start to look for a dropped toy, but if it doesn't quickly reappear, they will forget about it. By 9 months they will remove an obstacle to uncover a partially hidden toy (Sharma and Cockerill, 2014). This suggests that they recognise that part of an object represents the whole object (Bloom and Lahey, 1978). At 12 months the child is capable of reaching and searching for a fully hidden object if they see it being hidden.

Cause and effect

The newborn baby is prompted by innate reflexes which are soon modified by their experiences. Things happen to the baby; they are picked up, fed, bathed, cuddled and rocked. At the same time they discover they have certain abilities of their own, for example, they can look and notice things; listen and hear sounds; touch and feel their blanket and their mother's body; move their arms, legs, head and body; cry and make interesting noises.

Between 1 and 4 months the baby is very concerned with their own body, and they begin to repeat physical movements – an early attempt to make things happen again. At this stage they do not distinguish themselves from their environment, or from their actions and the effects of their actions. The child's reflex movements sometimes cause enjoyable things to happen; for example, as they wave their hand, a brightly coloured mobile twists and turns. Through constant repetition of such 'accidental' activities, the child learns that their movements have an effect, and they begin to separate himself from their environment.

Between 4 and 10 months the child begins to repeat activities to make interesting things in the environment happen again. The child is beginning to coordinate information from two senses at once (Bee and Boyd, 2019) and is paying increased attention to objects and events in their immediate environment. The parents help to develop this awareness by directing their child's attention to toys placed near their line of vision and maintaining their attention by moving the toys, talking about them and helping the child to manipulate them. As children develop object permanence, their visual and tactile explorations become more systematic. They begin to recognise the connection between their own action and the interesting outcome; for example, they realise that grasping a dangling string swings a mobile or toy into view (Sharma and Cockerill, 2014).

From 10 to 12 months the child's actions become more purposeful as they develop the understanding of cause and effect. They now act with an end or goal in mind; for example, they pull the string because they want the toy that is on the end of it. The subtle difference between this child and the younger one is that the latter would pull the string even if there were no toy on the end. The 1-year-old child is able to combine two behaviours in order to achieve specific ends; for example, they can employ both gesture and vocalisation to gain somebody's attention and direct it to an external event. They use people to achieve their goals and satisfy their needs, thus developing their understanding of instrumental relations.

Early verbal understanding

The exploration of real objects in the real world gradually leads on to the symbolic representation of objects. We use symbols, such as toys, pictures and words, to stand for objects, ideas and events. The use of symbols is basic to true language, which is a system of symbols that allows the individual to transcend the here and now in their communication and thought. The child must have reached at least the early stages of concept formation before meaningful language is possible, because words are symbols and symbols must be related to concepts and not to specific objects.

Situational understanding

Through the child's experiences with the real environment, they come to understand a good deal. Parents and caregivers often feel that their 1-year-olds understand everything that is said to them. Infants as young as 6 months will turn to a familiar voice, and by 9 months show understanding of "no" and "bye bye" (Sharma and Cockerill, 2014). Between 9-12 months infants are able to follow commands like "more juice" and "Where's mummy?" when used in daily routines (Buckley, 2003). In fact, the child understands few of the actual words and perceives them merely as part of the total situation. The child uses all the available contextual clues such as the parents'/caregivers' gesture and intonation, and their familiarity with the situation to interpret what is going on (Dockrell, 2019). For example, if a mother asks her child to sit down for dinner while pulling out the highchair and tying on their bib as food smells waft from the kitchen, they would be unlikely not to understand what they wanted.

Initially, talking is part of the whole situation, but gradually the child becomes aware of a familiar phrase emphasised by the parent/caregiver's clear intonation and stress pattern. Soon, the phrase heralds the event that is associated with it, and the child of 9 to 12 months shows anticipation and an appropriate response, which itself may become part of the familiar routine (Reynell, 1980). Gradually, the situational clues become redundant so that the child of 12 months starts to recognise the names of familiar objects, especially when a gesture is used at the same time.

Between 11 and 13 months the key words in the phrase are identified as the most significant; for example, 'cup' signals the arrival of orange juice or milk; later it is associated with the action of drinking, and finally with the object itself (Reynell, 1980).

Symbolic understanding

At 12 months the child understands real, familiar objects in relation to themselves and can demonstrate knowledge of their function by using them appropriately, for example, drinking from a cup. This is sometimes referred to as definition by use or functional play. Around 13 to 15 months, the child will play meaningfully with large dolls and toys. At this stage they may use some single words, usually situational ones such as "bye bye" (Reynell, 1980). At 15 to 18 months they will use real objects appropriately in relation to large dolls and to caregivers. This spontaneous meaningful play with these toys is the beginning of symbolic play and shows a developing awareness of symbolic representation. (See Chapter 3 for more detail on symbolic play development.)

Early vocalisations

Functions

Children use vocalisations to perform many functions from an early age. Halliday (1975) identified the following seven basic functions or purposes:

1 The instrumental function - to satisfy material needs; for example, to obtain an object like food or drink, or gain support of some sort such as being comforted.
2 The regulatory function - to control the actions of specific people; for example, requesting something or directing the behaviour of others.
3 The interactional function - to interact with those around to maintain social exchanges; for example, greetings and farewells.
4 The personal function - to express individuality and personal preferences; for example, expressions of pleasure, or to signal interest in an object.
5 The heuristic function - to obtain information to learn about and explore the environment; for example, asking questions.

6 The imaginative function – to play and create a world of fantasy; for example, sounds accompanying pretend play.
7 The informative function – to give information; for example, to state a fact or give a message.

The first four functions occur in parallel and relate to the use of language by the child between the ages of 8 months and 18 months. Developmentally they precede the heuristic, imaginative and informative functions. The heuristic function and the imaginative function appear around the same time at 13½–15 months, with the informative function appearing much later at around 21–22½ months (Halliday, 2004).

This list by Halliday describes the intentional behaviours of the child, but even before these functions are established the child's vocalisations are reflections of their different feelings and states, for example, hunger, pain, discomfort, pleasure and excitement.

Form

The first sound a baby makes is usually a loud cry. During the next few weeks they will also yawn, sneeze, belch and cough, which are mainly due to physiological activities such as breathing and feeding. These early vocalisations have no communicative intent but may still be interpreted as communication by many parents/caregivers, who respond with speech and play (Snow, 1977). Although there are individual variations in the rate and pattern of development between children, there is a clear progression from these early reflexive cries and vegetative noises to increasingly more complex vocalisations and babble (Morgan and Wren, 2018).

Between 2 months and 4 months, nonreflexive vocalisations develop, with laughter and other sounds of pleasure heard (Stark, 1980). Cooing or comfort sounds appear around about 3 months (Lang et al., 2019) and resemble the production of vowels like [ooo] and [aahh]. These vocalisations need more modification by the vocal tract than crying, which decreases as pleasurable sounds increase.

As the child develops increasing control over phonation and articulation the infant's approximation of vowels becomes more accurate, and new sounds appear such as raspberries and clicks (Nathani et al., 2006). To begin with there is no intention to communicate, and sounds are produced for pleasure and curiosity. The frequency and intensity of the infant's vocalisations are influenced by whether or not they are comfortable (Delack, 1976), stimulated or get a response (Weisburg, 1963).

By around 6 months, or at the very least just before the emergence of babbling, the child is able to combine vowels with consonants to produce canonical syllables (Oller, 2000), which contain one 'consonant-like' and one 'vowel-like' element, for example, [da] and [ba] (Lang et al., 2019). These are an important developmental stage for the child, as these canonical syllables form the basis for later production of spoken words.

Babbling

Around 7 months these canonical syllables are combined into repetitive consonant-vowel (CVCV) sequences known as reduplicative (or duplicative) babbling, for example, [dada] [mama] (Fagan, 2009). Canonical babbling mirrors processes found in early speech development; for example, there is a strong preference for syllables with an initial consonant (CV) over ones with a final consonant (VC) (Oller, 2000).

A more complex form of vocalisation is non-reduplicated or variegated babble consisting of a sequence of syllables with different consonant vowel combinations like [badeda] (Stark, 1980). Some researchers consider variegated babble a separate, sequential stage occurring after reduplicated babble, while others have argued that variegated babble occurs from the commencement of the babbling stage and develops in parallel (Morgan and Wren, 2018).

Babbling in the form of both reduplicated and variegated syllables continues to increase from babbling onset. However, there is a decline in the number of longer strings of repetitions in reduplicated babble towards the end of the first year as the child learns to understand and produce words (Fagan, 2009). In contrast, variegated babble appears to increase between 12 months and 14 months (Smith et al., 1989), forming part of the child's vocal repertoire alongside the production of their first words.

Between 9 months and 18 months the child may produce long strings of syllables with different consonants and vowels with varied stress and intonation pattern known as 'jargon' (Nathani et al., 2006). Although this appears to be a sentence-like structure, there is no linguistic or grammatical content. When first words appear, they may be embedded in strings of expressive jargon.

Early babble:

- Stimulates the child and brings them pleasure, with infants producing a large number of vocalisations even when they are alone (Nakazima, 1975; Oller et al., 2019).
- Satisfies an interest in producing and exploring sound (Fagan, 2009).

- Practises sound production and perception, as the baby experiments with moving their lips, tongue, soft palate and larynx, while listening to the results (Fagan, 2014).
- Attracts adult attention and brings responses and material needs (Snow, 1977).

Later stages of babbling:

- Maintain social interaction (Stern, 1977).
- Communicate feelings and needs, mainly through the nature of the intonation pattern (Halliday, 1975).

Protowords

Protowords or vocables are sound sequences, occurring between babbling and the first true words, that are not an attempt at adult words but are used consistently and frequently to signal different meanings. They tend to be idiosyncratic creations by the individual child in response to an object or social interaction; hence interpretation of meaning is usually restricted to adults who know the child, with protowords only becoming meaningful within a specific communicative context (Adamson, 2019). These vocalisations normally stand for functions rather than objects or people, for example, to make requests, indicate rejection, frustration or pleasure and express likes and dislikes. They are accompanied by gestures and actions that convey the gist of the message; for example, a child consistently says "der" whenever they ask for an object, pointing to the one they want (Carter, 1979). These sound sequences may consist of only a consonant and vowel, or even a single vowel, and can be difficult to distinguish from the first attempts at true words.

First words

Between 9 and 15 months the first recognisable words emerge and are often single vowels; reduplicated syllables such as 'dada' and 'mama'; or single syllables such as 'da' for dog (Fagan, 2009). There is a clear link between pre-speech vocalisations and these early words with the use of similar sounds (McCune and Vihman, 2001) and canonical (CV) syllables (Oller et al., 2019). A study by (Schneider et al., 2015) found that this early vocabulary included words referring to animals, games and routines, and that these results were consistent for both early and late talkers.

Gesture

Gestures or movements of the head, hands or other body parts are visual actions that express meaning nonverbally and form an important part of social interaction and communication. They include deictic gestures used to direct attention and representational or iconic gestures that illustrate an object, action or quality. The infant's comprehension and use of gestures is closely linked to their speech and language acquisition, with delays in the development of gesture an important predictor of later language delays (Lüke et al., 2017).

The use of gestures by the child occurs before the spoken word, with evidence of coordination between rhythmic movements and vocalisation occurring as early as the babbling stage (Iverson and Fagan, 2004). Between 8 and 10 months gestures with communicative intent emerge with the use of deictic gestures like giving, showing and pointing to direct the attention of others (Bates and Dick, 2002). These gestures enable the adult to follow the child's lead and provide language input related to the focus of their attention (Goldin-Meadow et al., 2007).

Other gestures, like shaking the head for 'no' and waving 'bye-bye', also appear around this time. These ritual gestures occurring during social interactions within a familiar routine. By 12 months the child is able to join with the adult in imitative gestural games such as peek-a-boo and pat-a-cake. Significantly, Rowe et al. (2008) found that the use of gesture by the parent or caregiver was positively related to the type and amount of gesture produced by the child.

At around 12 months, or just before the appearance of first words, the child starts to use actions associated with familiar objects known as recognitory gestures, for example, drinking from an empty cup. This coincides with the early stages of symbolic understanding. Later, the use of communicative gesture is combined with speech in the early single word period of expressive language (Esteve-Gilbert and Prieto, 2014).

Activities to promote early communication skills

Guidelines

Here are some practical tips to help you make the most of activities with your child.

- Reduce distractions during activities by turning off the television or background music.
- Respond to your child's interests by joining in with their play, and follow their choice of activities, games and toys.
- Follow your child's lead. Talk about what they are doing and respond to their communication.
- Keep activities engaging and enjoyable for your child and you. Make it fun!
- Make sure you are at the same level as your child so they can see your face and mouth.
- Use a lively voice to help gain and keep your child's attention. Babies and young children prefer slow speech that is higher pitched, with a sing-song rhythm.
- Be animated to attract and maintain your child's attention. Use a lively facial expression and gestures along with your spoken language.
- Be consistent in your responses so your child starts to make connections and understands events.
- Make sure your child has a quiet environment for some of the time during the day so that they can listen to their own sounds and those of their natural environment.
- Make communication activities a dummy-free time.

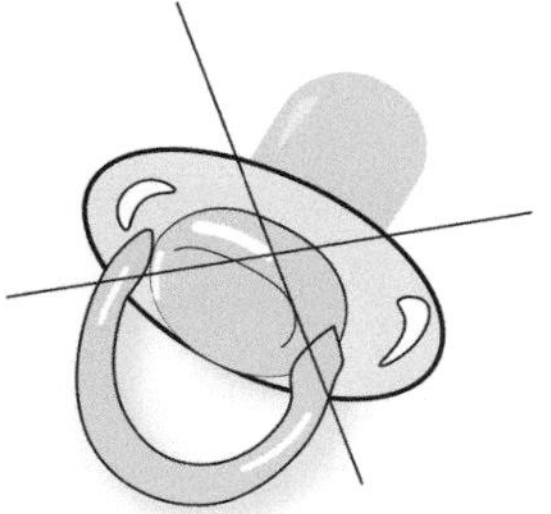

Remember when choosing toys to avoid small objects that might fit in the mouth and be a choking hazard.

Early social interactions

Your early social interactions with your child are an important foundation for the development of their language and communication skills. Here are some ideas about how you can connect and engage with your child during shared play.

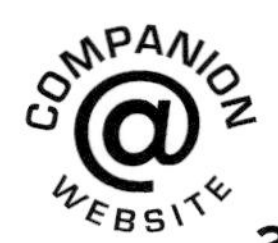

Share your child's interest

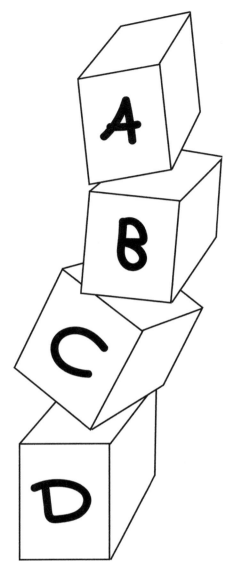

Follow where your child is looking and attend to whatever has caught their interest. Gradually create a connection between yourself and the object or activity. You might look at an object together, listen to the sound it makes, take turns in holding it or explore how it works. Remember to use this time to talk about it too, using simple words and phrases.

You can use any situation that presents itself, for example, your child playing with their toes, watching a moving or dangling toy, listening to music or the sound of rain, looking out of the window, playing with a toy or building with bricks. You can respond by tickling their toes, swinging the mobile, shaking the rattle and knocking down the bricks.

Follow your child's lead

During play sessions you can join in with whatever your child is doing and imitate their actions. This might be anything from smiling, looking, babbling, humming, clapping hands or making sounds. Build on an activity by introducing another familiar activity into the routine; for example, if you and your child are smiling at each other, maybe you can start a peek-a-boo game.

Start a 'conversation'

Incorporate into games like 'peek-a-boo' the actions and vocal features that are a normal part of conversations. Attract your child's attention by making eye contact and using nods and gestures along with an animated facial expression, such as smiling and raising eyebrows. Keep their interest by using a lively voice and exaggerated up-and-down intonation. Leave spaces for your child to join in with the conversation in whatever way that might be, from a gurgle to a sound or a word.

Exploring objects

Your child needs to gain hands-on sensory experience of an object in order to maintain their interest in it and learn about its properties.

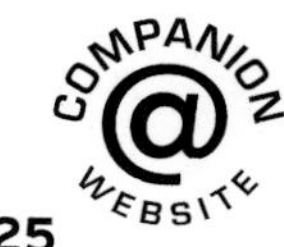

Rattle

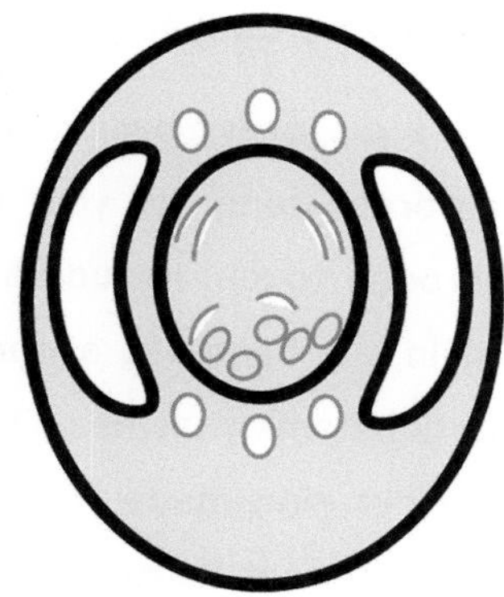

Your child may start to reach and grasp spontaneously, but sometimes they may need a little prompting. Attract your child's attention with a lightweight rattle. Place the rattle in their hand and help them shake it. Next, hold the rattle a very little way away and guide their hand to it. Make sure they grasp it, and help them to shake it. Start the reaching movement off for the child by prompting them by touching their arm. Gradually move the rattle further away, and then to your child's side so they have to turn their body to grasp it.

Hanging toys

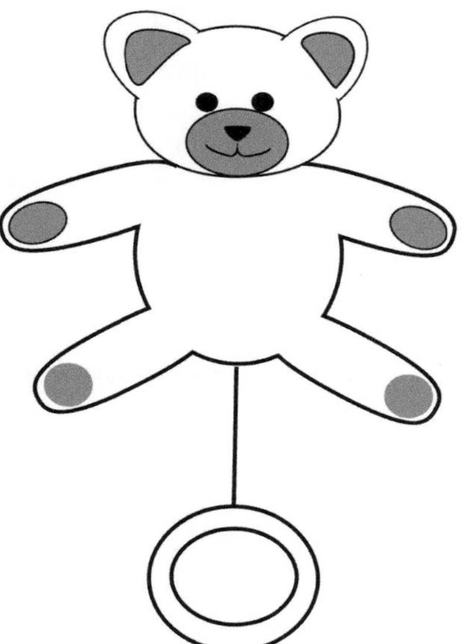

Hanging toys will encourage your child to reach, touch and grasp. Use thick elastic thread to securely attach the toys, and include items that vary in shape, size and texture. The best toys to start with are those that your child can manipulate easily to produce a result. Always give plenty of demonstrations, and when your child is attentive and enjoying the result, help them to manipulate the toys for themselves; for example, hold their hand around a string or handle to pull a toy towards them.

Sound-making toys

Sound-making toys offer an extra auditory reward for reaching out and grasping an object. Try squeaky toys, soft blocks that rattle or tingle, balls with a bell inside, and shakers. You can make your own home-made shakers from small tins, bottles or jars that have lids. They can be filled with water, sand, beads, buttons, pebbles, rice or lentils. There are endless combinations.

Just make sure lids are secure by gluing or taping them shut.

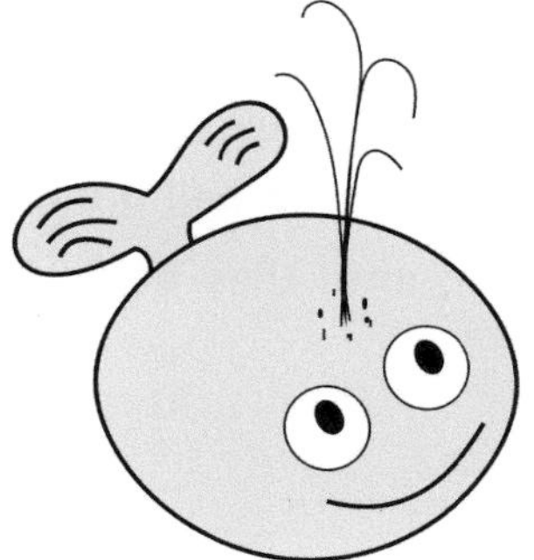

Bath time

Add lots of soft bath squirter toys in different shapes and sizes. Gently squeeze to fill with water, and then encourage your child to squirt away.

Discovery basket

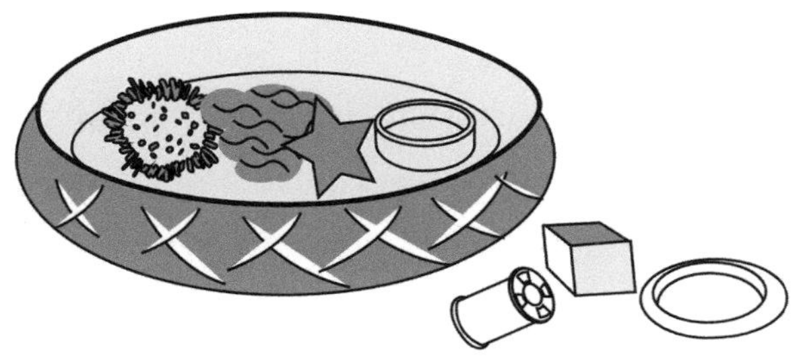

Fill a discovery basket with a variety of different items for your child to explore through touch. Include small items that fit in one hand like a wooden block, and larger items that need two hands like a teether ring made from natural rubber. Use different textures and weights, so your child experiences grasping soft and hard; light and heavy; rough and smooth items. Try multisensory activity balls, textured balls, fabric blocks and stacking rings. Homemade items might include mini scrunchies, shower puffs, sponges, wooden shapes or puzzle pieces, cotton reels, scrunched up paper and cardboard tubes cut into rings.

Supervise play at all times.

Looking and following

Children enjoy the fun and surprise of objects that appear and disappear. Start with games where objects or toys move out of your child's line of vision but are still visible.

Tabletop games

Roll a ball or other toy along a tabletop and encourage your child to watch the moving object. As it falls off the end of the table, bring their gaze down and show them where the object or toy is lying. Let your child pick it up and then repeat the activity. When you have their total interest, help your child roll the object along the table, continuing to show them where it has landed, if necessary.

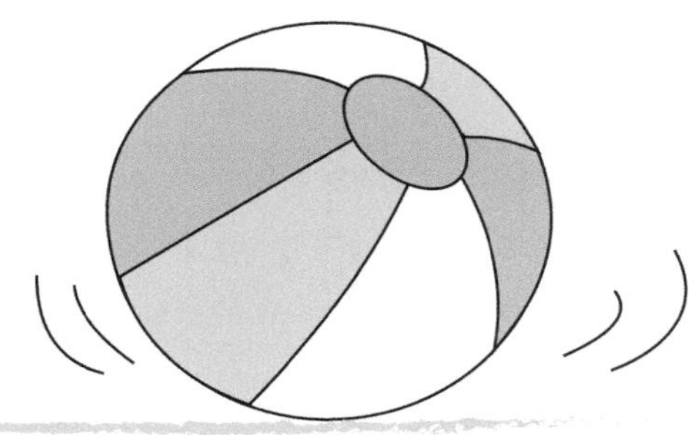

Floor games

Sit on the floor and roll a ball between you and your child. Then roll it behind your child a little way; help them to turn around and find it. Later you can roll the ball behind yourself and keep moving so that they can see where the ball is, until they begin to look for it.

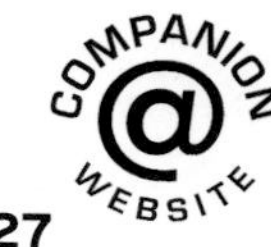

Dropping games

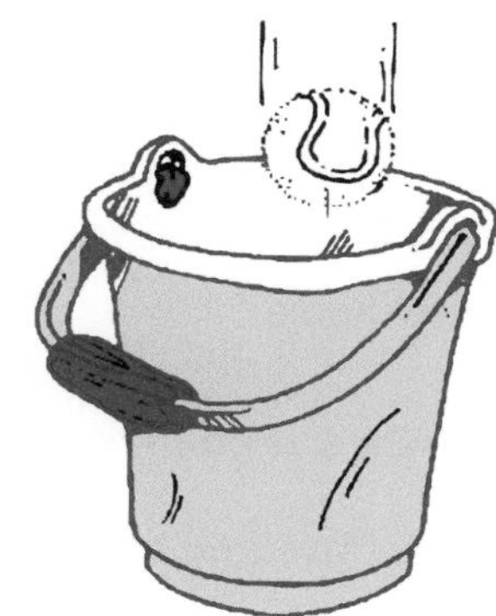

When your child drops a toy out of their cot or highchair, help them look to see where it has gone. Play games where you and your child take turns to drop small objects like wooden bricks into a posting box. Any container big enough to allow your child to put their hand in and retrieve the object will do. Try using boxes, baskets, buckets and cardboard tubes.

Push and pull toys

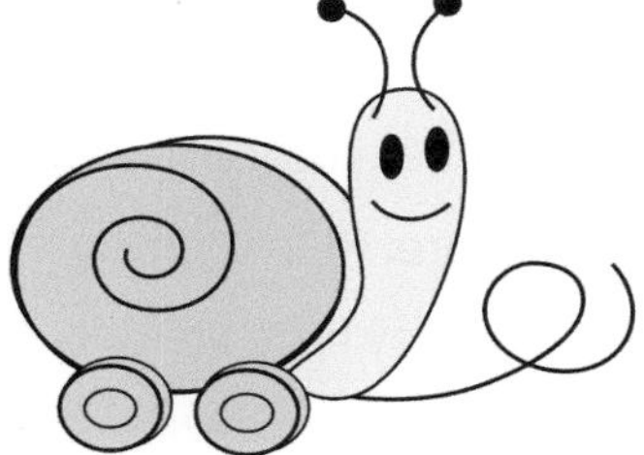

Push and pull toys can be used to attract your child's attention and then be gently moved to encourage your child to look and follow their movements.

Posting games

Play a game of posting where your child will see an object disappear and then reappear quite quickly. For example, posting a range of small toys down a large cardboard tube. Add some fun by letting items fall into a box, sand tray or water in a bowl.

Hide and seek games

Hide and seek games help encourage your child's awareness that an object or a person continues to exist even when they can't be seen. They are also a great way to interact with your child, and they encourage looking and listening skills too.

Everyday situations

Use naturally occurring situations to encourage your child's awareness that a person or an object continues to exist even when it can't be seen; for example, comment upon people leaving the room and coming back again. Help your child to anticipate somebody's reappearance, for example, a sister coming home from school. Comment on things outdoors that your child sees regularly, such as a shop or a funny sign that they pass on the way to the park and then see again on the way home.

Hide-di-hi

Play peek-a-boo games. Hide yourself behind a door or curtain and help your child by peeping out and calling their name.

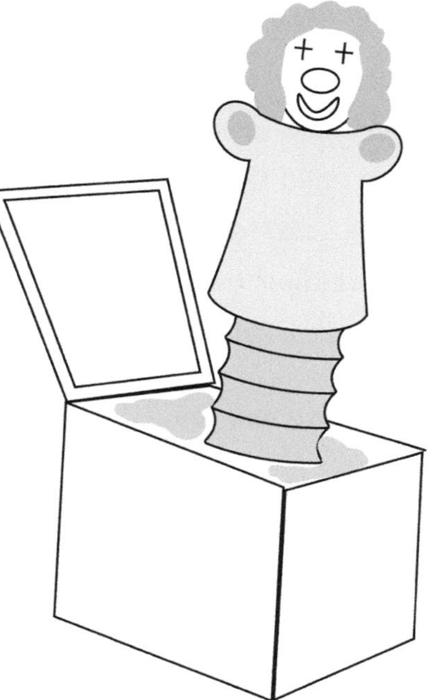

Where's it gone?

Use a favourite toy or object to play a hiding game. Help your child to cover just the edge of the toy with a scarf or cushion, and then encourage them to remove it again. Make a big show of surprise at seeing the whole object once more. Help them cover more and more of the object until the toy is completely hidden, and again prompt them to remove the cover. Vary the activity by using a toy or object that makes a sound even when it is hidden.

Pop-up toys

A jack-in-the-box is a classic game where Jack is hidden and suddenly appears at the press of a switch. Push down the lid, and Jack disappears again. Other pop-up toys, especially ones incorporating push-down flaps, are also suitable.

Two Little Dicky Birds

Two Little Dicky Birds is a great little rhyme that involves two little birds that fly away and disappear, only to reappear when you call "come back".

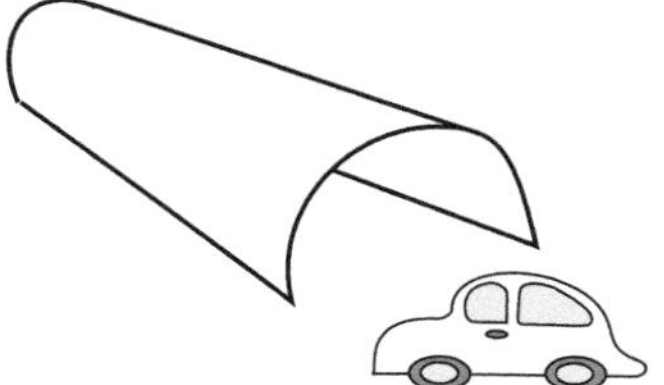

Tunnels

Show your child how a car or a train vanishes as you push them through a tunnel. As it reappears on the other side, make a big show of surprise.

Cause and effect

Lots of your child's early spontaneous activities teach them about the connection between their actions and the world around them, like how a cry will elicit a response from you. There are also several toys that do something as the result of an action upon them, which are excellent for helping your child to explore the relationship between their actions and an object.

Bang bang

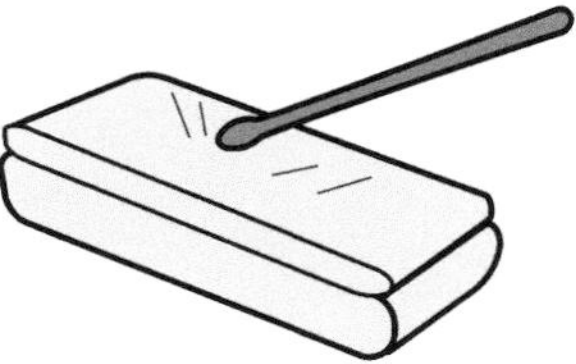

Take advantage of your child's interest in banging objects. Give them a stick and provide lots of different objects to hit. A hard wooden brick will feel different from a soft cushion. An empty tin will sound different from a full one.

Roly-poly toys

Let your child have a selection of rolling toys to explore their different movements. Objects can be as varied as balls, toys with wheels, or even apples and oranges.

Make a noise

Find toys that make a noise as a result of some action by you or your child. Inflatable roller toys with noise makers inside are easy to roll. Drums (or upside-down saucepans) can be beaten with a stick. A rattle can be shaken.

Pop-up toys

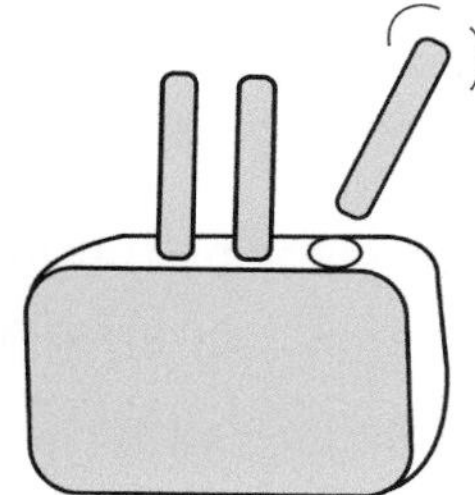

Use pop-up toys that the child releases by performing a certain action, for example, jack-in-the-box and other pop-up toys like Galt *Pop Up People*.

Hammer away!

Simple hammer benches are a great way for your child to pound away at a peg with a hammer. Once the peg goes through the bench, your child can turn it over and start again.

Spinning top

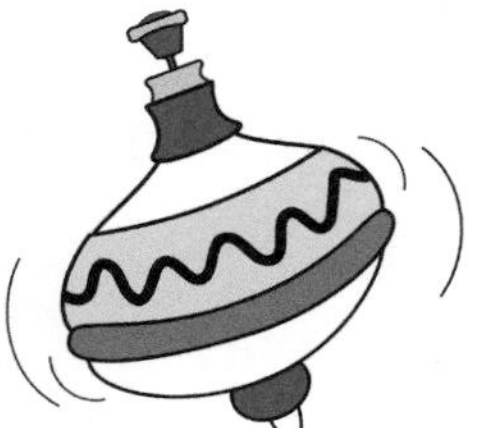

Help your child press down on the spinning top and see it spin.

Simple turn-taking games

These social games encourage some focused time for you and your child to play together. They support the development of important skills like turn taking and sharing, as well as providing an opportunity to introduce words and phrases to your child.

Games of give and take

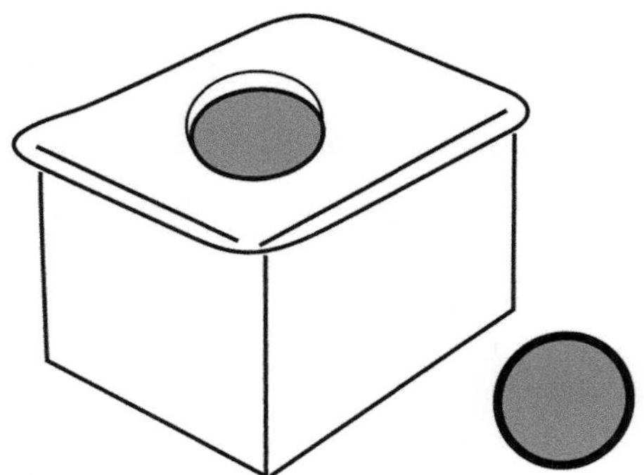

Give your child a toy and hold out your hand for it back, using accompanying language such as "here y'are" and "give it to me". Encourage your child to hold out their hand or to reach for the toy. These games can become more purposeful; for example, your child hands you a toy to post in a box. Take it out of the box and give it back to your child to help them do the same.

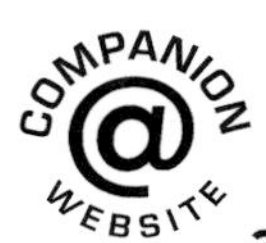

Games of back and forth

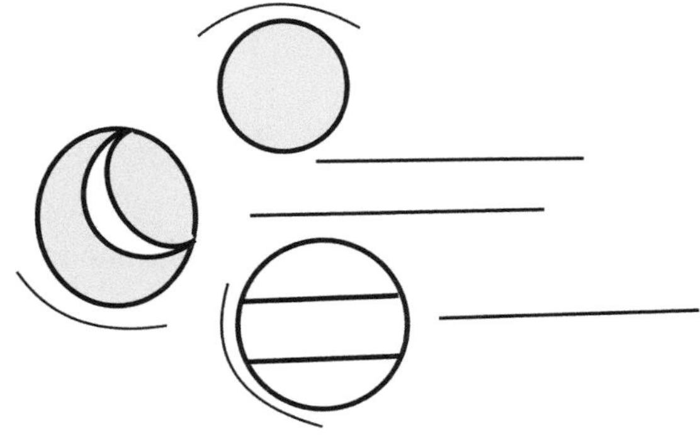

Sit opposite your child for some back-and-forth games. Roll a ball to your child and encourage her to roll it back to you. Introduce turn-taking language using names rather than pronouns like 'you' such as "Mummy's *turn*" and "Molly's *turn*" into the sequence. Comment on what is happening "*Molly* is rolling the ball – here it comes," "*Mummy* is rolling the ball". Play the same game by pushing cars, trains and other toys on wheels to and fro.

Clapping games and finger play

Try clapping routines like *Pat-a-cake*, or finger play with *This little piggy*, *Walkie round the garden* and other tickling games. Your child will enjoy the sensory experience of touch combined with rhythmic movements and singing.

Peek-a-boo games

You and your child can take turns to hide your faces in your hands and then peek out with a loud "boo". Try hiding behind a book or pull a large hat down over your eyes. You can also play 'peek-a-boo' with different parts of the body, so when your child is getting dressed you can make a big fuss when a hand reappears from a pyjama sleeve.

Early play

These early play activities will help your child understand that objects can be used in a symbolic way to represent other objects, so a toy cup can be used in the same way as their real cup. It also provides an opportunity to introduce associated language and practice the words and phrases they hear in everyday activities.

What's in the bag?

This game encourages your child to carry out actions with real objects. Hide some of your child's everyday items like a cup, bowl, brush and flannel in a bag. You can have a special colourful bag just for this activity, but any opaque bag will do. Attract your child's attention to the bag by shaking it and asking, "What's in the bag?" Take out one of the objects with a great show of surprise – "Look, brush" – before handing it to your child, as this will help engage them in the activity.

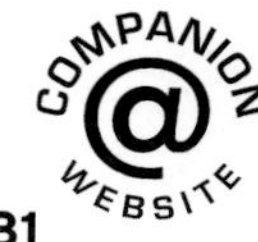

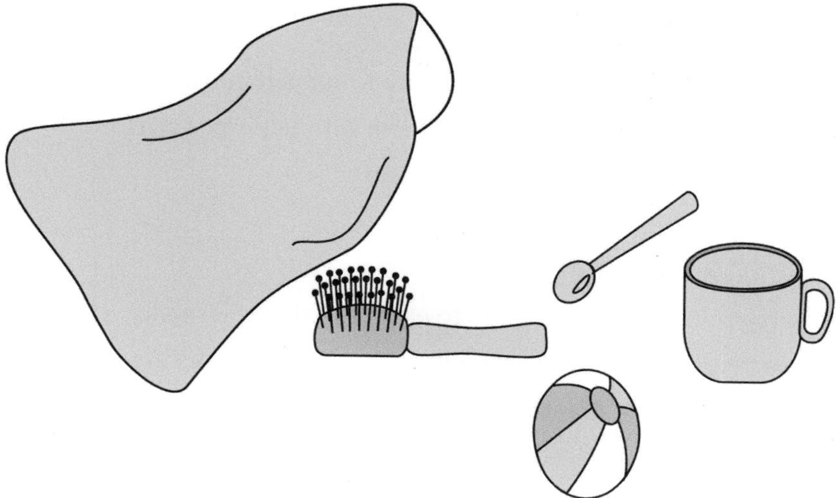

At first your child may bang or mouth the object; help show your child how to use the object both on yourself and the child, for example, brushing your hair and then your child's hair. Let them have the object again and continue to encourage their play. When your child carries out an action, reinforce this by imitating them and talking about what they are doing – "brush" or "brush hair". Let your child take a turn in pulling out an object from the bag.

Daily routines

Your child will love to copy everyday activities they see going on in the home. At first, they may need to use real items alongside real activities, for example, helping wash up beakers in the sink. But you can also incorporate similar actions and routines into a play activity, for example, a wooden spoon is a great way to explore making sounds on a saucepan, but it can also be used for stirring or eating pretend food. And you don't have to have any food for this game either! It's all about the objects and the actions.

Large doll play

Help your child to recognise the symbolic nature of large dolls by including your child's favourite doll or teddy in daily routines. Use them in the same ways that you interact with your child yourself; for instance, when you bathe them, give them their dinner and play with them, include the doll in these activities. You will probably have to perform actions on the doll yourself, telling your child what you are doing all the while, for example, "Now we wash *your* (or use child's name) face, then we wash *dolly's* face". Encourage your child to take their turn at washing dolly, always using real objects at this stage. If preferred, teddies or similar stuffed animals like a bear or monkey may be used instead of a doll.

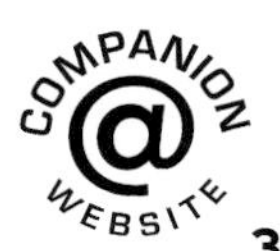

Listening to everyday sounds

Develop your child's awareness of the sounds around them in their daily environment. Learning to recognise sounds and associate them with objects, actions and events will help develop your child's attention and listening skills.

Everyday situations

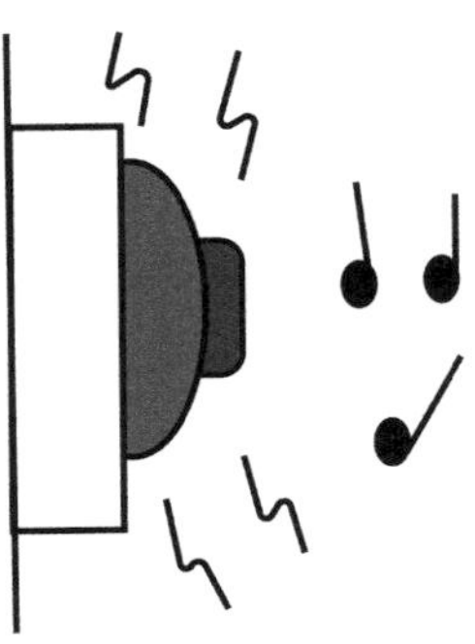

Help your child to anticipate and respond to events that are normally signalled by a particular sound; for example, when the bath taps are running it must be time for a bath; when the doorbell rings there must be someone at the door. Talk about the event, drawing attention to the sound, and then take them to see what are happening.

Out and about

Draw your child's attention to the sounds and noises you can hear when you go to the shops or sit in the park. Make your own sounds by kicking through leaves or splashing in puddles.

Sensory toys

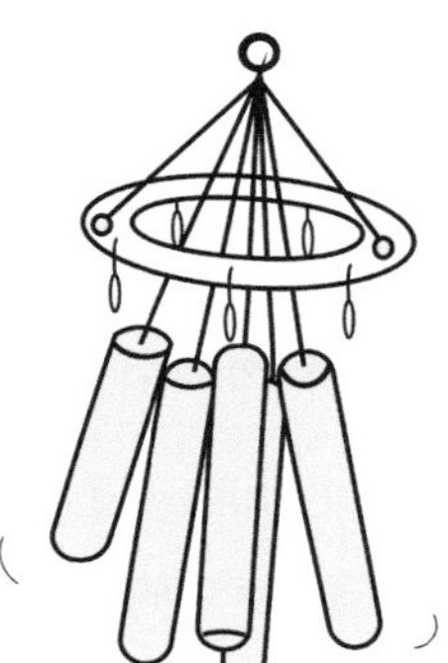

Interest your child in listening to sounds using toys that combine sound with visual and tactile stimuli, such as light-up music boxes, musical mobiles, LED garden wind chimes, balls with bells or fabric activity toys like soft cubes and crinkle-cloth books.

Homemade music

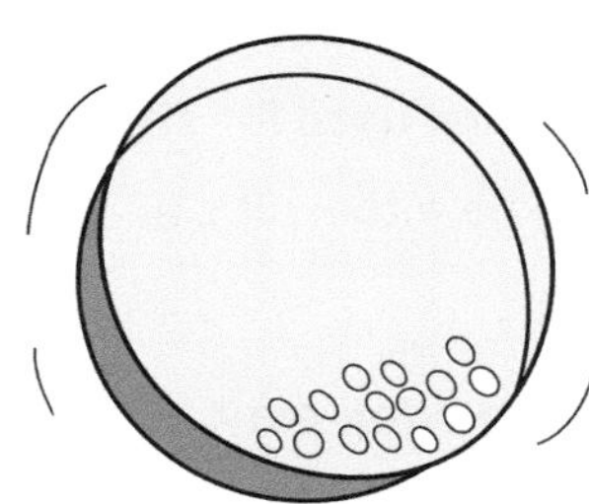

Make music at home using homemade sound makers. Bang a saucepan, a tin, or a wooden box with a wooden spoon; bang two objects together – plastic egg cups or two sticks; or make a repetitive rhythm using a squeaky toy or rattle. Show them how to make quiet sounds and noisy sounds. Use noise or sound words like 'pop', 'crash' and 'bang' to accompany actions.

Musical toys

Musical toys for babies and infants are an early introduction to music. Help your child to make music with a xylophone or drum; shake a rattle; or watch the cascading beads as you roll a mini wave drum or rainmaker.

Listening to symbolic sounds

Symbolic sounds are speech sounds or noises that are associated with the object or things they represent, so we know 'woof' refers to a dog and sounds a little like their bark too.

Symbolic sounds are often used in a repetitive way and are usually easier to say, so games involving these sounds will also encourage your child to vocalise.

Action sounds

Make sounds to accompany your child's actions, so say "splish-splash" as they pat the water during bath-time, or "wheeee" as they come down the slide.

Splish

Splash

Describe a sound

As you play with a noisy toy or a musical instrument, describe the sound, for example, "Where's the one that goes squeak squeak?" "Here it is" or "What noise does the drum make?" "bang, bang". Help your child to make the action as you say the sound, so banging the drum as you say "bang, bang".

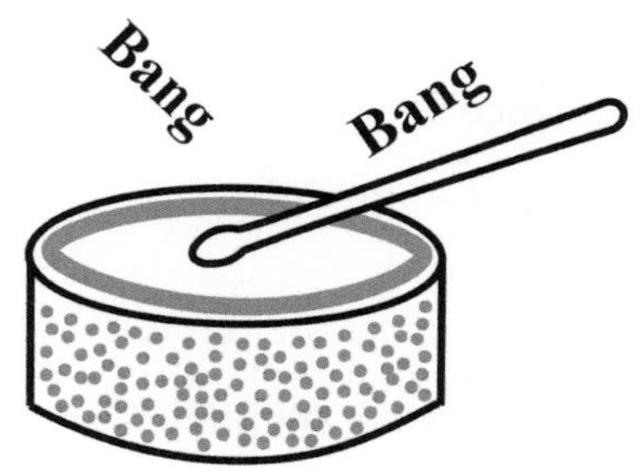

Animal sounds

Show your child pictures of animals in books like *Old MacDonald's Farm* and *Can You Say It Too? Woof! Woof!* by Sebastien Braun. Use board books with holes, books with flaps, or books with peepholes that reveal different animals. This will help your child to focus on particular animal sounds. You can make the sounds for your child, or books like *Listen to the Jungle* by Marion Billet or *Dear Zoo Noisy Book* by Rod Campbell have buttons to press for animal sounds.

Noisy traffic

Make traffic noises when playing with cars, trains and trucks, like 'beep' and 'broom-broom'. Encourage your child to join in and copy you. Books like *Listen to Things Go* by Marion Billet have real life sounds at the press of a button.

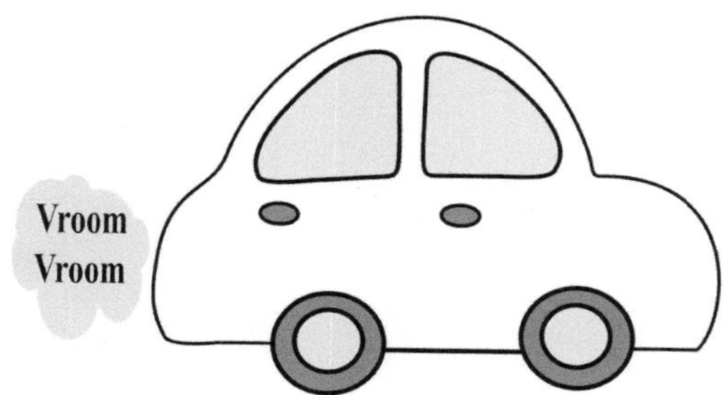

Note these books and similar items should be supervised by an adult due to the small parts related to the sound mechanism.

Listening to early words and phrases

There are lots of ways to introduce language into your child's daily life:

Have a daily natter

Place your child where they can see you and watch what you are doing so that you become the focus of their interest. Make sure they can see your face and mouth clearly, as this helps build their understanding of facial expressions and how sounds are made. Talk to your child about what you are doing, "Mummy's brushing her hair", or talk about what you are planning to do "We're going to the park, Nana will be there".

Chat and play

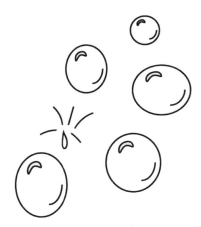

During play you can respond to your child's vocalisations and actions with comments like "Hello smiley" and "Pop! *Milo* burst the bubble". Take turns so you talk about what you are doing too, "Bubbles", "Mummy burst the bubble". Use pauses to give your child a chance to respond, whether that's a sound, gesture or an attempt at a word.

Follow your child's interests

If an object attracts your child's attention, then let them look at it and help them explore it through touch where possible. Say the name of it, repeating the word a few times in different ways – "*dolly*", "Hello *dolly*", "Let's hug *dolly*", "Aaahhh". Keep your sentences simple, with the focus on the key word.

Face-to-face games

Your child can be sat on your knee while you play tickling games, finger plays and bouncing games, in which you make your child bounce up and down and suddenly fall down. This helps them look at your face, and in particular your mouth. Singing songs and nursery rhymes can also take place in this position. Encourage your child to take a more and more active part.

Books

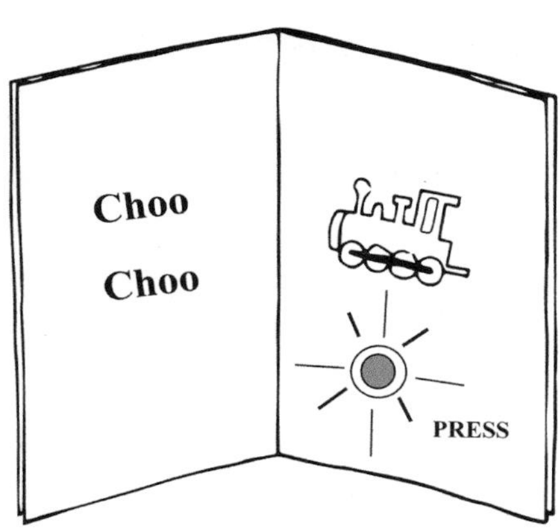

Sharing books with your child will help develop their attention and listening skills, language and literacy. Books are the perfect all-rounder for stimulation and learning. Talk about what you can see rather than reading the story word by word.

Books also offer the opportunity to combine a sensory experience with listening and talking.

Encourage your child to interact by helping them:

- Press buttons to play different noises in a 'sound' book.
- Explore different textures using 'touch and feel' books.
- Look at books with eye-catching features like bright, colourful pictures, shiny mirrors and 'lift the flap' options.

Singing

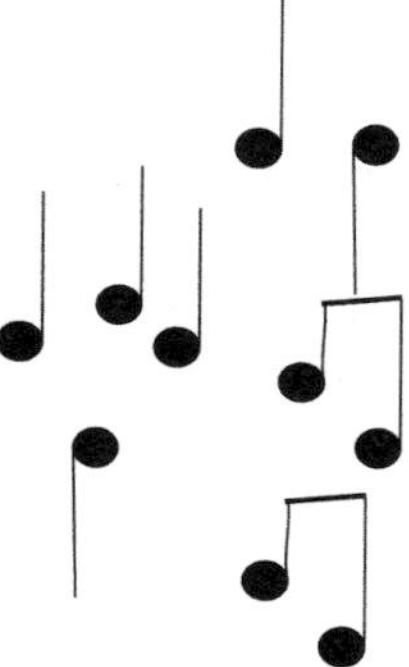

Singing is a great way to interact with your child and will set the foundations for later speech and literacy skills. It helps develop your child's listening skills, sense of rhythm, vocabulary and understanding of verse. You may want to sing using different languages if your home is bilingual.

Singing a lullaby

Singing a song or a lullaby to soothe your child is a great way to interact with them.

Action songs

Choose songs that include rhyming words, actions and simple phrases with lots of repetition. Try *Wind the Bobbin Up*; *The Wheels on the Bus;* and *Twinkle, Twinkle Little Star*.

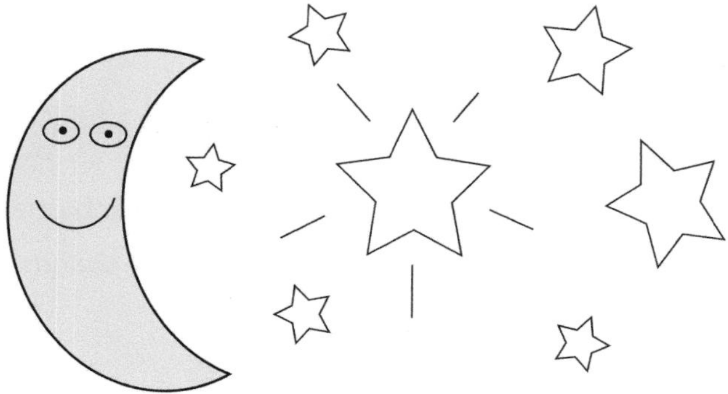

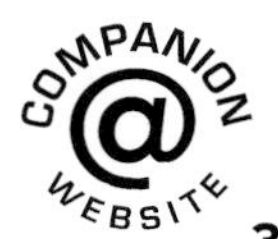

Songs with sounds

Sing songs with simple word-like sounds like 'pop' in *Pop Goes the Weasel* or the animal sounds 'moo' and 'baaah' in *Old MacDonald's Farm*.

Movement and singing

Nursery rhymes and songs are often accompanied by rhythmical movements such as swaying, rocking and knee bouncing. This helps develop rhythm and spatial awareness and combines language and social interaction with movement.

Row, Row, Row Your Boat

Row, Row, Row Your Boat is a great rhyme for combining singing and movement along with turn taking. Sit opposite your child on the floor, hold hands and gently rock back and forth singing the song. Introduce other movements as you repeat the chorus, so your boat can rock side to side or bounce up and down on the waves.

Lap play

Try combining the following songs with lap play – *This Is the Way the Ladies Ride* (knee bouncing to different rhythms); and *Pop a Little Pancake* (up and down, tickles, cuddles and kisses).

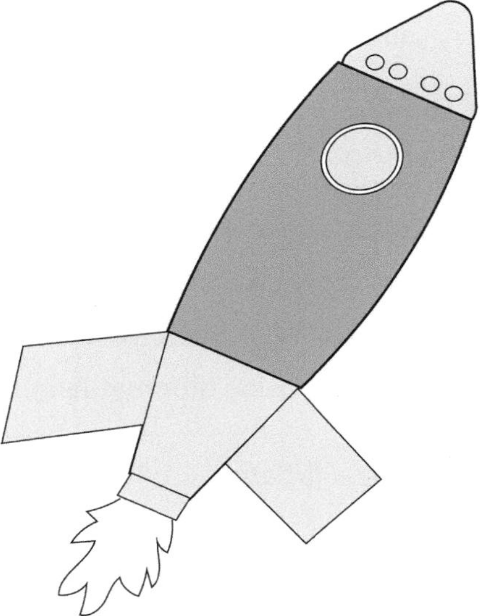

Build anticipation

Draw out key words like 'up' or use pauses with *Zoom Zoom We Are Going to the Moon* (rocking side to side, big lift up); and *Up Like a Rocket* (up and down, forwards and backwards).

Sound play

Encourage sound play through games and activities that encourage your child to experiment with different noises and combinations of sounds that they can repeat over and over. Make this a dummy-free time.

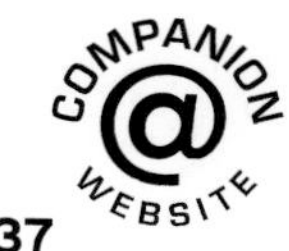

Feel a sound

Have fun with different sounds that your child can see, hear and feel. Try blowing a raspberry on their tummy or let them feel your lips as you hum.

Oooo

Aaaa

dadadada

bababa

Babble songs

Sing to your child using babble-sounds like 'la-la-la', humming, or nonsense sounds. Incorporate their coos and gurgles into your songs.

Babble conversations

Hold your child close and face to face with you so you both have good eye contact. Take turns to make sounds and babble. Follow your child's lead and imitate any sounds they make, and pause for a response. This shows you are listening, and they will enjoy the attention. When your child repeats a sound or makes a new sound, copy and leave a pause again.

Surprise toys

Use exciting toys and games to elicit sounds. Toys that provide an element of surprise, like pop-up toys, are the most likely to make your child vocalise. Whenever they do so accidentally or intentionally, respond immediately by copying their sound.

Mirror play

Use a mirror large enough for you and your child to see yourselves in and make silly faces and playful noises together, for example, cooing, blowing raspberries or making lip-smacking noises. Copy any sounds or facial expressions your child makes, and maybe add a few new ones of your own.

Feelings

Make sounds that are associated with feelings and emotional states in the appropriate situations, so say "ah" when bubbles or fireworks go up; "oh" when you hurt yourself or are surprised; "grr" when pretending to be angry, and so on. Accompany these sounds with the appropriate gestures, facial expression and exaggerated intonation.

Using sounds to communicate

When your child can make some sounds, help them to use them in a purposeful way. Use play situations and familiar routines to elicit spontaneous vocalisations. Your child only needs to vocalise or make an approximation of the word. These are the first steps in helping them to learn that they can use their voice to communicate needs and make responses.

Shaping sounds

Once your child is using sounds to communicate their needs, start differentiating between the different noises; for example, if they say [mu] associate it with 'Mum' or [bu] with a ball so that they begin to understand that language is meaningful.

Sounds in play

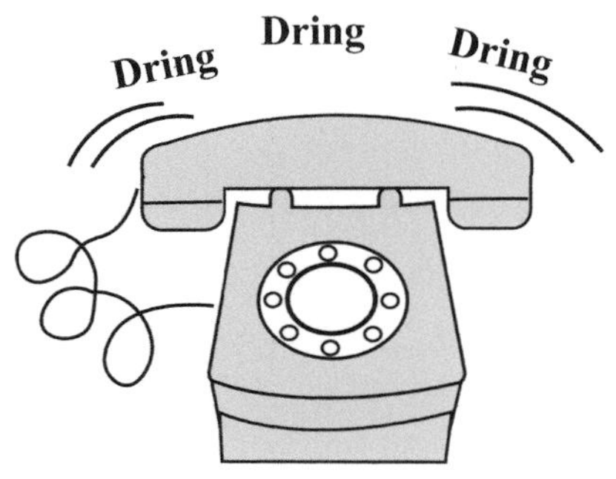

Incorporate sounds into a play routine so you are able to model the sound over and over. A ringing toy telephone like the Fisher Price Chatter Telephone may be useful in prompting imitation of sounds and attempts at chatter. Model the sounds of a ringing phone with a "brr-brr" or "ding ding", leaving a pause for your child to join in. Accept your child's efforts even if they are not quite there with the sound; instead, just repeat the sound back to them clearly: "*brr-brr*". Respond to your child's vocalisations by picking up the phone receiver. Hand them the phone as you make a sound.

Using sounds in play

Use a sound that your child is already making as part of a play routine. If they are saying [uh] encourage its use in activities where it can be shaped into the word 'up'. For example, bounce your child on your knee while singing along to *Up Like a Rocket*, pause and say "up" before lifting them up. Encourage your child to copy you before you lift them up. This way your child will start to learn that they have to say the sound at a certain point to be lifted up.

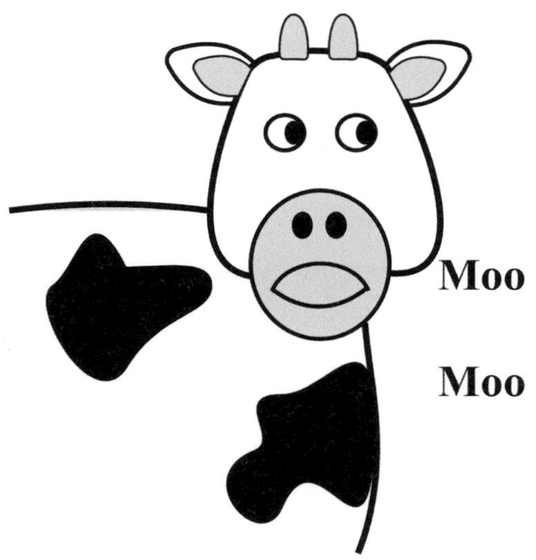

Copy the sound

Symbolic sounds like animal sounds and vehicle noises are usually easier to say, so games involving these sounds will also encourage your child to vocalise. As you play with a toy or look at a picture, make the appropriate sounds: "Moo, moo." Use the sound in comments like "The cow says moooo. She must be hungry. Mooo". Leave a gap for your child to join in – "the cow says ...". Accept your child's efforts even if they are not

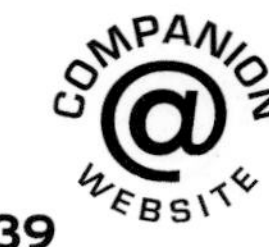

quite there with the sound; instead, just repeat the sound back to them clearly: "*Moo*, Yes, the cow says *moo*".

Encouraging first words

Your child will learn words more readily if they hear words in association with what they are doing or seeing. Avoid trying to make your child say a particular word by asking questions like 'What's this?' or asking them to copy or repeat words after you. If they say a word incorrectly, just repeat the word back clearly.

Offer a choice

Offering your child a choice may also prompt them to attempt to vocalise, for example, asking "Would you like *water* or *juice*?" Make the link between the word and object clear. As you say "*water*" hold out a beaker of water, and then as you say "*juice*" show your child the carton. This association between what your child is hearing and seeing is very important for learning sounds and words. It also makes it easier for your child to indicate their choice, whether this is with a word, a sound, a reach or a point to the desired object.

The success of this exercise depends upon consistently and regularly responding to your child's attempts at *communication*. You can model words once they indicate a choice: "You want *juice*" "Here's your *juice*". The objective is not to turn the situation into a battleground, however, so be light-hearted and give your child lots of good examples and encouragement.

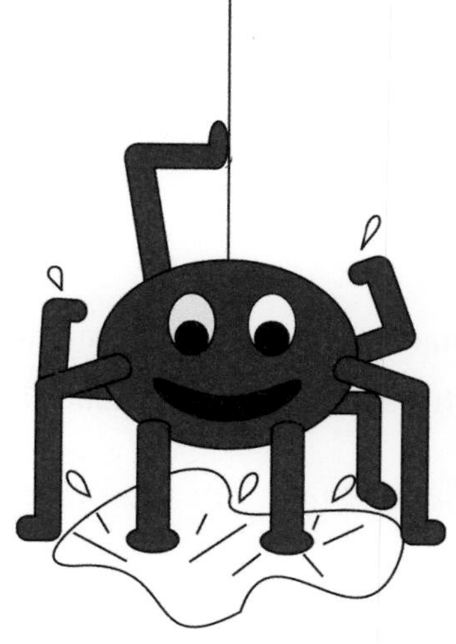

Nursery rhymes and action songs

Sing simple nursery rhymes and action songs together. When your child is very familiar with a nursery rhyme or song, you can leave a pause for them to join in at key moments by making the appropriate action, sound or word. Rhymes with repetitive choruses are best for this. Try *Incy Wincy Spider*, *The Wheels on the Bus*, *Twinkle, Twinkle Little Star* and *Hey Diddle Diddle*.

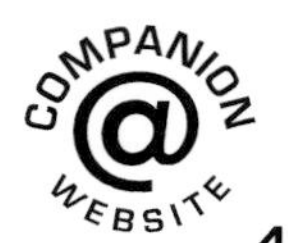

Naming objects

Name objects that attract your child's attention. For example, "Bubbles", "Look at the bubbles", "It's going up", "bubbles". Comment and expand on your child's attempts at words and phrases. So you might respond with "Yes, bubbles" "bubbles" to your child's attempt of "bubu".

Everyday routines

Make the most of everyday routines to introduce different vocabulary. For example, use bath time to build on your child's natural curiosity about the body by introducing the names of body parts and action words like splash and wash. Let your child help you to tidy up by putting clothes in drawers or in a washing basket. Give your child one article of clothing at a time as you name it, for example, "Now, the *coat*".

Picture books

Choose books with simple, repetitive stories and bright colourful pictures. Talk about the pictures rather than reading the story word by word. This will help your child associate the words with what they can see. This might be about the characters, actions or objects. Follow your child's lead by talking about things they seem interested in and copying any sounds or words they make. You can also expand on what they say; for example, your child says "bear" and you reply "big bear".

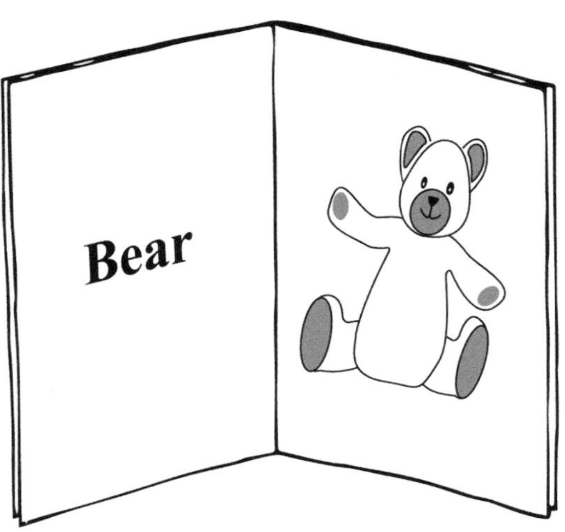

Your child's name

From very early on it is important to help your child learn their name. Use your child's name during daily routines to get their attention. Make it meaningful and positive by using it before a tangible reward, like offering a drink or a toy.

Include your child's name in turn-taking games. Help your child to make the connection by looking and pointing to them as you say their name. You can even add their name to rhymes and songs.

2

ATTENTION AND LISTENING SKILLS

DOI: 10.4324/9781003031109-3

Introduction

Attention control refers to the ability of an individual to attend to a stimulus and sustain that attention even when confronted with other distractions. It is a complex cognitive skill essential for various forms of learning including problem solving (Choudhury and Gorman, 2000) and information processing tasks (Ebert and Kohnert, 2011), and for language acquisition (Gomes et al., 2000). Attention control is a form of self-regulation and as such is thought to be essential for the development of executive functions (Hendry et al., 2016). Attention and listening skills also play a critical role in social communication, social development and social adaptation.

Factors affecting attention and listening skills

There are many factors that might affect the development of a child's attention and listening skills.

- **A sensory impairment:** A sensory impairment affecting hearing or vision is likely to impact on a child's attention and/or listening skills.

  Examples include:
  - *Hearing loss:*
    - Children with a permanent hearing loss were found to have delayed functional auditory skills, such as following instructions or hearing in noise, when compared to peers with typical hearing (Nassrallah et al., 2020).
    - A conductive hearing loss related to otitis media with effusion (glue ear) may cause the child to have difficulties in speech perception, particularly in noisy environments (Cai and McPherson, 2017).
  - *Vision impairment:*
    - Children with a vision impairment may have delays or atypical development of joint attention; for example, a child with a visual impairment may not engage in reciprocal eye-gaze and pointing but instead may have a range of idiosyncratic responses (Ross, 2017).
- **An underlying neurodevelopmental disorder:** Delayed or impaired development of attention and listening skills is associated with a number of neurodevelopmental disorders:
  - *Developmental Language Disorder* (DLD)*:* Children with DLD are likely to have a range of difficulties with attention and listening. These include problems with sustaining

attention to a task over time (Ebert and Kohnert, 2011), processing information and shifting attention between different stimuli (Aljahlan and Spaulding, 2019).

  - *Autism (Autistic Spectrum Disorder, ASD):* The development of attention skills is impaired in children with autism. For example, young infants show reduced and delayed development of joint attention skills (Naber et al., 2007).
  - *Attention-Deficit and Hyperactivity Disorder (ADHD):* Children with ADHD typically present with shorter attention spans, impulsivity and hyperactivity (Barkley, 2006).

- **Auditory Processing Disorder (APD):** APD has "its origins in impaired neural function" and is characterised by difficulties hearing speech in noisy environments and problems with attending to and remembering spoken instructions (BSA, 2018, p. 6). However, it should be noted that there is continued debate regarding the existence of APD as a discrete clinical entity in children (Neijenhuis et al., 2019). Rather, developmental APD may occur alongside other conditions that include attention problems, speech and language difficulties, learning disorders and cognitive delay (Moore, 2018).
- **Emotional and behavioural disturbances:** Emotional disturbances and behaviour disorders may negatively impact on a child's concentration and communication skills (Ogundele, 2018).
- **Physical and physiological disturbances:** Physical illness, tiredness and medication may cause the child to lack concentration.
- **Noisy home environment:** The child's home or learning environment may have led them to ignore certain stimuli; for example, they have accommodated to a noisy environment (Heft, 1979).
- **Noisy learning environments:** Environmental distractions can be too strong for the child to attend to the activity in hand (Erickson and Newman, 2017), and chronic noise exposure in learning environments can have a detrimental impact on attention, concentration and listening skills (Shield and Dockrell, 2003).

Always seek professional advice where there are concerns regarding delayed or atypical development.

Models of attention

Levels of attention control

Cooper et al. (1974) and Reynell (1980) established clear stages in the development of attention control. Within each stage there is considerable variability, because attention depends upon the situation and the nature of the activity and is influenced by a multiplicity of factors.

Level 1 (0 to 1 Year): This is characterised by extreme distractibility, when the child's attention flits from one object, person or event to another. Any new event, such as someone walking by, will immediately distract them.

Level 2 (1 to 2 Years): The child can concentrate on a concrete task of their own choosing but will not tolerate any intervention by an adult, whether spoken or visual. They may appear obstinate or 'wilful', but in fact their attention is single-channelled, and they must ignore all extraneous stimuli in order to concentrate upon what they are doing.

Level 3 (2 to 3 Years): Attention is still single-channelled in that the child cannot attend to auditory and visual stimuli from different sources. They cannot therefore listen to an adult's directions while they are playing, but they can shift their whole attention to the speaker and back to the game, with the adult's help.

Level 4 (3 to 4 Years): The child must still alternate their full attention, visual and auditory, between the speaker and the task, but they now do this spontaneously without the adult needing to focus their attention.

Level 5 (4 to 5 Years): The child's attention is now two-channelled, so they are able to understand spoken instructions related to the task without interrupting their activity to look at the speaker. Their concentration span may still be short, but they can be taught in a group.

Level 6 (5 to 6 Years): Auditory, visual and manipulatory channels are fully integrated and attention is well established and sustained.

From the age of 4 to 5 years, children are expected to be able to listen to verbal instructions and attend to individual and group activities in a classroom that is often noisy, is full of children and has dozens of competing and distracting stimuli. However, many language-delayed children are not at a mature enough level of attention to cope with these demands. Cooper et al. (1974) found that many language-delayed children manifested attention problems and that activities directed to these also helped their language development.

Conceptual frameworks

Researchers have offered a number of different conceptual frameworks to account for the cognitive processes underlying the development of attention control. There is general agreement that these cognitive processes are multidimensional and can be subdivided into

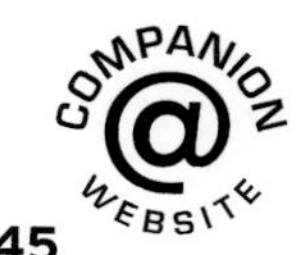

attentional domains. A model proposed by Posner includes the three attentional networks – alerting, orienting and executive (Petersen and Posner, 2012; Posner, 2016). Alerting refers to the ability to attend to and sustain that attention over a period of time. The ability to shift this attention focus evolves throughout early childhood and employs the orientating network, whereas the ability to pay selective attention in the face of competing distractions falls under the executive network. The work of Mirsky et al., 1991 in identifying discrete attentional processes they labelled focus, sustain, shift and encode provides a useful model for shaping the focus of intervention approaches.

Activities to promote attention and listening skills

This chapter covers the development of attention and listening skills from 0–60 months and contains a wide range of practical activities to support the development of these skills. These activities are designed to develop the child's ability to attend to visual and auditory stimuli, sustain attention to a task and develop the selective attention and listening skills necessary for dealing with competing demands in the learning environment.

Activities for attention control:

The aim is to consolidate the child's skills at their level of attention and to take them on to the next stage. The materials listed are suitable for children in that age group; for older children, it is best to use age-appropriate materials if possible. For example, with a 3- to 4-year-old at Level 1 of attention control, glove puppets, small cars and miniature dolls could be used to attract and sustain their interest. Activities for older children are also provided for all levels.

Activities for listening skills:

Listening skills are an integral part of many of the attention activities and reflect the growing auditory competence of the child as they progress through the attention levels. Activities are provided that target specific auditory skills such as sound location and auditory discrimination.

Activities for memory skills:

Activities are provided for practice with visual and auditory memory.

This chapter should be read in conjunction with Chapter 1 "Early Communication Skills" and Chapter 4 on "The Development of Verbal Comprehension" to gain a broader understanding of the child's development of attention and listening skills.

General guidelines

- Reduce ambient noise in the room by turning off background music (Manlove et al., 2001), and address any factors increasing noise levels. This could be as simple as using soft cups on chair legs to stop scraping sounds and lining storage tins and bins with fabric.
- Improve room acoustics by installing sound-absorbing soft furnishings like bean bags, curtains and carpets (Dockrell and Shield, 2006). Fabric is an easy solution to use for wall displays and to cover tables and cupboard tops. Even hanging mobiles can help improve room acoustics.
- Avoid visual distractions by removing unwanted clutter from the table or floor space.
- Choose materials of interest to the child that are also age appropriate. The materials and resources listed are suitable for children at that developmental stage; for older children, it is best to use age-appropriate materials if possible.
- The activity must be developmentally appropriate for the child, taking into account their level of functioning in other areas, such as symbolic understanding, language development and performance skills.
- Use clear, simple language that is appropriate to the child's level of understanding.
- Ideally rewards should be inherent in the game or activity itself, for example, the satisfaction of completing a puzzle or the joy of discovery – a toy hidden inside a set of nesting barrels.
- If intrinsic rewards are insufficient, then other rewards, whether material (stickers, charts) or social (smiles, praise) must be immediate and consistent, so that the child learns to associate them with the task.

Recording observations

Observe and record the child over an extended period of time in a variety of situations within the learning environment. These include spontaneous or child-initiated play, engagement in individual and group learning activities, as well as interaction with other children and adults. Observations from parents or caregivers are invaluable in gaining a broader understanding of the child's level of attention control and listening skills.

Make a note of:

- the type of stimuli that interests the child (e.g., environmental sounds, musical instruments, vocalisations, spoken language, toys with movement or visual effects, digital images);
- responses to auditory stimuli (e.g., stilling, head turn, vocalisation, preferences);
- responses to visual stimuli (e.g., tracks, fixated, preferences);

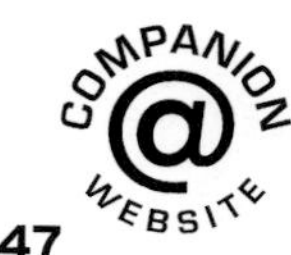

- the type of activity that attracts and sustain the child's attention;
- how long the child is able to sustain attention;
- the context (e.g., quiet one to one play with an adult, noisy outside play);
- who or what distracts the child (e.g., background noise; movement; outside events);
- how children or adult's gain the child's attention (e.g., calling, touch or showing);
- how the child gains the attention of another child or adult (e.g., calling, touch, or showing);
- the type and length of spoken instructions the child is able to follow appropriately (make a note of whether they seem to be looking and following other children);
- how the child is able to integrate competing auditory and visual information (e.g., can they follow instructions whilst engaged in a task; can they listen in a noisy environment);
- responses by the child to spoken instructions (e.g., body language, gestures/signs or spoken language);
- frequency of responses (e.g., sometimes, often, rarely).

Attracting and sustaining attention to people

Encouraging eye contact

The ability to make eye contact with other people is an important skill for the development of speech, language and communication. The listener gains extra cues about the content and tone of a spoken message from the speaker's facial expression and lip patterns. These cues are particularly important for understanding spoken language in children who have delayed language skills. Eye contact and eye gaze are also important for regulating communication, as it helps to initiate and maintain successful social interactions.

Aims

To encourage the child to initiate and sustain eye contact with adults and other children.

Outcomes

- Initiates eye contact with an adult or another child.
- Maintains appropriate eye contact with an adult or another child.

Strategies

- Be sensitive to cultural differences in eye contact, and never force a child to look at you.
- Incorporate eye contact as a natural part of an event or activity rather than relying on instructing the child to 'look at me'.
- Remember to model appropriate eye contact; for example, face the child when talking.

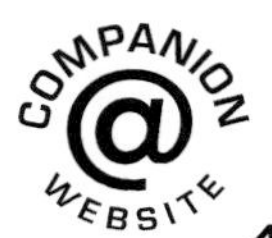

- Get down to the child's eye level where they can easily see your face rather than physically turning their head to look at you.
- Support the child's posture if necessary, to ensure good head control.
- Get the child's attention by calling their name, and use a lively intonation and a higher pitched voice to maintain their interest.
- Vary your facial expression and use lots of social rewards like smiles and vocalisations.
- Adapt your expectations. Looking at the face or forehead might be an acceptable compromise for those who struggle with eye contact, for example, children with ASD.

Suitable materials and resources

Dressing up materials like colourful floppy hats, tinsel wigs, funny glasses, false moustaches and clown noses; washable face paints; paper fans; lace; net; fancy dress or masquerade eye masks; cheerleader pom-poms and face masks. Musical instruments and sound makers like rattles, maracas, bells and squeaky toys.

Activities to encourage eye contact

Everyday routines

Use the natural proximity offered by everyday routines like getting dressed and undressed, mealtimes or bathing to make eye contact. Incorporate some fun games into the activity to maximise your interaction with the child. Pulling clothes on and off is ideal for playing peek-a-boo, and bubbles are great fun and less messy in the bath.

Playtime

During play make use of opportunities for eye contact, for instance, occasions like pushing them on a swing (from in front) or catching them as they come down a slide.

Play peek-a-boo

Start with see-through materials like net and lace; move on to more opaque materials and items that cover your face. Once the child is understanding the game try hiding behind the brim of a large floppy hat, peeping through a tinsel wig or waving colourful cheerleader pom-poms.

Funny faces

Place your face close to the child's and make very exaggerated lip shapes; pull faces; waggle your tongue; zoom your face in and out; chatter or sing with exaggerated intonation.

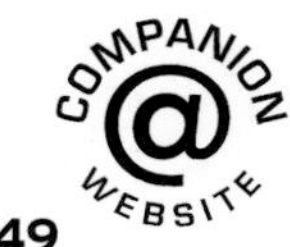

Put on a mask

Choose masks with holes for the eyes and mouth so you can attract the child's attention by batting your eyelashes or sticking your tongue out and wiggling it. Masquerade eye masks accentuate the eyes, and those with a handle allow you to quickly lower and raise the mask.

Flutter a fan

Use colourful paper fans to attract the child's attention. You can hide behind it, then peep out from above or to the side of it.

Dressing up

Put on a silly hat, false moustache, clown nose or funny glasses – anything to get the child looking at your face.

Make a sound

Hold a rattle close to your face and shake it to make a sound. Stop the noise and wait for the child to look before you continue. Alternate with other sound makers like maracas, bells, and squeaky toys.

Freeze

Lots of physical games allow for natural eye contact to occur. Help the child bounce on a big ball or small trampoline. Be on the same eye level as them. If they look away, 'freeze'; continue bouncing when you get eye contact.

Activities for older children

- Encourage older children to use eye contact with younger family members by playing peek-a-boo or singing nursery rhymes and songs like *Row, Row, Row Your Boat*.
- Choose activities that focus on the face like:
    - face painting or face decoration with face jewels and glitter, face paints and temporary tattoos;
    - taking family selfies with face stickers and photo booth props;
    - having fun with novelty glasses – try giant, colourful sunglasses or fancy dress eyewear, or go scary with glasses that have pop-out springy googly eyes;
    - making and decorating their own masquerade eye-masks.
- Introduce eye signals into physical play by using eye movements to give instructions, for example, look up for a 'jump', look left for a 'step to the left' and look down for 'a crouch'. Have fun with children inventing different eye movements and commands; less obvious ones are rolling eyes around for a spin or blinking rapidly for bunny hops.

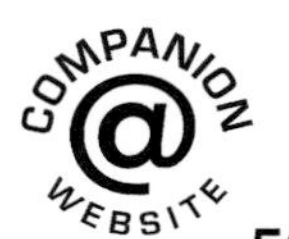

- Use a mirror to encourage the child:
    - to look at and talk about the reflection of their face in a mirror; they can outline key features by drawing on the mirror with a wipe-off marker;
    - to draw a self-portrait using what they can see in the mirror;
    - to copy the facial expressions of a partner.

      (Make sure you encourage an awareness and emphasis on the eyes.)
- Choose traditional board games that require players to sit opposite each other like draughts or chess. Vertical 'board' games like *Connect 4* (or *Four in a Row*) and *Jenga* are even more useful as the game is at eye level.

Attracting and sustaining attention to people

Attention to voice

These activities provide opportunities for the child to attend to voice and will help them to become familiar with the sounds and rhythms of language. Encouraging the child to engage in reciprocal games, rhymes and songs is also important for the development of social interaction skills.

Aims

To encourage the child to listen and respond to the different intonations, rhythms and sounds of spoken language.

Outcomes

- Attends to and enjoys rhythmic patterns in rhymes and songs.
- Joins in with actions, sounds or words.
- Creates own actions and movements as a response to a song.

Strategies

- Encourage attention to the face, and particularly to the mouth.
- Use a lively voice with a higher pitched voice to maintain their interest.
- Choose rhymes and songs with repetitive phrases to help the child begin to recognise particular sounds and words.
- Use facial expression, gesture and movement alongside spoken language.
- Make use of props to engage the child's attention.
- Incorporate songs and music from the child's home language.

Suitable materials and resources

Familiar rhymes, action songs, call and response songs with repetitive sounds, words and phrases. (For English as an additional language (EAL) children ask families to record lullabies, songs and music from home.) Homemade or bought puppets and other props to accompany singing.

Activities to encourage attention to voice

Rhymes

Use your fingers to attract the child's attention in rhymes; stroke their cheeks; place their own fingers where they can see them and play *This Little Piggy Went to Market, Round and Round the Garden* and so on.

Action songs

Songs with actions encourage attention to key words and changes in the rhythm. Actions involving the hands and face will also encourage the child to look at your face. Try *This is the Way we Wash our Face, Head, Shoulders, Knees and Toes* and nursery rhymes like *Incy Wincy Spider*. Emphasise key words and use gestures to encourage the child to join in with the sounds and actions.

Finger games

Sit opposite the child to play finger games using rhymes like *Pat-a-Cake*; *Two Little Dicky Birds*; *Ten Little Fingers*; and *This Little Piggy*; or hold hands as you move back and forward to *Row, Row, Row Your Boat*.

Ring-a-Ring-O'-Roses

Rhymes that use sounds to build up anticipation will also encourage the child to look at your face. For example, the sneeze in *Ring-a-Ring-O'-Roses* can be drawn out to increase the tension: aaaaaaaahhhh – tisshoo! Find out about similar songs in the child's home language and incorporate these into song time.

Puppet conversations

Encourage attention to your face by playing with a hand puppet of the child's favourite animal or story character. Hold it close to your face as you make it move, nod its head, wave and clap its hands or paws. Have little conversations where the puppet whispers in your ear, and then looks at your face to see your reaction.

Lullabies

As you pick the child up, hold their head close to yours while you sing their favourite lullaby, or chat to them with lots of melody and vocal inflection. Gently sway to the rhythm together. Leave pauses for them to respond with gurgles and sounds of their own.

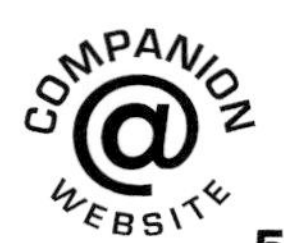

Nonsense words

Read rhymes and stories with nonsense words like *Mr Brown can Moo! Can You?* or *There's a Wocket in my Pocket* by Dr Seuss. Let the children have fun by encouraging them to join in with some of the sounds and words.

Activities for older children

Learning a song is a fun way to provide listening practice for words, sounds and phrases. It also helps with turn taking, listening, language and communication. Singing as a group supports children in learning the lyrics and the melody, as peers can be models for them to copy. Many songs can be accompanied by percussion instruments or adapted to include actions, movements and dances, so all children regardless of language ability are able to participate.

- Sing songs that involve actions so children who are struggling with saying sounds or words can participate by making an action. Try different gestures and body movements in songs like *Clap, Clap, Clap Your Hands, One, Two, Three*; *If You're Happy and You Know It;* and *Grand Old Duke of York*.
- Sing call and echo songs that require children to listen to a phrase sung by the adult and repeat it back. Examples include *Charlie over the Ocean*, which also has a chase game element, and *Boom Chicka Boom*, a familiar campfire song.
- Once children are familiar with call and echo songs, introduce songs where the chorus response is different. This might be one where the chorus is different from the lead singer, but is repeated throughout the song, or one where the chorus is different for each verse.
    - Adapt *Charlie over the Ocean* by introducing some objects so children can choose an object and introduce a different phrase for each new verse. So instead of *Charlie caught a big fish* you have *Charlie caught a boot* or *Charlie caught a stick*.
    - *Toom-bah-ee-lero*, a song written by Ella Jenkins, can be accompanied with various percussion instruments, but drums like djembe, tambour and bongo work particularly well with the rhythm.
    - *The Hokey Cokey* combines loud cheerful singing with actions and movements.
- Learn some songs in different languages to help children explore new sounds and experiment with different ways to use their voices. This is a good inclusive activity for EAL children, as it means all children start from the same point regardless of their first language. For example, *Jambo Bwana* (Kenya), a traditional greeting song in Swahili; or *liăng-zhi-lăo-hŭ* or *Two Tigers*, a traditional song from China.
- Combine singing with movement. Try out the BBC Bring the Noise *Robot Song*, where the children can dance and talk like robots. The children can sing the full lyrics or just

say the robot noises. Use percussion instruments to beat out the rhythm, which is based on 'long' and 'short'.

See:
www.bbc.co.uk/teach/bring-the-noise/eyfs-ks1-music-play-it-bring-thenoise/z4sq92p

Attracting and sustaining attention to people

Response to own name

Calling a child's name is a good alerting strategy to gain their attention, so it makes sense to help the child learn their name and the names of their peers early on. Recognising when their name is called will help the child attend to the speaker and be more able to listen to language directed at them.

Aims

To encourage the child to recognise and respond to their own name.

Outcomes

- Responds consistently when their name is called by looking or turning their head.
- Recognises when name is used, for example, in a simple rhyme or song.

Strategies

- Use the child's name to communicate in a meaningful way. Avoid just teaching them to respond to their name for no purpose.
- Link positive rewards and experiences (something they like to do) with calling the child's name.
- Avoid *overusing* the child's name to get their attention to say 'no', make demands or give other disciplinary rebukes.
- Use cues like pointing, eye contact and gesture to help the child recognise when you are saying their name.
- Some children may respond better when their name is called using a higher pitched, sing-song rhythm. Explore incorporating the child's name into rhymes and songs.

Suitable materials and resources

Toys for playing give and take games like balls, bean bags and wheeled toys. Greetings and farewell songs. Sensory balls (available from specialist manufactures) add extra interest by having different textures, and some light up or have sound.

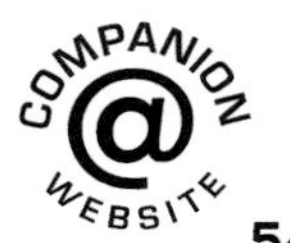

Activities to encourage a response to own name

Everyday routines

Use the child's name during everyday routines to get their attention. Make it meaningful and positive by using it before a tangible reward like offering a drink or a toy.

Roll, Roll, Roll the Ball

Sit opposite the child and gently roll a ball to the child saying the child's name in simple phrases sung along to the tune of *Row, Row, Row Your Boat*.

Roll, roll, roll the ball
Roll the ball to (child's name)
(Child's name x 4) roll the ball to me

Sing my name

Make up songs that include the child's name. Help the child to make the connection by looking and pointing when you say their name.

Greetings and farewell songs

In a group situation sing greeting and farewell songs to help children get to know each other and the adults.

Some examples are:

- *Hello, Hello, What's Your Name?* sung to the tune of *Frère Jacques*:
  Hello (child's name), Hello (child's name)
  How are you? How are you?
  It's really good to see you!
  It's really good to see you!
  Here at (name of nursery or school)
- *Good Morning to You* sung to the tune of *Happy Birthday*:
  Good morning to you
  Good morning to you
  Good morning (child's name)
  Good morning to you
- *Farewell* sung to the tune of *Twinkle, Twinkle Little Star*:
  Goodbye, goodbye little (child's name)
  Goodbye, goodbye little (child's name)
  We are sorry to see you go

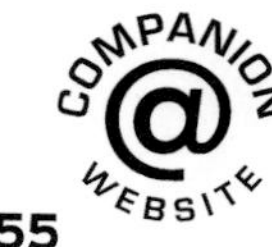

Beanbag game

The children sit or stand in a circle. They must call another child's name and throw a beanbag to them.

Activities for older children

- Two or more children and adults can play this adapted game of 'Simon Says'. Players take it in turns to give instructions using names. So "Aliyah, clap your hands". Aliyah then instructs another player "Toni, jump up and down".
- Adapt a story to include the child's name. Tell the story once, and then repeat it, explaining that they must put up their hand when they hear their name.

For small groups of children:

- Tell a simple story replacing the characters with the names of the children. Ask the children to put up their hand when they hear their name in the story. Call the names of the more able children first, to act as models, or use looks and pointing to cue children to respond.
- Try varying the activity by asking all the boys to stand up when they hear the name of a boy, and all the girls to stand up when they hear the name of a girl called out.
- Avoid allocating children to negative or bad characters in a story. Choose simple stories that allow for a series of actions by different characters. Stories based on a shopping trip, farm visit or seaside outing provide lots of opportunities, for example, "Billy saw a crab", "Chen found a shell".
- Maintain interest by adding in the names of teachers, assistants and so on.

Attracting and sustaining attention to objects

Attention to objects

Most children have an innate curiosity about themselves and their world, and infants soon discover that objects and people exist apart from themselves. Children start to understand and make sense of their environment through sensory exploration of the objects that surround them. The child responds to these stimuli through simple motor reflexes like sucking and grasping and moves on to develop fine motor actions like squeezing, pushing and pulling.

Aims

To attract and sustain the child's attention to objects and events in their environment, in order to encourage sensorimotor exploration and social interaction.

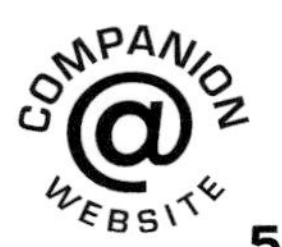

Outcomes

- Sustains interest in a toy or object for increasing periods of time.
- Explores a range of toys and objects through sensory exploration.

Strategies

- Choose visually engaging objects and materials that appeal to the child.
- Stimulate all of the child's senses as far as possible with toys that are multisensory, using sound, light, colour and texture.
- Help the child to play with an object or toy in different ways by exploring all of its properties through their different senses.
- Do not continue with something the child has lost interest in, but wait a while before introducing another object.
- When a child gets bored with a toy, try presenting it in a different way, for example, hiding it in a feely bag or box.
- Gradually extend the duration and complexity of activities.

Suitable materials and resources

Spinning discs, sun catchers, windmills, jack-in-the-box, pop-up toys, wind-up and clockwork toys, bells, rattles, wind chimes, squeaky toys, musical instruments and other sound makers; anything that catches the child's interest.

Activities to encourage attention to objects

Rattle

Shake a rattle to one side of the child's face, varying the intensity of the sound and movement. Shake it on the other side, and when they turn place it in their hand, bring their hand into vision and help them to shake it. Repeat using bells, squeaky toys and other sound makers.

Spinning patterns

Twirl a patterned disc on a string so that its pattern revolves and changes. Hang a sun catcher in the window to reflect light and colour. Spin a spiral sun catcher and see it shimmer and shine.

Light-up toys

There are a huge variety of toys that light up, from bath toys, musical instruments and balls to soft toys and teddies. Use these to attract the child's attention to an object, and then extend their play through exploration.

Wind toys

Wind toys combine movement, colour and sound. Enjoy the colours of a spinning whirligig or handheld windmill. Hang wind chimes that jingle as they move.

Action toys

Action toys encourage the child to be an active partner by engaging with the object through levers, buttons or dials. Try pop-up toys, clockwork and wind-up toys, and any cause-and-effect toys like a jack-in-the-box or a humming top that move or make a noise at the press of a button or a lever.

Sound makers

Encourage the child to explore different sound makers and musical instruments. Allow the child some space and time to initiate their own actions with the sound maker. You can then follow their lead and help to extend their play by showing them how different actions make different sounds. For example, a slow roll of a rattle compared with a rapid shaking movement.

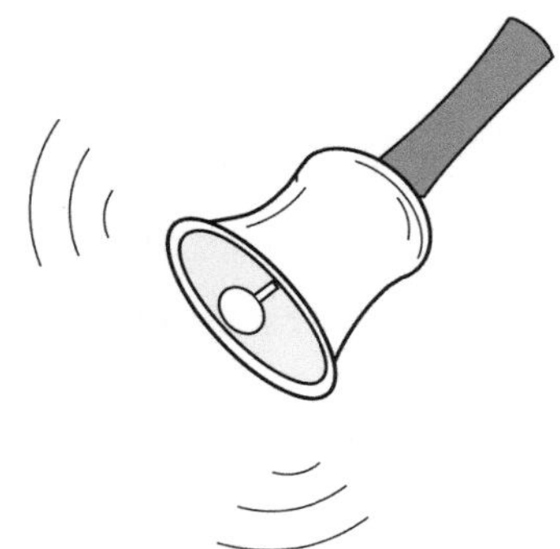

Multisensory toys

These toys are available from specialist manufacturers and will stimulate all the child's senses, encouraging exploration using different sounds, colours, light, textures, weight and density. Bubble tubes also provide a multisensory experience with stimulating light effects, changing colours and gently rising bubbles. Interact through touch or voice to change the colours and flow of the bubbles.

Activities for older children

- Make feely boxes or bags and fill with natural items (cones, shells, pebbles, sponges), everyday objects (brushes, plastic graters, spoons) or materials with different textures (silk, sandpaper, card, carpet). Make sure items are safe to touch with no sharp edges.

Link to the curriculum by focusing on:

- different attributes like colour, shape or size;
- mathematical concepts like length, weight and number;
- items starting with the same letter and so on.

Attracting and sustaining attention to objects

Visual tracking

Once you have gained the child's visual attention to an object, encourage them to track its movements. The ability to visually track an object enables the child to sustain attention to an object even when it starts to move out of their field of vision. This is essential if the child is to form adequate concepts about the world. It also forms the basis for later visual skills required in reading and writing.

Aims

To encourage the child to visually track a moving object even when it starts to move out of their field of vision.

Outcomes

- Visually tracks a toy or object within sight.
- Visually tracks a toy or object as it moves out of immediate sight.

Strategies

- Support the child's posture if necessary so they are able to easily track objects by turning their head.
- Some children may have difficulty with balance and head control, so seek the advice of a physiotherapist or occupational therapist on supporting the child's posture.
- Once the child is attending to a toy or object, encourage them to track its movements.
- If they don't do this spontaneously, they may have to be gently helped to turn so that they learn they can keep the toy or object in their sight.
- Stop moving the toy or object if the child's attention wanders and recapture their interest by starting to move it again.
- Remember that side-to-side movement is easiest at first, then try up-and-down movement and finally vary the direction.

Suitable materials and resources

Push along carts and wagons; wheeled toys on string; toy cars, trains and planes; skittles; giant bubble blowers; maracas with LED lights; a ball with a bell inside; musical instruments.

Activities to encourage visual tracking

Favourite toy

Hold a favourite object or toy in front of the child until you have their attention and then move it slightly, first to one side and then to the other. This gradually extends their field of

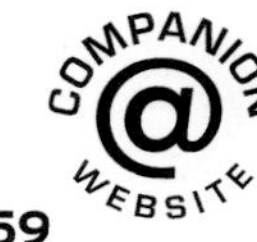

vision. To begin with it may be necessary to move the child's head so that they look in the right direction.

Moving objects

When the child is able to follow slow, simple, side-to-side movements, begin to vary the speed and direction. Other moving objects that would be useful at this stage include a puppet on a stick; balloons; balls and extending toys such as Christmas paper-chains.

Sound makers

Use sound makers to attract the child's attention. Shake a rattle, bell or other sound maker to one side of the child's face and gradually move it across their field of vision. When they turn, shake it again and give it to them, helping them to manipulate it. Carry out similar activities with a variety of sound makers, preferably ones that the child can manipulate easily themself.

Blowing bubbles

Blow bubbles to watch them rise and fall, burst them or pretend to catch one. Let some burst on the child. Help the child to pop a bubble. Can they catch one too? Have fun outside with bubble blowing machines and giant bubble wands.

Roll a noisy ball

Let the child explore the ball and draw their attention to how the bell inside makes a noise. Roll the ball across the floor or table, so it appears in front of the child before it disappears out of sight. Encourage the child to follow the ball.

Incy-Wincy Spider

Use your hands to act out the action of the spider slowly climbing up the spout, then tumbling down again. Make sure you move your hands up high above the child's head and then low down to the floor to encourage them to look up and down.

Bumpy ride

Push a large car from side to side in front of the child and encourage them to push it. Show the child how different surfaces affect its movement. For example, a thick carpet will slow it down, a bumpy surface will make it go up and down and a downward slope will speed it up.

Toys on strings

Use large, wheeled toys on string that you can push away from and then pull back towards the child. Encourage them to hold the string and pull the toy towards them.

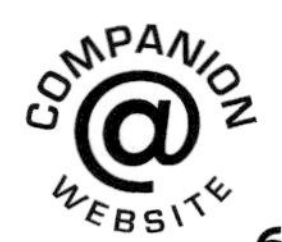

Skittles

Make your own skittles using plastic drinks bottles weighted down with some sand in the bottom. Spread out your skittles and have some fun using a giant beach ball. The child can track the rolling ball. (Other toys that can be knocked down are a tower of bricks, cartons, cardboard tubes and boxes.)

Activities for older children

- Ball games – keeping track of the ball is an integral part of any ball game, from a simple catch and throw game, through volleyball, to bat and ball games. For children who have difficulty catching small balls, use a balloon, soft beach ball or a chiffon scarf instead.
- Music and movement – actually fun for all ages! Props encourage looking and following too. Try incorporating jingle sticks with streamers; chiffon scarves; streamers and stretchy bands. Pair or group children for copying games.
- Scanning and tracking – older children may need practice with scanning and tracking items on a page. Practice this with worksheets with multiple items that the child has to scan in order to find and mark a target item; dot-dot pictures; and colour by number.

Attracting and sustaining attention to objects

Shifting attention between objects

It is important that the child can shift their attention from one object to another so that they can explore all aspects of a large object or make choices and comparisons between objects.

Aims

To facilitate the child to shift their attention from one object to another.

Outcomes

- Looks back and forth between two objects.
- Relates two similar or two different objects together.
- Uses two different objects in a similar way.

Strategies

- Use favourite toys or other objects of interest to the child.
- Avoid having too many toys out at once.
- Start by focusing on the same toy or activity as the child.
- Introduce items by playing alongside with a similar object.
- Allow the child to lead before gradually introducing another object.

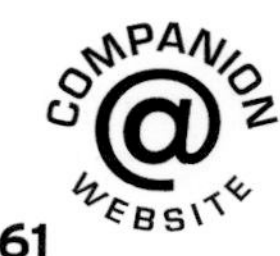

Suitable materials and resources

Bricks; blocks; Duplo bricks; water toys; cars; and any take-apart toys.

Activities for shifting attention between objects

Bang together

Show the child how to relate two similar objects together using simple fine motor movements. You can bang two bricks together; knock one plastic beaker against another; or crash a toy car into another car.

Hammer together

Show the child how to relate two different objects through play with hammer and pounding sets.

Little ducks in a race

Have fun with water spray bottles and plastic ducks in a tub. The squirts of water make the ducks move across the tub. Try accompanying the race with *Five Little Ducks*.

Tap together

Have a treasure basket with items that make a sound when tapped together: two shells; two rhythm sticks; or claves. Try different movements and different sound makers, for example, rubbing two sand blocks together or banging cymbals together. Let the child experiment, so they can tap a shell with a stick.

Beat out a rhythm

Encourage the child to explore making sounds with musical instruments and different beaters. So a wooden stick can be used to tap a guiro or beat on a drum. Extend the child's play by showing how you can make different sounds by scraping the guiro with the beater.

Making sounds

Show the child how different musical instruments might be used to make a sound in a similar way, so you can shake a tambourine in the same way you might shake a rattle.

Take apart, and put back together

Use a large toy that has easily removable parts. Encourage the child to take off the part and put it back. Examples include take-apart airplanes, trains, cars and animals like dinosaurs.

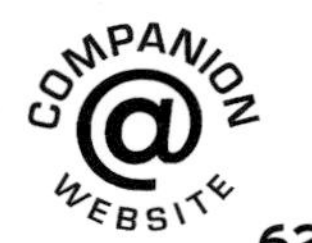

Doll play

Use a large doll, wearing a large hat. Remove the hat with a big show of surprise and put it on your head, then the child's head. Redirect attention to the doll by putting its hat back, saying "There!"

Gone fishing

Encourage the child to relate different objects to each other by using tools with toys in a water tray; for example, use a net to scoop up seashells or a magnetic fishing rod to catch toy fishes or frogs. Try singing along to the game with *Five Little Seashells*; *Once I Caught a Fish Alive*; or *Five Speckled Frogs*.

Activities for older children

- Water play – let children explore relating items in water play. They will have fun pouring water from one container to another; filling bowls and buckets using funnels and jugs. Provide pipe builder sets with funnels, cogs and water wheels that can be slotted together to create water carrying systems. Link with STEM curriculum by exploring concepts like flow, motion and gravity. Introduce related vocabulary like *full, empty, pour, fill, through, down, up.*
- Sand play – the properties of sand make it an ideal material for children to explore the effects of different tools in creating texture.
    - Children can make marks and patterns with rakes, lollipop sticks, combs, wheeled toys, seashells, hands and fingers. Help them to compare the effect of size and density with similar items that range in scale, material and shape, like a rake, fork and comb.
    - Provide pipes or pieces of plastic guttering for children to add water deep into the sand to create rivers and pools. Encourage imaginative play with various natural materials and objects that can be added to create land and seascapes. Link with topics about nature and the environment.

Developing joint attention

Joint attention occurs when the child and adult show interest in and interact with the same object. There is a mutual focus of attention that is characterised by triadic interactions between the "child, adult and other" (Sharma and Cockreill, 2014, p. 87). Importantly there is a shared understanding between the child and the adult that they are both interested in the same object or event. The child is able to follow eye gaze or pointing by the adult, or in turn directs the adult's attention using gestures or vocalisations. Joint attention supports the development of social interaction, communication and language development.

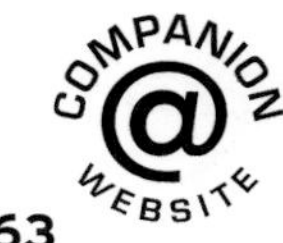

Aims

To facilitate joint attention to an object or event of shared interest and encourage the use of gestures, vocalisation or speech to direct attention.

Outcomes

- Responds to the adult's attempts to establish joint attention.
- Switches attention between the adult and an object and back again.
- Attracts adult attention to an object by vocalising, pointing, showing or looking.

Strategies

- Create opportunities for a shared experience with the child.
- Choose visually engaging objects and materials that appeal to the child.
- Position yourself to be on the level with the child to make eye contact.
- Being face to face makes sustained interaction easier for the child.
- Use gestures like pointing and showing to help direct the child's attention.
- Make the link between pointing and the object clear. Avoid vague points to objects across the room.
- Be consistent in responding to attempts from the child to direct your attention.
- Have a balance between turns between yourself and the child.
- Allow the child time to respond, leaving pauses for them to fill.

Suitable materials and resources

Interactive toys and games; multisensory toys with sound, light, colour and texture; and picture story books.

Activities to develop joint attention

Follow the child's lead

Generate opportunities for a shared experience by following the child's interests and attending to objects and toys that capture their attention. Help them explore objects, commenting on them and pointing to interesting features.

Bubbles

Most children love chasing after the bubbles to pop them. Wait for the child to look at you or make some sort of signal before blowing more bubbles. Help the child blow bubbles for you to pop. Large bubble blowers are useful for children who find smaller bubble wands difficult.

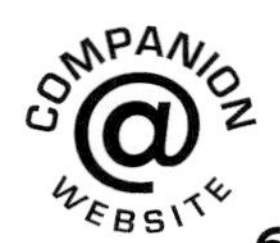

Sensory toys

Sensory toys with different visual effects will attract the child's attention. Have a duplicate so you can copy the child's actions. Try looking at glitter tubes, ooze tubes, liquid cell timers and spiral liquid tubes.

Shape-sorting box

Place the shape-sorting box between you and the child. Take off the lid and encourage the child to take out the shapes and place them on the floor. Put the lid back on and hand a shape to the child. Encourage the child to post it through the correct hole by pointing and commenting "Look, try this one". Take a shape and hold it near your face, asking "Where shall I put this one? In here?" pointing at the matching hole. Continue to take turns with the child.

Copy me

You will need a pair of identical plastic bowls and wooden spoons to play a 'follow the leader' game. With the bowl turned upside down start with beating the bowl, beating faster, then louder. Then turn the bowl right side up and stir with the spoon, fast and then slow. Can the child do some actions for you to follow? Make this more complicated by using musical instruments and creating rhythms and tempos.

Shared books

Look at books together helping the child to turn pages. Point at something of interest and make a sound or action, "Look a cat, miaow". Prompt the child to stroke the cat. Follow the child's eye gaze or points to comment on anything that interests them or catches their attention. Books with interactive elements are particularly useful, like pop-up pictures, lift the flap, peep holes, sound buttons and tactile elements.

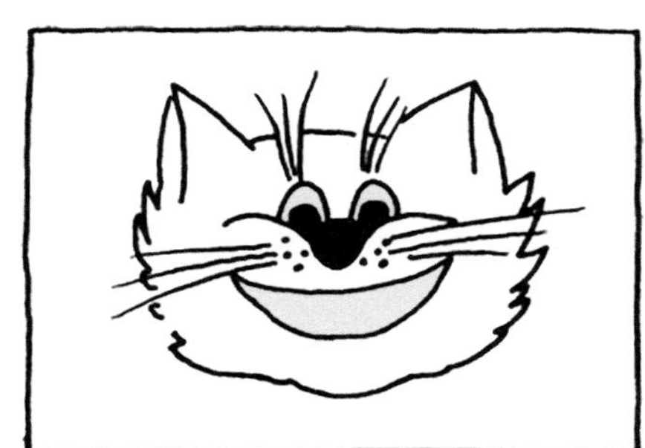

Activities for older children

Older children may benefit from continued support and practice with following directions, giving directions to others, turn taking and social interaction. Suitable activities will be found in the later sections on listening skills and in Chapter 3 "The Role of Play".

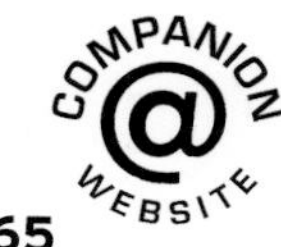

Attending to adult direction in play

These activities help the child to tolerate adult direction in extending their play choices and encouraging greater flexibility in how they engage with different activities. They are suitable for shifting children from Level 1 to Level 2 of the Reynell Levels of Attention.

Aims

To help the child tolerate the adult's presence and involvement in an activity of the child's own choosing.

Outcomes

- Comfortable with adult playing alongside.
- Tolerates adult involvement in an activity.
- Attends to adult directions within the activity.

Strategies

- Allow the child to play with an activity of their own choosing and follow their lead.
- Reduce visual distractions by removing extraneous materials and toys.
- Choose a quiet time when background noise is reduced.
- Position yourself so you are on the same eye level as the child. This makes it easier to get their attention and to interact.
- If at first the child cannot tolerate you sharing their toys, have a duplicate set handy.

Suitable materials and resources

Simple picture puzzles; take-apart toys; balls; bricks; shape-posting boxes; nests of beakers; musical instruments; hammer, pound or tap toys.

Activities for encouraging attention to adult direction in play

Parallel play

Use a duplicate set of toys to sit beside the child and play alongside. At first copy the child's play and any sounds or words they use. However, the focus is on play rather than language input at this stage, as the child will be unable to assimilate spoken language when engaged in an activity.

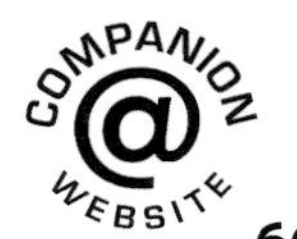

Demonstration

Begin to extend the child's play by demonstration without intervening in what they are doing; for example, if they are playing with bricks, build a small tower with your bricks. They may respond in one of these ways:

- appearing not to notice but beginning to imitate your actions;
- stopping their play and watching you with interest;
- knocking over your tower! In any case contact has occurred and you have caught their attention.

Generalisation

Generalise with plenty of games and activities, extending the child's exploration of toys as you play alongside. See if the child can copy you.

- Shape-posting box: take your shape and try it in several holes before finding the right one.
- Nests of beakers: pile them on top of each other and use them as containers, as well as fitting them together.
- Floor toys: show how lorries and trailers can be linked up, cars raced and bumped together.
- Water-play: demonstrate pouring from one container to another.
- Musical instruments: show how to make loud and quiet sounds.

Encourage shared play

When the child can tolerate your presence and begins to imitate, you can make small modifications to their play. You can push the correct jigsaw piece in front of them; add a brick to their train or tower; or encourage them to use different coloured crayons when scribbling.

Give instructions

Talk about the task by commenting on what the child is doing. Accompany your actions with integral spoken instructions, for example, "The brick goes on top"; "Let's turn it over"; or "Try a red pencil".

Finally, allow the child times during the day to play alone or alongside other children. Solitary play will encourage concentration skills and allow the child space to explore and experiment by themselves.

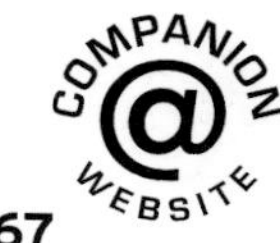

Activities for older children

Some older children may continue to show rigid attention to an activity or demonstrate repetitive play behaviours. Try the following:

- Provide resources like Lego or building blocks that encourage sharing of materials, but also allow the child to play on their own. The use of a personal tray, bucket or bag allows the child to select items to play with from a shared pile to then use in solitary play.
- Provide resources for children to work together like floor jigsaws, construction kits, sand and water play.
- Help children extend their play by providing opportunities for the child to change the rules in a game or make up some rules of their own. Examples include inventing new card games; setting up obstacle courses; organising physical play with footballs or other similar items; and creating homemade board games.

Shifting focus of attention

Children with single-channelled attention prefer to focus on an activity of their own choosing. They find it difficult to listen to instructions when engaged in an activity and may not respond when you talk to them. This will help children move from Level 2 to Level 3 of Reynell's Levels of Attention.

Aims

To establish the child's own control over their focus of attention in order to be able to shift attention from an activity to an adult, and then back again.

Outcomes

- Shifts attention from task to focus on adult directions.
- Shifts attention back to their own activity.

Strategies

- Use child-initiated play where possible or provide simple activities that engage the child's interest.
- Position yourself so you are on the same eye level as the child. This makes it easier to get their attention and to interact.
- Call the child's name and establish eye contact before you give instructions.
- Give simple, short and clear instructions before the start of the activity, when the child's full attention is on you.

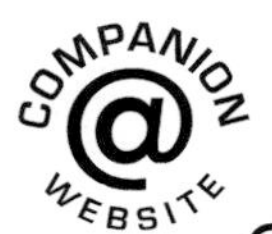

- Relate instructions to the activity.
- Use gesture, symbols and other visual cues to help the child understand your requests and instructions.
- You may need to use prompts to help the child refocus back on their activity.
- Gradually reduce adult support until the child is able to focus their own attention.

(Eye contact is important, so you may need to work on this – see earlier section for ideas.)

Suitable materials and resources

Skittles; stacking beakers; balls; car ramps or marble runs; water play equipment; cooking items; plasticine and dough for modelling.

Activities to help shift focus of attention

Ready steady go

The child has to wait for the instruction "go" before they carry out an action. The element of anticipation builds tension and will attract the child's attention.

Try the following:

- Knocking down a tower of bricks or beakers (encourage the child to build these first);
- Rolling a ball to knock down skittles (again, encourage the child to set these up first);
- Car ramps or marble runs.

Pancakes

Help the child to beat together eggs, flour, milk/water to make a batter for pancakes. As the child is busy beating and stirring, give instructions about adding extras like chocolate chips or mini raisins. Have these ready to hand to the child.

Water play

As the child is playing with toys in a water tray, you can help them add food colouring and then some baby shampoo. Provide a whisk for them to make some bubbles.

Creative art

Give the child different soft materials to explore like dough or clay. Help them to flatten and squash it into different shapes. Have a supply of materials like pasta, sequins, seeds and sticks. Give instructions like "Find a button" and "push" to encourage them to press it into a shape. Later they can tear apart the dough or clay and collect up the buttons.

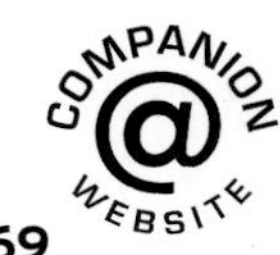

Follow-my-leader

Play imitation games with the adult leading on actions. Keep instructions very short to begin with, for example, "clap hands".

Everyday routines

Use the ideas outlined in strategies above to give instructions to the child during everyday routines and activities.

Activities for older children

- Play the parachute game *Merry-Go-Round*. Children stand sideways to the parachute holding on to it with one hand. As they walk around in a circle, the chute will start to look like a merry-go-round. Have a cue word that signals a change in direction. Switch directions every now and then.
- Reinforce the importance of looking and listening for spoken instructions, for example, looking at the adult during circle time and at other children during 'show and tell'.

Building concentration span

The ability to focus and sustain attention underpins all other attention and listening skills and is a vital skill for successful learning.

Aims

To increase the child's ability to sustain attention to adult initiated tasks.

Outcomes

- Sustains attention to a task of their own choosing.
- Sustains attention to an adult-led task.

Strategies

- Reduce background noise and remove visual distractions.
- Have one activity out at a time in a clutter-free area.
- Start with child-initiated play activities and gradually move to more adult-directed tasks.
- Prompt the child to stay on task and ignore distractions (Kannass et al., 2010).
- Practice with games and toys that have a natural start and finish.
- Combine adult-led tasks with a favourite activity as a reward on completion.
- Use 'back chaining' (see the 'Introduction' for an explanation of this technique) so the child only has to complete the final one or two stages of an activity.

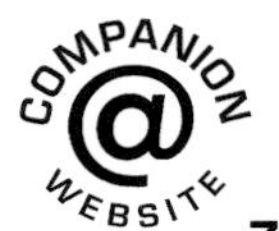

- Gradually increase the length of time the child spends on activities.
- Gradually increase the complexity of the activities.

Suitable materials and resources

Puzzles, shape sorters, shape posting boxes, simple construction toys and tabletop games.

Activities for building concentration span

Tabletop activities

Simple puzzles, shape sorters and posting boxes have a clear start and finish. This encourages the child to continue until the task is completed.

Early construction kits

Simple construction kits for building a car, robot or dinosaur provide the child with a concrete result for their efforts in concentration.

Start/finish boxes

Use start and finish boxes (or other receptacles) to help the child visualise the concept of starting and finishing. Activities are placed in the start box, and once completed they go in the finish box. Using a colour code on the boxes will also help, for example, green for start and red for stop.

Bag it up

Keep items in a bag. The child must return items to the bag and put it away each time. Bags can contain books, puzzles and other toys.

Be active

Children who tend to be fidgety and easily distracted are likely to be more engaged with active play. This can be movement to music, 'Simon Says' games or action songs.

Musical chairs

In a group play 'musical chairs'. Each child sits down when the music stops. Real chairs are not necessary; the floor will do nicely!

Pass the parcel

Play this traditional game where the child unwraps a parcel when the music stops and must pass it on when it starts again. Keep the wrapping simple so the parcel moves swiftly round the circle.

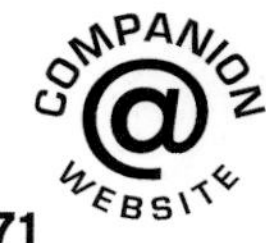

Musical statues

The children move around as the music plays; when it stops, they must stand still like statues, otherwise they are out. Alternatively, they can do an action like stamping their feet, clapping or waving their arms, so everyone is engaged all the time.

Animal sounds

Read a story or sing a song about a dog or a cat, and whenever the animal is mentioned the child must make the appropriate noise or mime the particular animal.

Activities for older children

- Give visual cues to indicate how long the child needs to stay focused on a task. Sand timers are ideal for this.
- Be unpredictable – avoid predictability in group activities. So maybe give one person two turns, go backwards and forwards and not just clockwise, or vary the order of children for answering questions so everyone stays focused on instructions.
- 'Follow the conductor' – Engaging children with simple music activities is a great way to improve attention. In this activity the children have to watch and respond to the cues from the conductor.

See: www.bbc.co.uk/teach/bring-the-noise/teaching-rhythms/zbwbscw

Simple listening skills

Listening is a complex, multidimensional skill that involves audition, attention, verbal understanding and memory. Often children are required to integrate information from both auditory and visual channels as they follow instructions and carry out tasks, frequently with competing stimuli from background noise. The ability to develop and sustain selective attention is crucial for successful language development.

Aims

To develop skills in simple listening tasks involving one or two key elements of information.

Outcomes

- Identifies one or two words presented within a phrase.
- Follows simple instructions with one or two key words.
- Listens to others in one-to-one situation or a small group of two or three.

Strategies

- Give the child time to focus their attention before giving instructions.
- Position the child so they can see your face if required.
- Reduce background noise and remove visual distractions (see the 'General Guidelines' section earlier in this chapter for more information on creating a good listening environment.)
- Vocabulary should be familiar to the child. These are listening activities and not comprehension ones.
- The length and complexity of the command will be dependent on the child's receptive language level.
- Keep instructions within the child's level of comprehension (see Chapter 4).
- At first accompany spoken language with lots of visual and contextual cues, gradually reducing these until the child is relying on listening alone.

Suitable materials and resources

Picture books; stories; picture cards; remote control cars or floor robots; and everyday objects.

Activities to develop simple listening skills

Simon Says

Ask the child to point to body parts or carry out simple actions. Encourage them to join in and give you instructions.

Action songs

Sing familiar action songs with the child that have repetitive words and phrases. Can the child complete the phrase with the final word, for example, "the wheels on the...(bus)"?

Posting objects

Create a fun posting box and collect together several pairs of different objects. Start off with one-word commands, for example, "Post the *ball*". Add some similar objects that vary in size, colour or shape. Gradually increase the length of the commands, for example, "Post the *red ball*" and "Post the *big shoe*".

Everyday commands

Practise the sorts of commands that the child will have to follow in class, for example, "Put the *pencils away*". In a group, ask each child to give something to another child, for example, "Give the *book* to *Michael*".

Listening to requests

Encourage the child to choose which of two or three toys they want. Show them each toy as you ask, "Do you want dolly, teddy or train?" etc. Emphasise these key words. Then try with a spoken request only.

Birthday presents

Prepare several picture cards of different items that might be used as gifts, for example, a teddy, train set, car, book and shiny shoes. Make up a story about a child's birthday and all their different presents. As the child hears the presents mentioned, they collect the appropriate picture. Afterwards read the story again and help the child to check that they have all the right presents.

Follow the trail

Set up a 'trail' in the outside play area for children to follow instructions like "Go round the bench" and "Touch the tree".

Simon Says

- Ask the child to touch two to three body parts.
- Ask them to touch or hand you two related objects, for example, the table, a chair.
- Ask them to touch or give you two unrelated objects, for example, shoe, book, which is slightly harder because they cannot guess the second object.
- Give them simple actions to do when they hear a sound, for example, when they hear you beat a drum, they must clap their hands. This will need some demonstration first.

Activities for older children

- Repeat the 'Simon Says' activity but with a group of children so they each have to listen to others give instructions.
- Give directions using more complex vocabulary like 'through' 'around' 'behind' to children racing remote control cars or floor robots. Set up a track with various obstacles that need to be negotiated before the finish line. Create some dead ends and circular routes in the style of a traditional maze.

Complex listening skills

Following complex instructions requires more processing of language by the child than remembering single items. Complex instructions might be simple, complex or single- or multi-part, requiring sequential completion.

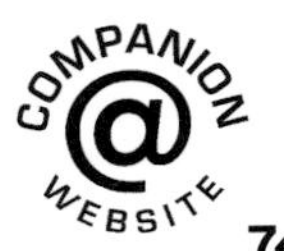

Aims

To support the child in listening to complex information in both single and multi-part instructions.

Outcomes

- Follows complex instructions involving three or four key words.
- Follows a sequence of instructions in the correct order.

Strategies

- Give the child time to focus their attention before giving instructions.
- Position the child so they can see your face if required.
- Reduce background noise and remove visual distractions (see 'General Guidelines' earlier in this chapter for more information on creating a good listening environment.)
- Vocabulary should be familiar to the child. These are listening activities and not comprehension ones.
- The length and complexity of the command will be dependent on the child's receptive language level (see Chapter 4).
- At first, accompany spoken language with lots of visual and contextual cues, gradually reducing these until the child is relying on listening.
- At first you may need to break down longer instructions into shorter chunks.
- Alternatively, wait until the child has completed one part of a sequence of instructions before giving them the next part.
- Always give instructions out sequentially in the order in which you wish the child to carry them out.
- Gradually introduce longer and more complex commands.
- Encourage the children to use visualisation and rehearsal strategies to help remember instructions (Gill et al., 2003), for example, imagining carrying out an activity or repeating back an instruction. Be sensitive to the child's abilities in speech and expressive language.

Suitable materials and resources

Picture books; stories; picture cards or photographs of objects; equipment for obstacle course; barrier game screen; magnetic books and boards; Fuzzy-Felt; and assorted playmats with miniature toys.

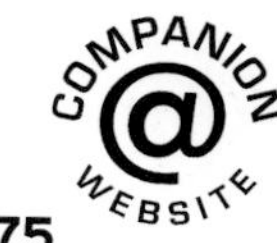

Activities to develop complex listening skills

Simon Says

Pointing to body parts – if the child understands 'my' and 'your', give commands such as, "Point to *your* ear, *your* knee and *my* neck", emphasising the possessives. Otherwise use children's names and make it a group activity.

Posting objects

Have up to four different coloured posting boxes and several coloured objects. Start off with simple commands, for example, "Post the ball". Gradually increase the length of the commands, for example, "Put the ball in the yellow box" and "Post all the red toys in the blue box".

Everyday commands

Practise the sorts of commands that the child will have to follow in class, for example, "Hang up your *coat* and fetch the *peg-boards*". In a group, ask each child to give something to another child, for example, "Give the *book* and *pen* to *Michael*".

Spot the missing information

Read stories familiar to the child with one or more pieces of information or words omitted. Can the child fill in the missing information?

Obstacle courses

Obstacle courses are good fun. Use tables, chairs, mats, play tunnels, steps, play barrels, hoops and benches to create the obstacles. Tell the child a series of actions to perform, for example, "Jump over the mat, crawl under the chair, and touch the wall". In a group this can be made into a race.

Barrier game

Two children sit on either side of a screen, each with a large sheet of paper and crayons. They take it in turns to tell each other what to draw, for example, "Draw a *house*. Put a *red roof* on it. Make *three windows*". At the end both drawings should look the same.

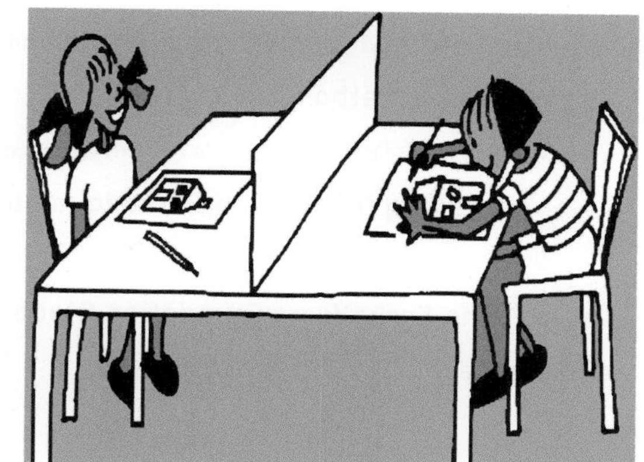

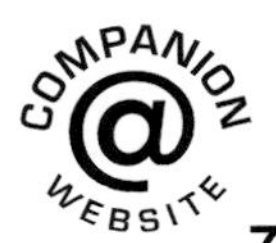

Create a picture story

Give instructions to the child on how to create a picture story by placing toys or pictures on a large illustration of a farm, zoo, street or park. Some ideas are:

- *Magnetic Books and boards* – place magnets on a range of different backgrounds. For example, *Magnetic Books* by Janod have several different games including *Boys/Girls Crazy Faces*; *Boys/Girls Costumes*; and *Animals*. The *Four Seasons* game is particularly useful for children working in pairs, as one child can give instructions to another child about how to replicate the four seasons scene cards.
- *Fuzzy-Felt* – ask the child to place *Fuzzy-Felt* pieces onto various scenes that include my house, a farm, under the sea and a picnic in the park.
- *Playmats* – these large floor mats are based on the idea of road maps and depict different scenes like towns, farms and seaside areas. Instructions can be given about where to place toy objects, vehicles, people and animals.

Activities for older children

- Create a scene with the child using a magnetic board or game like *Fuzzy-Felt* (see previous section). Recount a short story woven around the scene. Afterwards ask the child to retell the story using the pictures to help as a reminder.
- Use stories that focus on listening. *The Listening Walk?* by Paul Showers is a great book that has all sorts of different sounds that the children will have fun in recreating, for example, how to reproduce the sounds of the dog's toenails on the pavement! The story also introduces the idea of silence versus noise, and the importance of listening.
- Set up a themed project around sound and hearing. Activities might include:
  - Listening to music and sounds with their hands over their ears, while wearing woolly hats or headphones, and through ear-trumpets.
  - Using a stethoscope.
  - Playing shouting and whispering games.
  - Listening to and comparing loud and soft noises; pleasant and discordant sounds.

Link with the Early Years Foundation Stage (EYFS) curriculum on Understanding the World and Science.

Auditory skills

This section contains activities that focus on the general auditory skills of sound location and auditory discrimination. They provide practise in sustained attention and careful listening and help the child to recognise, compare and differentiate between auditory stimuli.

It is essential that you are aware of the child's hearing levels before attempting these activities.

Sound location

Sound location is the ability to identify the direction from which a sound originates and pinpoint the source. If a child cannot tell where a sound is coming from, they may have difficulty making a meaningful association between a sound and its source. This is important for relating sounds to objects and for orienting oneself to a speaker. Sound location is also vital for basic safety reasons; for example, a car approaching us from behind will be heard before it is seen.

Children with a unilateral hearing loss where one ear has reduced hearing will find it very difficult to locate sound. Modifications may need to be made to these activities, and one way is to increase visual prompts, so the child is not relying on auditory information only.

Aims

To practice identifying the direction of a sound and locating its source.

Outcomes

- Turns towards a sound.
- Accurately locates a sound by pointing to or naming the sound source.

Strategies

- Ensure there is a good listening environment with ambient noise reduced.
- Vary the direction of sounds; in front is easiest, with sounds to the side and then behind the hardest.
- Gradually increase the distance between the child and the sound source.
- Gradually reduce the volume of the sound.
- Use fewer repetitions of the sound.

Suitable materials and resources

Sound makers, musical instruments, ticking clocks and music boxes.

Activities to develop sound location

Sound-making toys

Some children may need support in starting to turn and look for a sound source. Shake or squeeze a sound-making toy in front of the child and allow them to take the toy and

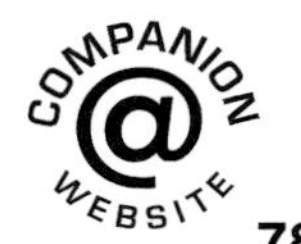

play with it. Encourage them to turn to the sound by shaking it slightly to one side, again allowing them to play with the sound maker. Gradually introduce different locations behind them and then slightly above their head.

Find the sound

While the child shuts their eyes, hide a sound maker like a wind-up toy, loudly ticking clock or music box in the room. The child will need to be quick before the sound stops. Start with locations close to the child and gradually move further away. Using sound makers in this way is more fun for the child and eliminates the need for them to understand or use language.

Listen for the sound

One child is chosen as the listener. Two children are given a musical instrument each and are asked to sit on either side of the listener,* who is blindfolded. The children take it in turns to make a sound, and the listener identifies whether it is to the right or left by pointing. Increase the demands on the listener by moving from rattles and sleigh bells that have a continuous sound to single beats on a chime bar or a drum.

* Alternatively use empty shoeboxes with one side cut out so the sound maker can be hidden away so negating the need for the blindfold. Small egg shakers would be an ideal instrument. This way the middle child can keep their eyes open.

Hide and seek!

Play this traditional game with adults and children. Two or more hide in different places and call to the child who is the seeker. Tell them to find one particular adult or child first. A variation would be to give the hiders a sound maker or musical instrument. The seeker is asked to find one particular instrument by its sound. As this is a sound location activity, the seeker needs to be staying in one place and not searching around the room as you would in the traditional game.

Point to the sound

Give the child a fun item like a magic wand or colourful pointing stick. Blindfold the child or ask them to close their eyes and make a noise fairly close to their head. Ask them to point to the noise and keep still. This way they can see how close they were in pinpointing the sound when the blindfold is removed or they open their eyes. Gradually increase the distance and angle, making sounds higher or lower than ear level. (This game may need two adults – one to make the sounds and one to hold the child's hand in place while the blindfold is removed.)

Always be extremely cautious when carrying out activities where the child has their eyes closed or is blindfolded. Some children may find this distressing, so use other methods like asking them to close their eyes, look down or cover their eyes with their hand. Some alternatives to blindfolding are also suggested in the activities.

Activities for older children

- Play 'Listen for the Sound' (see the previous section) and introduce listening for speech by getting the children to call the child's name. To make it really difficult, you could set a rule that the child only responds to certain words, so the name of a fruit or the name of an animal. You may need to use picture cues to help the two assistants in generating vocabulary.
- Take the child or a group of children on a listening walk. Talk about the different sounds they can hear and ask them to find where the sound is coming from.
  - Introduce vocabulary like near, far, loud, quiet, above, below, side, noisy, pleasant, screechy.
  - Identify different types of sound and classify into different categories like environmental, human, animal and nature.
  - Help the children create a sound picture to represent their walk. Discuss how sounds can be above us from an aeroplane, under our feet when we splash in a puddle and to the side from a bird in a bush.
  - Help children describe the sounds using concepts like rhythm, tempo, pitch and volume. Invent musical notation for the different sounds so the children can produce a musical version or soundscape of the walk. You may want to link to songs like George Gershwin's *Rhapsody in Blue* or *The Little Train of the Caipira (finale)* by Heitor Villa Lobos.

Auditory discrimination

Auditory discrimination involves the perception of similarities and differences between sounds. Very early on the child distinguishes between human and other sounds and between speech and non-speech. They are able to differentiate between similar sounds, so they are able to recognise that the ring of the doorbell is a distinct and separate sound from the one made by a phone. They will learn to recognise the voice of a family member and distinguish this from other voices, like that of the next door neighbour. The ability to discriminate between and identify sound sources in this way is essential to the development of the child's listening and speech skills.

Aims

To help the child recognise the difference between a range of sounds and learn to associate a sound with the sound maker.

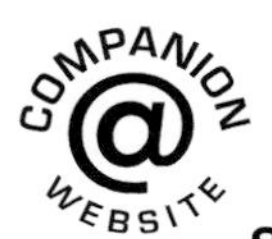

Outcomes

- Identifies when sounds are the same or different.
- Discriminates between two or more similar/dissimilar sounds.
- Identifies a sound maker from its sound.

Strategies

- Make sure that the child can associate a sound to a sound maker through lots of demonstration and play.
- Always let the child see what you are doing when introducing a new activity.
- When the child can successfully discriminate between sounds using both visual and auditory skills, let them attempt a purely auditory task.
- If the child is unsuccessful at their first attempt, it is essential to repeat the task exactly, as it is all too easy to confuse the child by changing the original stimulus.
- Start with very dissimilar sounds and then gradually introduce ones that more similar to each other.

Suitable materials and resources

Sound makers; musical instruments; shakers containing a range of materials; identical pairs of musical instruments and sound makers; music box; and recordings of everyday sounds.

Activities for auditory discrimination

Sounds the same

Activities that help draw the child's attention to the way two identical sound makers make the same sound is a good way to start with auditory discrimination. If the child makes a sound with an object, try to make the same sound. So if the child drops a brick, show them how you can make the same sound by dropping another brick. Try this activity with various items like shaking a bunch of keys or rattling clothes pegs in a tin.

Musical instruments

Lay out two or three musical instruments in front of the child. (Allow some free play initially to help familiarise the child with the sound of the instruments.) While they shut their eyes, make a sound. Can the child find the correct one and play a sound back?

Everyday sounds

Lay a number of everyday objects before the child – for example, keys, bell, a spoon in a cup and a wind-up toy – and while they shut their eyes, make the associated noise. They must correctly identify the object.

Sound lotto

Play sound lotto or bingo games – matching sounds to pictures, using recordings of everyday sounds, for example, a running tap, boiling the kettle, the doorbell ringing, and familiar classroom sounds and familiar voices. In the last item, the child points to the person whose voice he hears.

Gift boxes

Fill pairs of identical 'gift' boxes with different items that make a noise when shaken. For example, pegs, toy bricks, shells, small pebbles or dried pasta. The child has to find the two that match and open them. You can also use small toys that will rattle about and give the child something to play with when the box is opened.

Noises in the room

Ask the children to take turns to be the listener and shut their eyes. Make a familiar noise in the room, for example, shut the door, ring a bell or use a pencil sharpener. Ask the child to find the objects and make the same noise. Let other children take the role of making the noises for the listener. This is a game that is easily played outside too.

Matching animal noises to pictures

Have three or four pictures of familiar animals. Make an animal noise and get the child to identify the correct picture of the animal which would make the noise.

Actions to music

Use music with groups of children to help them recognise and respond to different musical instruments and musical elements.

- Ask the children to walk around the room while you play one of two instruments, for example, the recorder and the drum. They must march like a soldier to the drum and dance like the Pied Piper of Hamelin to the recorder. Tell them stories to illustrate these characters.
- Children act out or pretend to be various objects, events or creatures when they hear different musical instruments, for example, tiptoe like rain drops to a glockenspiel or slither like a snake to a rattle.
- The children walk around the room while you play on the drum. They take giant steps when they hear a loud beat and pixie steps when they hear a soft one.
- Play musical pieces with different tempos to encourage children to compare slow and fast dance movements.

Identical shakers

Place several identical pairs of shakers before the child and ask them to choose one and shake it. They must then shake all the others until they find the shaker they think sounds the same. They can check if they are right by opening them to see if the contents are the same. This can be extended into a matching pairs game.

Activities for older children

- Discrimination with musical instruments
    - Simple discrimination: show the child two dissimilar sound makers or musical instruments, for example, a drum and a rattle. When they are settled, demonstrate each sound until they know which sound belongs to which toy. Ask them to shut their eyes or hide the instruments behind a screen. Make one of the sounds, and they must either point to the correct sound maker or make the same sound with a duplicate set of sound makers.
    - Complex discrimination: repeat 'Simple Discrimination' but gradually increase complexity. Either increase the number of dissimilar sound makers or, keeping to two objects, make the noises more alike. The child should eventually be able to discriminate between several fairly similar sounds.
    - Fine discrimination: use a pitched percussion instrument like a xylophone to encourage fine discrimination. Play all the notes on a xylophone, and let the child have a turn too. Ask the child to close their eyes or turn away. Play one high note and one low note and ask the child if they are the same or different.
- Similarities and differences – introduce games where the children need to identify similarities and differences related to various features.
    - Categories: children identify the sound that is the odd one out in a group of related sounds, for example, a car horn amongst two or three animal noises.
    - Sounds that go together: purring and a meow; bath with a running tap and water draining down the plug hole.
    - Rhymes: children collect rhyming pairs of words.
    - Initial sounds: sound lotto or bingo games using words with the same initial sound or phoneme.

Memory

There are three types of memory – short term memory (immediate recall), working memory (where information is acted upon) and long-term memory. Working memory is responsible for encoding, storing and processing information during cognitive tasks (Baddeley, 2007) and plays a vital part in speech and language development.

Although the tendency is to divide tasks into visual memory and auditory memory, it is by no means certain that these are separate. Many perceptual tasks involve memory, and a child's failure in such tasks could be due to limits on their memory rather than an actual perceptual difficulty. Auditory tasks also have a memory load; for example, in order to discriminate between two hidden musical instruments a child must retain both the visual representations of the instruments and the sounds that they make.

General guidelines

- Memory involves an awareness of past events. The best way to help the child to remember everyday events is to talk about them beforehand, while they are taking place and then again afterwards. By talking about an outing or event beforehand you alert the child and help them to take in subsequent information and make sense of what they see.
- Role play can help the child to relive and remember incidents.
- Use prompts to help children who have difficulty recalling information such as saying to the child, "I saw a tiger", "Tell me all the animals you saw". Cues can gradually be faded out, or if necessary, they can be employed by the child in their everyday life.
- Imaginative use of iPad book creator apps that capture images, video and sound can help create visual memories of outings and trips.
- A task should always be within the child's ability with a little effort on their part and help from the adult. The child should experience and be aware of early success.
- Teaching should follow a developmental sequence.
- Keep spoken instructions appropriate to the child's level of comprehension.
- Tasks and materials should be varied, as children cannot be expected to stick to the same task for long periods.

Visual memory

Visual memory is the ability to recall or remember details of a visual experience, whether this is images, events or words. The child needs to process, store and retrieve this information if they are to recognise and make sense of what they see. In order for this to take place, they need to attend long enough to assimilate the visual information.

Aims

To provide practice in attending to a task in order to remember visual information presented in different forms.

Outcomes

- Able to recall one or more visually dissimilar items.
- Able to recall one or more visually similar items.

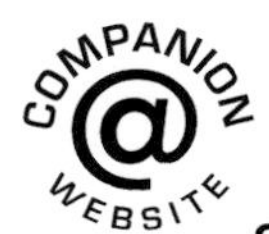

Strategies

- Allow the child time to become familiar with a new activity; for example, practice at posting pictures in a box before asking the child to remember items.
- Allow the child time to become familiar with new materials; for example, let them handle objects before you start the activity.
- Some children may need to have an option to give a nonverbal response.
- Give the child plenty of time to familiarise themselves with the visual information.
- There may be several ways the child can demonstrate visual recall, including naming an item, finding a duplicate or similar item, or making an appropriate gesture.
- Tasks may involve several skills rather than one 'memory' skill, and the child may need support to complete the activity as required.
- Be aware of learners who may be colour blind or have a colour vision deficiency. They may have difficulty distinguishing red/green, or blue/yellow, or may see no colour at all. See www.colourblindawareness.org for more information.
- Use cueing strategies:
    - Point to each item the child has to recall.
    - Tell the child to keep a picture of it in their mind.
    - Encourage the child to say the name of each item out loud, or do this for them if more appropriate.
    - Encourage the child to make associations between items (Brady et al., 2019).

Suitable materials and resources

Familiar objects from the home or learning environment; pictures or photographs of these items; small toys and figures; construction toys like bricks, interlocking cubes, and Lego; and matching and sorting sets for colour and shape.

Activities for visual memory

Activities requiring nonverbal responses

Beakers

Place two beakers in front of the child and put a toy under one of them. With their back turned or eyes closed, shuffle the beakers around and then ask them to find the toy. When they can do this, let the child see as you hide two different toy animals under two different beakers. Show the child a duplicate animal to find by searching under the beakers.

Duplicates

- Show the child two objects or different-coloured bricks. Hide them and have the child find duplicates from a box of bricks.

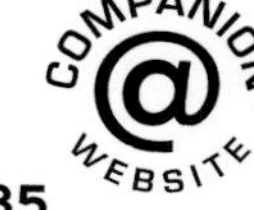

- Show the child two toys. Produce a duplicate of one of them, hide it and ask the child to point to the correct original.
- Show the child a sequence of two wooden shapes. Ask the child to recreate the sequence using duplicate items. Use increasingly longer sequences of shapes.

Three in a row

Show the child three objects in a row. With their back turned or eyes closed, shuffle the objects around, and then ask the child to put them back into the correct order. (It is best to have a model available so the child can compare their effort with the original!)

Picture book

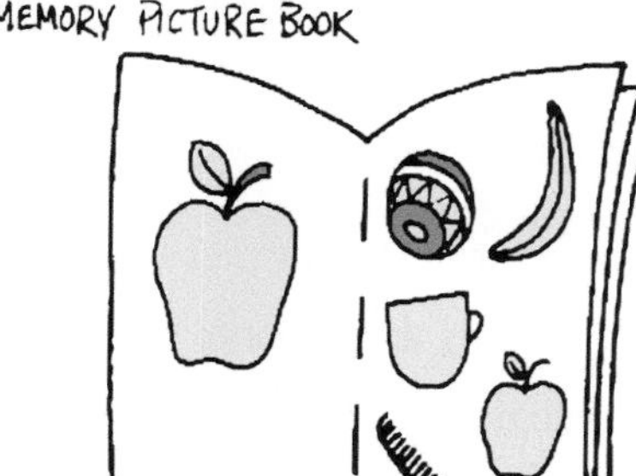

Make a picture book with a large picture of an animal or toy on each alternate page. On the intervening pages stick a number of smaller pictures, including a small version of the large picture on the preceding page. Show the large picture to the child, and then ask them to find the smaller image without referring back to the large one.

Hiding games

Hide a small toy in one of your hands – see if the child can remember which hand it is in. When they can do this, put your hands behind your back for a moment and see if they can still remember where it is.

Hide and seek

Let the child see where you hide before they come and find you. Gradually make them wait longer before they come to seek you out.

Pairs or Pelmanism

Lay several pairs of picture cards face down and take turns with the child to collect identical pairs by turning them over, two at a time. Encourage the child to remember the positions of different pictures.

Snap

Use shape, colour or picture cards and lay them face down as they are played so that the child has to remember what and where they are.

Board games

Play a simple board game and ask the child to remember what colour, shape or number was on the dice each time they throw it.

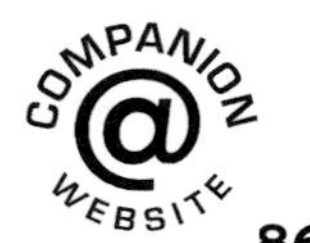

Activities requiring 'naming'

Remember the picture

Show the child a picture of an object. Turn it over and ask the child to name the object. Gradually increase the number of pictures.

Postman

You or the child post objects into a toy postbox. The child recalls what they are by naming them or finding duplicates. He can then lift the lid of the box to check that they are right. Homemade postboxes can be easily made from cardboard boxes.

Missing one

Place three toys or pictures in a row: ask the child to shut their eyes and take one away, leaving the gap as a positional clue. The child names the missing item (or finds a matching item from a duplicate set). Repeat the activity but this time remove the positional clue by moving the items together or jumbling them up. Lotto, Snap and Pelmanism cards are also useful for this game.

Shopkeeper

Show the child pictures of things they have to 'buy' from the 'shop' – a visual shopping list. They can either fetch these items from the shop (good for children who may struggle to name items), or ask for them from another child, who can play the shopkeeper.

Kim's game

Place a number of objects on a tray and allow the child several minutes to memorise them. Cover with a cloth and ask them to remember as many items as possible. It may help to trigger their memory if the objects are all in the same category, for example, all toys or all utensils. Variations of this game include removing one or two toys and the child must say what is missing or adding a new item for the child to identify.

Colour patterns

Use coloured Unifix cubes that fit onto the finger. Use the following hierarchy to build up the child's memory:

- 2 cubes the same colour – red/red
- 2 cubes of a different colour – red/yellow
- 3 cubes the same – red/red/red
- 2 cubes the same, 1 different – red/red/yellow
- 1 cube the same, 2 different – red/yellow/yellow

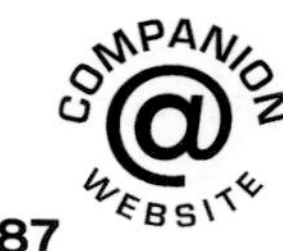

- 1 cube the same, 1 different, 1 same – red/yellow/red
- 3 cubes different – red/yellow/blue
- 4 cubes the same – red/red/red/red

Present these combinations, hide them and have the child reproduce them from memory*. They make good quick-fire group tasks too. This activity can be carried out with a range of different materials, for example, pegs, threading-beads, daubs of paint, building-bricks, coloured sticks or pencils.

* Always refer back to the model so that the child can check that they are right.

Activities for older children

- Help children understand and plan for daily activities with a visual timetable or visual time line. Use photographs, images, symbols etc. to represent different tasks and events during the day.
- Use memory aids such as mnemonics, colour coding for important information and mind maps.
- Encourage children to understand which memory aids help their learning. (This will be personal to each child.)

Auditory memory

The child needs to attend to, process, and store what they hear and be able to retrieve this information, if they are to recognise and use spoken language in a meaningful way. Many listening tasks have a memory load; for example, when following a two-sequence instruction, the child must remember all elements and the sequence in order to respond correctly.

Aims

To provide practice in attending to a task in order to remember auditory information presented in different forms.

Outcomes

- Points to or fetches one or more items.
- Recalls one or more spoken items.

Strategies

- Avoid asking the child to remember lists of words without a context. Instead make language functional by relating it to a task or communicative situation, for example,

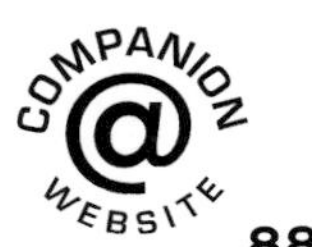

incorporating items to remember into a story, or following instructions as part of a game.

- Ensure that the child recognises and has prior experience of the objects and materials in an activity.
- Use familiar vocabulary and phrases so the focus is on memory and not comprehension (St Clair-Thompson and Holmes, 2008).
- Allow the child time to become accustomed to a new activity; for example, let them explore items in a shopping game by maybe preparing and laying out the shop.
- Remember that it is easier for a child if they can see the objects and pictures that you want them to remember, as they may then use visual memory to help them, for example, items of food in a shopping game. If you want them to rely on auditory clues alone, keep the objects hidden from view.
- Organise information into meaningful groups, so have objects from a single semantic category like food or animals (Black and Rollins, 1982).
- Encourage active listening so the child is asked to look at the speaker, take turns and pay attention to others.
- Use physical prompts, gesture and signs alongside spoken instructions, or cue cards with pictures, signs or text if appropriate, but gradually remove these so the child is relying on auditory memory.
- Some children may need to have an option to give a nonverbal response, for example, pointing at or fetching an item rather than naming it. For those children who can name encourage them to rehearse key words by repeating them.
- Provide a visual indicator of the number of items the child has to recall, for example, having two boxes ready for two selected objects.

Activities for auditory memory

Shopping list

Lay out a pretend shop with several toy items or have real vegetables, fruit and canned foods. Read out items from a shopping list for the child to fetch from the shop.

Shopping bag

Use a real net bag (expandable) and gather together several different items. Ask the child to put a series of objects inside. Gradually increase the number of objects displayed and requested.

Stick and peel books

Ask the child to select various images from the sticker sheets to build up an illustration.

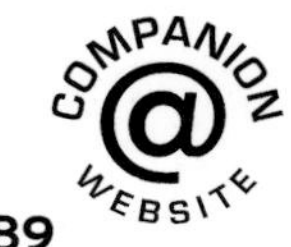

Playing in the tree

Draw a large tree and stick pictures of various items on and around it by using a reusable adhesive like Blu-Tack. These might include a bird, a butterfly, an apple, a kite, a balloon, a flower, a leaf, an acorn, a rope swing, a ladder, a bird box and a spider's web. Name the items the child must remove. Other pictures might be a house, boat or shop with topic-related items.

Treasure hunt

Ask the child to collect a list of various items from around the room in a treasure hunt. This game can also be played outside, where there is scope to have a lot of fun with a treasure island, pirate's boat and sunken chest in the water tray.

Fantasy

Introduce a fantasy element, for example, "You're going to a desert island and you need a bottle of water, a torch and a swimming costume". Ask the child to choose these objects from a selection. Alternatively use pictures, which will allow for a wider choice of items like an axe, a rope or a tent. Further fantasy ideas include space travel, superheroes and fairy tales.

Dressing up

Have a pile of clothes and ask the child to put on different combinations of items, for example, "a hat and one sock". (If numbers are used be sure the child understands them.)

Pack the suitcase

Have a real holiday bag and some real clothes or large doll-sized ones. Ask the child to find items to pack in the bag. Start with one or two and gradually increase the number of items.

Draw a washing-line

Ask the child to 'hang up' a series of small pictures of clothes on a pretend washing line.

Everyday instructions

During the normal course of the day the child can be asked to fetch things for activities.

Activities for older children

- Story recall – read or tell the child a simple story which mentions objects, animals or actions. Afterwards list the ones the child can recall, and then reread the story or let

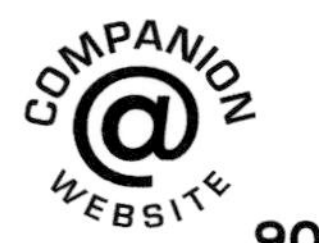

them see the pictures to find out how many they have got right. Stories such as *The Golden Goose* and *Chicken Licken*, which slowly build up the list of characters, are easier to remember.

- Can the child spot the 'odd one out' in a series of words? This can be based on a number of different features:
  - dog cat orange (semantic difference)
  - cake make tuck bake (rhyming difference)
  - ball bush bone toy (initial phoneme difference)

  (It may be useful to start with similar words and talk about the connection between the items before attempting the odd one out.)
- Encourage the use of self-cueing strategies:
  - Encourage the child to gesture the object or trace its outline in the air, or do this for them.
  - Tell them to make a picture of the object and keep it in their mind (visualisation).
  - Model rehearsal techniques – for example, repeating a list of items to buy in a shopping game.
  - Give the child pictures to name as a reminder of items given orally as a shopping list.
- Encourage the use of clarification techniques like asking for repetition.

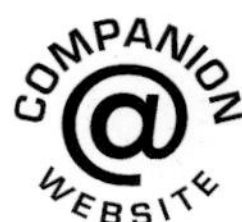

RECORD SHEET

Attention and listening skills

Name: **Review date:**

Outcomes	Comments

3

THE ROLE OF PLAY

DOI: 10.4324/9781003031109-4

Introduction

Children's play takes many different forms and serves many different functions. Its significance to the child's development is stated by Vygotsky: "Play is not the predominant form of activity, but in a certain sense, it is the leading source of development in pre-school years" (1977, p. 76). It is through the medium of play that the child is able to develop new skills and practise those already acquired: skills that range from motor dexterity to social competence (Jeffree et al., 1977).

Play is a voluntary and usually a pleasurable activity that enables the child to experiment with alternative skills and roles without the fear of failure (Howard, 2019). The child sets their own goals and makes their own rules. Play is an area of development that is of major importance in the child's development of cognition and language (Whitebread et al., 2017). It helps to develop the prerequisites that are essential to language development – listening, observation, imitation, concept formation and symbolic understanding. It is important to remember that the many types of play are interdependent, and progress relies on consolidation of all these skills.

Functions of play

- Play allows the child to develop new skills through observation, exploration, discovery, conjecture and imitation.
- Guided play by the adult supports language development (Weisberg et al., 2013).
- A child is able to practise language skills already acquired and learn newly introduced vocabulary.
- The child's symbolic understanding and concept formation develops through their play experience.
- Play is a pleasurable activity that relieves boredom and frustration and allows for a release of physical energy.
- The child is able to learn about and understand other people's roles through make-believe and sociodramatic play.
- Sociodramatic play provides an opportunity for expressing negative emotions of fear and anger in a harmless manner.
- Social play provides a medium for developing communication and negotiation skills.

Factors affecting the development of play

There are many factors that might affect the development of play. They include:

- **A sensory impairment:** A sensory impairment affecting hearing or vision is likely to impact on the development of play skills, in particular social interaction skills.

  Examples include:
  - *Hearing loss:*
    - A study by DeLuzio and Girolametto (2011) found that children with a severe to profound hearing loss were likely to be excluded from peer interactions during play. Despite evident competence in initiating and responding to social contacts, it appears it was their delayed speech and language development that led to difficulties with social interactions (Massey-Abernathy and Haseltine, 2019).
  - *Vision impairment:*
    - Children with visual impairment are more at risk of difficulties with social interaction (Caballo and Verdugo, 2007), as they are less able to make use of the usual visual cues from gesture and facial expression during cooperative play with peers.
- **An underlying neurodevelopmental disorder:** Play may be delayed or have areas of deficit. Some examples are:
  - *Autism (Autistic Spectrum Disorder, ASD):* A study by (Thiemann-Bourque et al., 2019) found children with ASD showed strengths in functional play skills but deficits in areas of symbolic play. Specifically, they were less interested in symbolic doll play and less likely to use a doll to act upon an object.
  - *Down's syndrome:* Children with Down's syndrome tend to exhibit repetitive play behaviours and engage less with exploratory play with objects (Venuti et al., 2009).
- **Environmental factors:** Factors in the home or learning environment may influence the development of play skills (Rettig, 1998). The child may lack the opportunities to play because of insufficient toys and play materials that are appropriate for their age and ability; may lack playfellows, because parents and caregivers are unable to play with the child or the child has no companions of their own age and ability; or may have no indoor or outdoor space for play and exploration.

Types of play

Piaget in 1962 outlined three main types of play – practice play, symbolic play and games with rules, which broadly reflect the sensory, motor and cognitive development of the young child. Practice play occurs during the sensorimotor stage (ages 0–2) of Piaget's theory of cognitive development, and it supports the development of the object concept or object permeance. Symbolic play marks the transition to the preoperational period (ages 2–7), as the child has growing awareness that objects and words can stand for or symbolise something else. His third category represents a growing understanding of rules and logical thinking and aligns with his concrete operational stage (ages 7–11). Similar categories have been identified by other researchers, with Whitebread et al. (2017) proposing that play can be divided into five fundamental types of play referred to as physical play, play with objects, symbolic play, pretence or sociodramatic play, and games with rules. However, it should be noted that here the term 'symbolic play' is used with reference to play with symbolic or semiotic systems like language, music and drawing.

In this chapter the focus is on the following types of play:

Object play

Most children have an innate curiosity about themselves and their world. They discover that objects and people exist apart from themselves. Exploration provides the means for the child to find out the properties and qualities of these other entities. It requires a combination of motor, perceptual and cognitive skills.

Imaginative play

Imaginative play is also known as pretend play, symbolic play and make-believe play. Fundamental to this type of play is the use of objects or gestures to represent other objects or events that are not present (Jeffree et al., 1977); for example, the child knows that an object is a banana but chooses to substitute it as a phone (Leslie, 1987). Pretence gradually becomes more elaborate and complex.

Functional play

At 12 months the child understands real, familiar objects in relation to themselves and can demonstrate knowledge of their function by using them appropriately, for example, drinking from an empty cup. This is sometimes referred to as demonstrating 'definition by use' of everyday objects. At 15–18 months the child will use these objects functionally on a caregiver (Sharma and Cockerill, 2014).

Large doll play

From 18 months the child will use real objects appropriately in relation to large dolls, feeding dolly with a cup, for instance. This marks the beginning of symbolic play (Sleigh, 1972) with

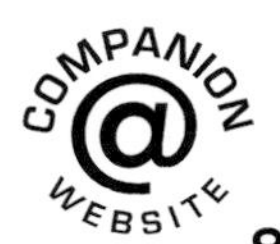

the development of pretence. By 2 years the child is able to sequence two or three actions in a simple make-believe routine. There is also development of object substitution, so using a toy brick as a cup to give dolly a drink.

Small world play

From 18 to 20 months the child recognises small and miniature toys and relates them to each other, for example, feeding a small doll with a miniature bottle, although they may also use the objects on themselves. From 2½ years the child acts out meaningful sequences with small toys, such as a doll's tea party. However, these sequences tend to be an imitation of familiar events to the child.

Role play

By 3 years old the child engages in make-believe play involving invented people and objects. At 4 years of age the child is able to plan events and use language to describe their play, for example, "My cat poorly" "The vet make better".

Social play

Interaction is a key element in the concept of social play and refers to the two-way process of give and take. This develops over time, as the child moves from play with parent/caregiver to parallel play and on to more cooperative play with other children.

Activities to develop play

These activities are designed to develop the child's object play, imaginative play and social play.

General guidelines

- The activity must be developmentally appropriate for the child, taking into account their level of functioning in other areas, such as attention and listening skills, language development and performance skills.
- Provide materials and resources related to the child's interests; for example, a love of dinosaur figures might be incorporated into role play.
- Design play environments that offer a safe space for children to explore and engage in both familiar and novel activities.
- Follow the child's lead and build on their efforts by showing them how to extend their play by introducing resources, demonstrating skills and modelling play behaviours.

- Use clear, simple language that is appropriate to the child's level of understanding.
- Introduce appropriate vocabulary to name objects and describe what the child is doing.
- Play is meant to be enjoyable. If a child does not want to participate in an activity, do not force them. A reluctant child will often join in when they see others enjoying an activity.
- Remember that a child needs time to play alone as well as with others. Let them play as they want to, and gradually try to direct them to more purposeful activity.
- Showing your pleasure in the child's play is a highly motivational factor. Value the child's efforts and the process rather than only rewarding successful outcomes.
- Allow for lots of repetition so the child can practise and refine newly acquired skills.

Recording observations

Observe and record the child's play over an extended period of time in a variety of situations within the learning environment. These include spontaneous or child-initiated play, adult-led activity, solitary play or engagement in cooperative and social play with peers and/or adults. Observations from parents or caregivers are invaluable in gaining a broader understanding of the child's play skills.

Make a note of:

- the context or situation (e.g., outside play; tabletop; playhouse);
- the type of play (e.g., exploratory; symbolic; imaginative);
- the material and resources that attract and engage the child's interest;
- prompts and cues used to engage the child with an activity;
- how long the child maintains interest in an activity (e.g., fleeting; sustained for several minutes; returns to activity over several days);
- the frequency of play activities;
- *object play:*
    - exploratory behaviours, (e.g., looks intently; pulling, tearing);
    - experimentation with materials (e.g., mixing paint colours; adds textures to dough);
    - how the child relates items in play (e.g., stacking bricks; pushes a toy inside a box)
    - what the child has made, constructed or created;
- *imaginative play*:
    - how the child uses items in an imaginative way (e.g., creates props; dresses up);
    - types of role play (e.g., familiar everyday experiences like cooking; occupations like a vet or teacher; fantasy characters like superheroes);

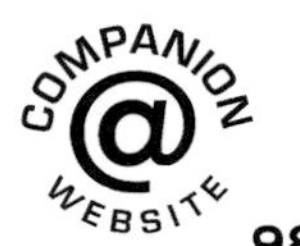

    - the content of dramatic play (e.g., themes like relationships, loss and bereavement);
    - the complexity of role play and dramatic play
- *social play*:
    - how the child interacts with other children (e.g., parallel play; cooperating in a task);
    - expressions of emotion (e.g., surprise, frustration, joy);
- the child's approach to play (e.g., curious; perseverance);
- how the play is planned and organised; (e.g., bricks spread across the floor haphazardly; play has a clear purpose with bricks selected and sorted);
- any decision making or problem solving (e.g., trial and error; predicting; testing out ideas; noticing links);
- any vocalisation, gesture and spoken language used by the child;
- ideas and thoughts expressed by the child in planning an activity, engaging with it or reviewing its progress or outcomes.

Object play

Most children have an innate curiosity about themselves and their world, and infants soon discover that objects and people exist apart from themselves. Exploratory play provides the means for the child to discover the properties and qualities of these other entities. This requires a combination of motor, perceptual and cognitive skills. Children use their sensory and motor abilities to find out the qualities and characteristics of objects by looking, listening, feeling, tasting, shaking, squeezing and dropping them. In this way the child begins to build up concepts about their world. This type of exploratory play with objects supports communication and language development (Orr, 2020). Later, exploratory play helps to extend and expand the child's knowledge of their world.

Functions

- To help the child discover objects and events through observation of the world around them.
- To help the child discover the nature and workings of objects, through their observation and manipulation of them.
- To acquire new skills, resulting from the child's discoveries.
- To practise these skills in different situations.
- To stimulate the child's curiosity, thus creating further desire and a need to explore.

Exploratory play

Exploratory play is a way for the child to find out about the properties and qualities of objects. This involves the use of all the senses combined with skills of manipulation to fully explore form and function.

Aims

To help the child discover objects and events through observation of the world around them.

Outcomes

- Explores a range of objects through sensory play and motor manipulation.
- Experiments with a range of materials to discover their different qualities and properties.

Strategies

- Provide a variety of objects and toys for the child to explore. The very young child needs the adult to bring experiences to them.
- Objects and toys should be related to the child's interests.
- Ensure toys are durable, as children may want to explore objects by banging, throwing and biting them.
- Use multisensory toys that provide experience of looking, listening, feeling and manipulation, as well as smell and taste.
- Demonstrate exploratory behaviours like pulling, stretching, and rolling.
- You may need to show the child how to explore an object with different senses; for example, smell a bar of soap yourself and then hold it for the child to smell.
- Let the child take the lead in activities. Your role is to extend and guide their play whilst continuing to present challenges to their learning.
- Be a partner in the child's play by helping them to hold a beater for a drum or showing them how to roll a musical ball.
- Vary materials and activities to maintain the child's interest.
- Interact with the child and ask open-ended questions.

Suitable materials and resources

Mobiles; bubble sets and lava lamps; sound makers and musical instruments; construction toys; Play-Doh; sensory balls and bricks; Koosh balls; smell pots; scratch and sniff books; and sensory bottles.

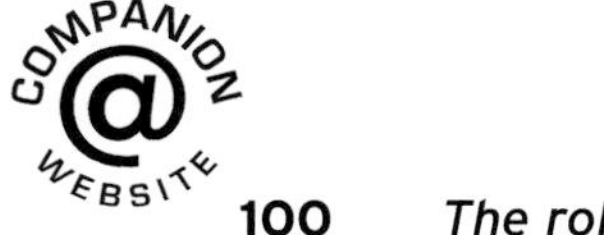

Activities to encourage exploratory play

Sensory bottles

Provide some sensory bottles for the child to explore different colours, shape and movement. Make your own bottles using clean resealable plastic water or drinks bottles. Always leave some room at the top of the bottle to allow for shaking the liquid, and glue lids on.

Fill with water and add:

- different food colourings;
- mini pompoms;
- some drops of glycerine combined with glitter and confetti;
- 3/4 liquid soap to a 1/4 of water, and add glass beads.

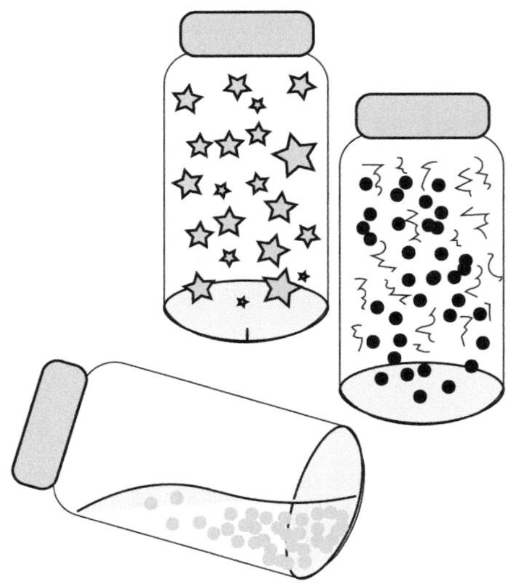

Musical instruments

Help children discover the different ways of making sound with musical instruments (shaking, tapping, hitting, plucking, blowing) by providing a range of instruments to explore. Show the different ways sound can be made from one instrument: for example, a tambourine can be tapped, softly scratched, shaken or hit with the palm of the hand. Vary movements by alternating between a soft and a hard blow; a slow roll of the wrist and a quick jiggle; or a loud tap versus a quiet tap. Use a stick to beat out a rhythm or strike the back of the tambourine against your knee or thigh.

Textures

Let children handle toys that vary in texture, for example, a hard building brick and a soft toy.

Squeezy, squeezy

Encourage sensorimotor exploration using Play-Doh. Manipulate it by squeezing, rolling and shaping it into different shapes. Try pushing it through different sized sieves or a garlic press!

Sensory bricks

The different textured surfaces of sensory bricks offer a tactile experience as they are held in the hand for stacking and building games. Help the child make connections between the texture and the visual elements. Try pushing the bricks into sand to make different imprints, or paint the bricks to use as printing blocks to create repetitive patterns.

Koosh balls

The colourful rubber filaments or strands of a Koosh ball are attractive and very tactile. They are easily gripped, and this helps children with learning to catch and throw.

Sensory balls

Use sensory balls that have different textured surfaces. Place a sheet of paper in a shallow cardboard box or plastic tray. Squeeze two or three different coloured paints on to the paper. Roll the balls through the paint to create different lines and patterns. Compare the different marks made by a smooth surface with those made by balls with a bumpy surface or the filaments of a Koosh ball.

Smell pots

These are small plastic pots with holes in the lid available from commercial suppliers. Alternatively, make your own by using recycled herb jars or covering old jars with perforated paper lids. Place different scented items inside for the child to explore using their sense of smell.

Scratch and sniff books

There are a vast array of scratch and sniff books available that provide an additional olfactory experience to accompany traditional nursery rhymes, and special events like Christmas and Halloween.

Balls

Children love playing with balls. Here are some multi-sensory ones:

- *Transparent jingling ball* – these large transparent balls can be rolled, pushed, and thrown. The jingle bells inside can be seen and heard as the ball moves.
- *Soft beach balls* – help the child to sit and bounce up and down on the ball (support them under the arms).

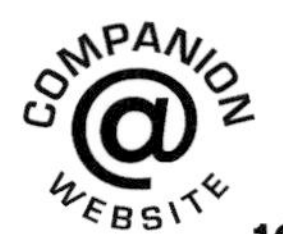

- *Squeaky balls* – show the child how to make a squeak by squeezing the ball.
- *Sensory reflective sound balls* – the shiny mirror surface of these stainless steel balls offers a distorted fish-eye lens reflection. Each one has a different sounding chime.

Sand-and-water play

Sand-and-water play present endless possibilities for exploratory play, for example, plonking toys into a water tray; floating toy boats; creating ripples by moving hands and feet to rock the boats; or making a lather (try whisking baby bubble bath or shampoo in a bowl), or filling a sand wheel and emptying it; building sandcastles and squashing them; and making patterns with rakes, shells and wheeled toys.

Activities for older children

- *Sensory bubble sets* are a colourful array of different liquid timers that show the passage of time using oil and water. Bubbles gently flow, cascade or bounce depending on the design of the timer, and some even have bubbles flowing upwards. Place on a light box for added visual stimulation. (Useful to link to curriculum with discussions about time, measurement, colour, light and gravity.)
- *Make a lava lamp* – Fill a quarter of a large empty plastic drinks bottle with water and top up with vegetable oil, leaving a gap of about three cm at the top. Wait for the water and oil to separate, and then add about ten drops of food colouring. Once the food colouring has mixed with the water at the bottom of the bottle, add some antacid tables. (Keep the lid off the bottle to allow the fizz to escape.) As the tablets dissolve, coloured bubbles will start to rise, and you will have a lava lamp! Play around with a torch to add light effects. (Useful to link to curriculum with discussions about density, diffusion and chemical reactions.)

Cause and effect

Learning about cause and effect is a continuous process which becomes more complex as time goes on. Lots of the early child's spontaneous activities teach them about the connection between their actions and the world around them, like how a cry will elicit a response from the parent/caregiver. Infants will use exploratory play to discover and test out ideas about causal links in novel toys (Schulz et al., 2007); and is crucial for later critical thinking skills like problem solving and the ability to hypothesise and make predictions.

Aims

To help the child explore the relationship between their actions and an object.

Outcomes

- Combines simple actions to cause things to happen.
- Experiments with different actions in a novel situation.

Strategies

- Some children may need plenty of demonstrations and help to manipulate the toys for themselves, for example, holding their hand around a string or handle to pull a toy towards them.
- Most children will benefit from time to explore cause and effect toys in spontaneous child initiated play.
- Use multisensory toys that provide experience of looking, listening and feeling as well as manipulation.
- Take advantage of the child's interests, so if they like banging objects, give them a stick and provide lots of different objects for them to hit (cushions, boxes, tins, drum).
- Appropriate language can be incorporated into activities with words such as 'on'; 'off'; and phrases like 'it's going', 'round and round' and so on.

Suitable materials and resources

Choose toys and everyday objects that do something as the result of an action upon them. Look for toys which make a noise, produce a picture or light up, have movement or open and close.

Toys that have sound

Rattles, shakers, squeaky dolls and toys, crying dolls, animal noise-makers, musical instruments, alarm clocks, music boxes, doorbells, balls with bells inside, pull-along toys with sound and inflatable roller toys with noise makers inside. These all make a noise as a result of some action by you or the child. Making sounds with the lips, cheeks, feet and hands also helps the child's understanding of cause and effect.

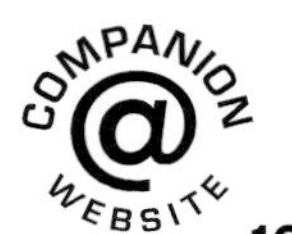

Toys that have movement

Peek-a-boo and pop up toys, jack-in-the-box or other 'in-the-box' versions, blow-windmills, push-and-pull toys, spinning tops, toys on strings, wind-up toys, clockwork train sets, bubble blowers, a toy cash register, hammer and pegs, a rocking horse, a see-saw, swings, toy cars, slides, sand or water wheels, water pumps and bath toys that pour, squirt or spray water.

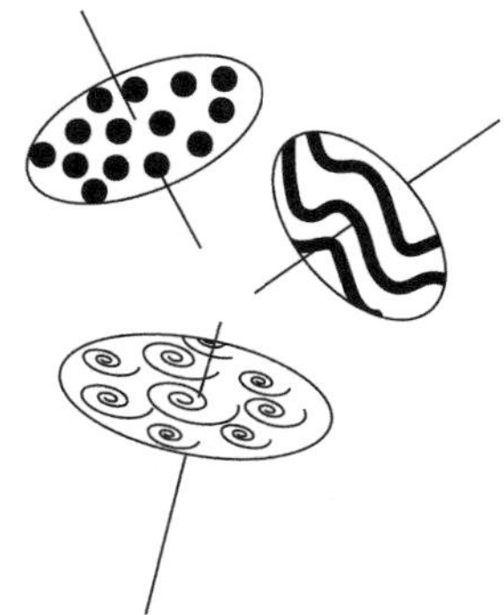

Toys that produce visual effects

Colourful boing balls, mobiles, picture-cubes with different colours or pictures on them and spinning-tops. Magnetic drawing boards, water doodle mats, draw tablets and discovery bottles. Torches: try helping the child to click the torch on and off; click fast and then slow; use a shadow torch or projector torch to show images on the wall.

Toys that open and close

Tins, boxes, beakers, jars, books, envelopes, bags, cases, purses, cooking pots, advent calendars, activity boards, toy furniture or doll's houses that have doors, windows, drawers and cupboards.

Toys that fit together

Nesting beakers, cups and barrels; nesting lunch boxes; chunky wooden inset boards, shape sorters and stacking toys; Lego Duplo; large toy knots and bolts; and Russian dolls. At first make sure lids or nuts are fairly loose and only require a little pressure to open. If the child is having great difficulty, then unscrew the item until it is almost off, and then let the child move it the last little bit.

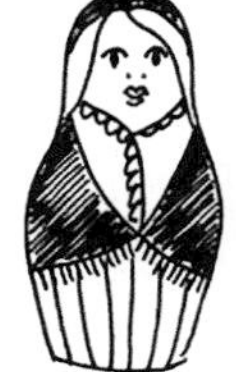

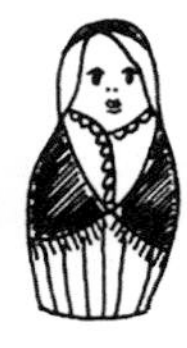

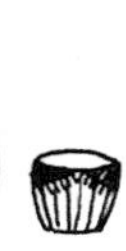

Activities for older children

- Pop-up picture books: the child is able to make the illustrations move by pulling tabs and turning cardboard wheels, for example, *The Haunted House* by Jan Pierikowsky.
- Explore different optical instruments that change the way we see things and talk about the underlying mechanisms. These might be kaleidoscopes, magic lanterns, slide-viewers, magnifying lenses, microscopes, three-dimensional glasses, tinted lenses, binoculars, telescopes and instruments like 'bug-eye' which multiply images.
- Experiment with changing the state of different substances – freezing water into ice cubes then letting them melt or making jelly from jelly cubes and hot water.

Imaginative play

Imaginative play is probably the most important type of play in encouraging children's language development (Quinn et al., 2018), as it deals with the child's ability to recognise and use symbols. There is a gradual development of the child's understanding of the purpose of objects followed by the emergence of pretend play characterised by nonliteral actions.

Functions

- To provide an opportunity for the child to represent their experiences in play.
- To help develop thought and language (Jeffree et al., 1977; Orr, 2020).
- Verbal comprehension cannot develop without symbolic understanding (Cooper et al., 1974).
- To provide the child with the opportunity to try out other roles, which leads to a greater understanding of others.
- To allow for emotional release through the acting out of fear and anger.
- To encourage creativity and imagination.

Functional play

At this stage the child's actions with objects mirrors those experienced in the home, where they learn by watching and copying the adults around them. Play is with real objects or realistic toy replicas and reflects the intended function or use of that object.

Aims

To encourage the use of real objects or realistic toy items in play that demonstrates understanding of their use or function.

Outcomes

- Imitates adult in carrying out simple actions with everyday objects.
- Demonstrates understanding through the playful use of familiar common everyday objects.

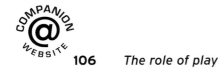

Strategies

- At first the child will need to observe lots of modelled behaviour before they will begin to copy actions with objects.
- Much of this experience will happen in the home, but some can be provided in an early years setting, for example, during mealtimes.
- Use real objects or realistic toy items at this stage.
- Help the child to focus on one object by presenting only a few items at a time.
- You should expect one self-directed action from the child, for example, drinking from an empty cup.
- Encourage and reinforce any attempts by the child to engage you in their play, for example, giving you a cup to drink from. This is a move away from a focus on self to other, and it is evidence of a development in their understanding.

Suitable resources and materials

Common household objects or realistic pretend play toys like a cup, a spoon, a plate, a flannel, and a hairbrush; a toy phone; pretend household tools; pull-along toys; and 'ride-on' cars.

Activities to develop functional play

Make-believe tea party

Use two or three life-sized items like a cup, a plate and a spoon in a simple make-believe tea party; for example, pretend to feed yourself from a spoon or drink from a cup. Encourage the child to copy you.

Surprise bag

Hide some everyday objects or large toy replicas in a 'surprise' bag or box, for example, a cup, a brush and a flannel. Play a game with the child where you or the child reach into the bag to find different items. Help show the child how to use the object both on yourself and the child, for example, brushing your hair and then the child's hair. Encourage them with lots of positive feedback and reinforce their actions with the object by imitating them. Talk about what you are seeing and doing, and what the child is seeing and doing – "brush", "brush hair".

Ride-on cars

Children love 'ride-on' toy vehicles. Look out for ones that have extras like a movable steering wheel, lights and a horn. Introduce traffic like signals for modelling vocabulary like 'stop', 'wait' and 'go'.

Toy telephones

Toy telephones provide children with endless fun. The Fisher-Price Chatter Phone has a spinning dial and a pull-along string and says "hello" and "goodbye". Alternatively use a toy replica of a smart phone. Encourage vocalisation and communication by having a two-way 'conversation' with the child.

Pull-along pets

Pull-along puppies encourage the child to mimic taking the dog for a walk. Other actions like stroking and petting can also be encouraged.

Pull-along and push toys

Use toys on wheels: push them along the floor and make car noises. Encourage the child to join in.

Activities for older children

Start to introduce smaller toy items into play:

- Place some small personal items like a mirror, a comb and a toy phone into a small bag or purse for the child to explore.
- Put a picnic cloth and some simple pretend tea party items like a cup or beaker, a spoon and a plate in a picnic basket. Encourage the child to use it in a pretend tea party.

Start to introduce dolls and teddies into play:

- Provide a range of dolls and teddies for children to pick up and carry.
- Have a doll and toy pushchair – a very familiar game, but one that helps the child act out what they see in their own family. This is also introducing pretend play and moving them towards acting out the role of a parent.
- Provide toy replicas of household cleaning tools like a vacuum cleaner for the child to mimic everyday activities they have seen at home. Vocabulary like 'on', 'off' and 'push' can also be introduced.

Large doll play

This involves simple pretend play where the child relates everyday objects or toy items to a large doll. These actions are still functional in nature and based on everyday familiar activities.

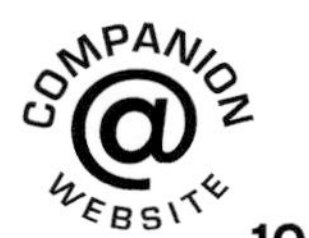

Aims

To encourage early symbolic play with large dolls and doll-sized material.

Outcomes

- Uses a real object in relation to a large doll or to an adult.
- Uses a doll-sized toy in relation to self, a large doll or to an adult.

Strategies

- Encourage the child to start relating objects to large dolls.
- If preferred, teddies or similar stuffed animals like a bear or monkey may be used instead of a doll. However, any substitution needs to have a movable head, arms and legs.
- Start with using real objects and gradually progress to doll-sized accessories.
- Provide the child with accessories that allow the child to copy familiar everyday activities with the doll.

Suitable materials and resources

Large dolls; teddies; puppets and soft toys like a monkey or a bear with a movable head, arms and legs. An assortment of large doll-sized accessories like a cup, a brush and clothing items.

Activities to encourage large doll play

Everyday routines

Help the child to recognise large dolls as symbols by using them in the same ways that you interact with the child during everyday routines; for instance, when you give them their dinner or play with them, include the doll in these activities. At first you will probably have to perform actions on the doll yourself, telling the child what you are doing all the while; for example, "Now we wash your (or use the child's name) face, then we wash dolly's face". Encourage the child to take their turn at washing dolly, always using real objects at this stage.

Playtime

Include dolly in games with the child, first as an 'observer' and then as a participant. Suitable games include rolling balls between you, the child and the doll; giving dolly a ride in a pull-along truck or train; dressing up; and sharing picture books.

Daytime routines

Let the child's routines become dolly's routines; for example, dolly has orange juice, face and hands washed, and sleep, just like the child. This also helps the child's understanding of their own daily routine.

Doll play

Slowly distance the doll's day from the child's day and help the child to carry out meaningful play with the doll. Use a large doll to carry out various actions with toy objects, for example, cuddling, washing, feeding and walking. Keep these actions simple at first. Give the doll to the child and encourage them to carry out the actions. If they use the items on themselves, then taking, for example, a cup, feed yourself and then the doll, saying "Now it's dolly's turn". Hand the cup to the child and encourage them to feed the doll. Give them lots of praise when they do.

Dolly's things

Gradually introduce doll-sized accessories, sticking initially to those possessions that the child is familiar with in everyday routines, such as dolly's 'own' cup, flannel and toothbrush. Continue to include the doll, now with its own items, in the child's routines.

Doll families

Introduce more dolls and give them roles to play in a pretend game, for example, mummy, nana and baby.

Dolly's favourite things

Introduce a wider range of familiar possessions, such as dolly's handbag, umbrella, hat and so on.

Activities for older children

- Provide doll accessories that might be used in a sequential sequence – flannel and towel or baby bottle and spoon. Encourage the child to sequence two actions, for example, feeding a doll with a bottle and then a spoon.
- Join in the child's play and encourage the child to relate the same action to you, for example, feeding using a spoon.

Early make-believe play with puppets

Puppets are a very versatile piece of equipment that can be utilised for all ages. They might be used by the child in a similar way to dolls for developing symbolic play, as a prop in a simple role play or as a character in a complex sociodramatic role play. Puppets help children relax (Kröger and Nupponen, 2019) and provide a way for children to practise communication skills with peers and adults in both structured interactions and in more informal child-initiated play. Children with limited language skills are able to engage with activities nonverbally through the use of actions and sounds.

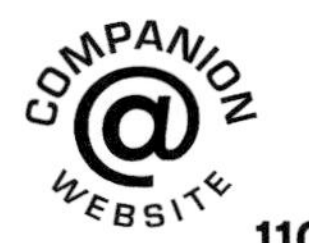

Aims

To provide structured interactions with puppets to improve social and communication skills.

Outcomes

- Engages in a communicative interaction with a peer, adult or group of children.

Strategies

- Choose puppets appropriate for the developmental level of the child.
- Choose puppets appropriate for the activity; for example, you will need a puppet with a mouth if the focus is on speaking.
- Puppets might be used by adults, for example, during story time, but remember to allow the children time and space to physically engage with the puppets too.
- Make puppets available alongside books so they can act out their favourite characters.
- Although the majority of children are fascinated by puppets, be aware that some children (and adults) may have a fear of puppets.

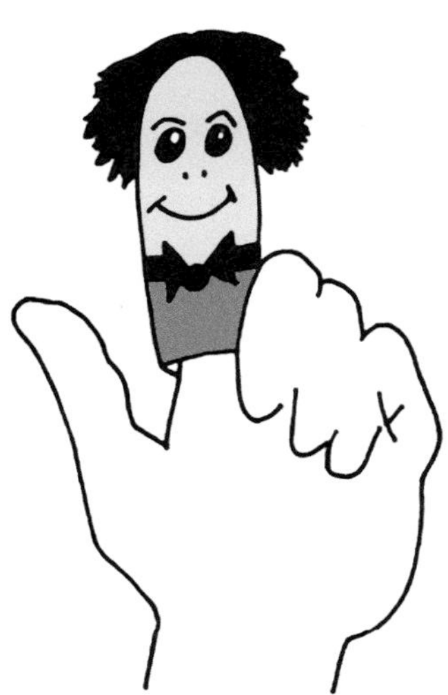

Suitable materials and resources

A range of puppets to include finger, hand, glove, string, marionette, rod and large people hand puppets. Puppets representing a range of ethnic groups are available from commercial producers.

Activities for encouraging early make-believe play with puppets

Peek-a-boo puppets

Use hand, glove or finger puppets to play peek-a-boo and hiding games.

Finger-play

Paint faces on your fingers and use them as puppets. Make them run, jump, dance and so on. Help paint faces on the fingers of the children.

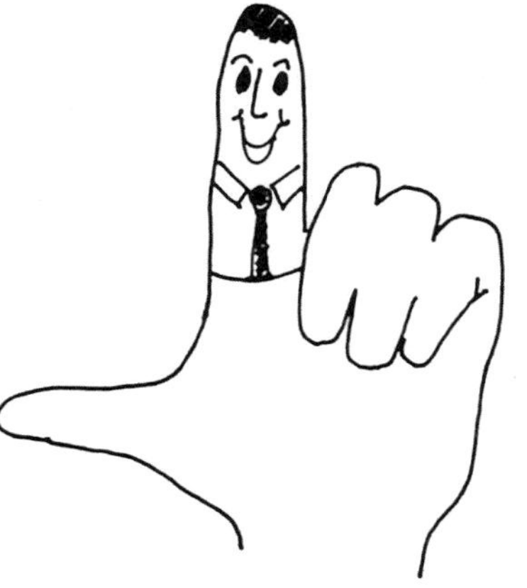

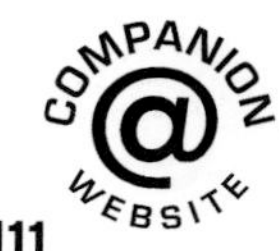

Finger puppets

Give the children finger puppets to wear as they recite nursery rhymes or finger play songs.

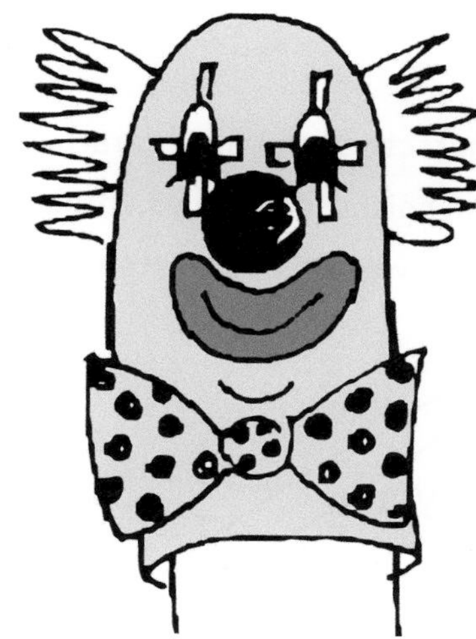

Hand puppets (glove puppets)

Hand puppets are great fun and are often very useful for the shy child. All puppets can be given a character with a voice to match.

Character puppets

Children can act out familiar stories from books using character puppets. These can be bought or home-made to use alongside story telling. Creating a puppet will prompt discussion around what the character looks like, so the three bears are different sizes, the three little pigs are pink and incy wincy spider has eight hairy legs.

Animal puppets

Animal puppets are useful for children with limited language as they can be encouraged to participate by making animal noises and acting out movements.

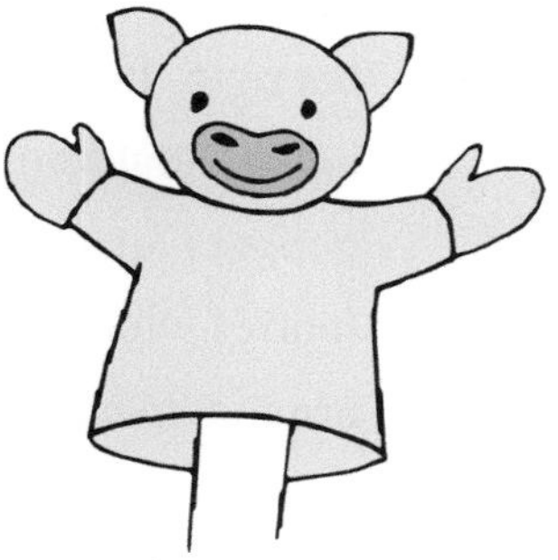

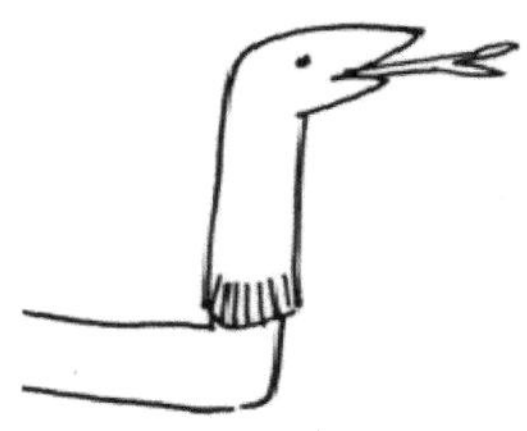

Make a puppet

Support children in making their own puppets by providing creative play resources and activities. Try creating the 'Sock Thing' character from *Kipper's Toybox* by Mick Inkpen or 'Pinocchio' from the *Elves and the Shoemaker* by the Brothers Grimm.

Large hand puppets

These puppets can be used in a similar way to dolls. They can wave goodbye, clap hands and usually feature a moving mouth, so are ideal to encourage social and communication skills. Use them to model language structures like greetings and farewells or to ask children questions in a non-threatening way.

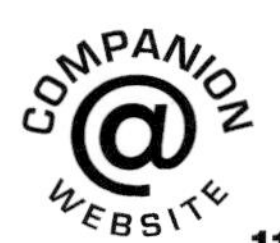

Demonstrate social interaction skills like taking turns and active listening using the puppet. Act out different scenarios where the children need to help the puppet improve their skills on looking, waiting for a turn, sharing and cooperating with others in play.

Activities for older children

- Children can create puppet shows, developing their own characters, plot and narratives. Allow children to engage at a variety of language levels from noises for animals, through to words and sentences. Storytelling and performance might involve simple sentences to much more complex and narrative language.
- Use stories to help children practice the use of social language; for example, a puppet who needed to make friends might ask – "Can I play?"
- Provide experience of the use of puppetry in different cultures. Examples include:
  - Kathputli are string or marionette puppets from the region of Rajasthan, India. Children can create their own puppets using traditional Indian printed fabrics. Vocabulary might be developed around colour, shape and pattern. Can be linked with the art and design curriculum for KS1 and 2.
  - Chinese shadow puppetry is a form of theatre art that uses jointed puppets made from paper, card or leather to cast shadows or silhouettes. A creative way to explore themes around the understanding of light and shadow. Links with the science curriculum, art and design, and drama KS1 and 2.
  - Wayang Golek are Indonesian puppets operated by wooden rods, which are accompanied by percussion musicians (*gamelan*). Children can experiment with different sound makers to create their own orchestra to accompany a puppet performance. Links with music in KS1 and 2.

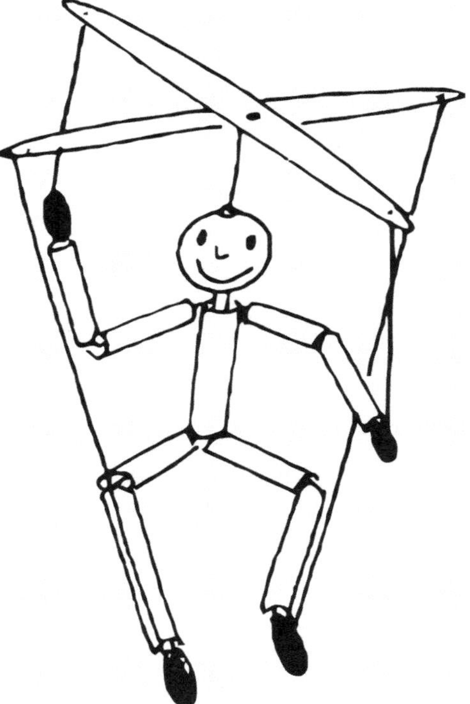

Small world play

Encourage miniature doll recognition as soon as the child is ready, as it allows for much more flexibility in symbolic play and other games. However, large dolls and home-corner play is still very important to the child and will continue to be for some time and therefore should not be discouraged.

Aims

To encourage imaginative play with small world materials to enable the child to recreate familiar everyday routines and to explore dramatic fictional scenarios.

Outcomes

- Relates small doll material in appropriate ways that reflect everyday experiences.
- Uses small doll material to act out dramatic scenarios in sequenced and complex ways.

Strategies

- Imaginative play should be fun, so do not give commands but join in and have fun.
- Encourage the child to talk about their play using self-commentary and parallel talk (see 'Introduction' for more information on these techniques).
- Provide lots of models of behaviour for the child to extend their play. Even imaginative children can get stuck in a play routine – your role is to provide stimulating materials and suggestions to help move children on.
- Provide character figures and materials so children can retell a familiar story or song.
- Introduce opportunities to practice language targets or learn new vocabulary.

Suitable materials and resources

Small world play sets like Playmobile, Lego Duplo World People, playmats, doll's houses, farms, railways and garages. A variety of miniature figures representing family and different occupations, creatures, animals, vehicles and buildings. Natural materials like sand, moss and twigs for setting a scene or recreating a particular environment. Junk material, scraps of material and construction items for improvised play.

Activities to encourage small world play

Doll play

Some children may need help to move from large to small doll play, so start to include slightly smaller dolls into large doll play. Gradually decrease the size of the dolls, and when they reach a certain smallness, it may seem only too obvious to the child that the doll needs its own set of small furniture and possessions. If it is not obvious to the child, then exaggerate the absurdity of the little doll wearing big shoes and clothes.

Small world themes

Set up small world play around different themes. These might be about familiar experiences for the child like the home, park or play group. Make sure there are also opportunities to explore real life events like a visit to a farm or to the seaside. More fantasy elements might be stimulated with a space scene or dinosaur park. Provide books for children to explore these themes further.

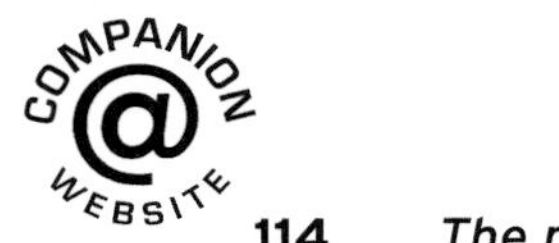

Occupations

Explore the roles of different occupations and help the child act out appropriate scenarios. So a fire fighter might put out a fire, but they may also visit a farm to rescue an animal. Encourage them to act out going to the doctors or taking their pet to the vets, where they can take on different roles.

Layouts

Miniature figures and small models can be used in conjunction with layouts to form a make-believe scene. Ideas for layouts include the seaside; a farm or zoo; a garden, street or town. Help the child to create their own using junk material. Materials like packaging, felt, gummed paper, sponge, corrugated paper, silver foil and scraps of material can be reinvented as a park. For example, trees can be cardboard cut-outs covered with green gummed paper, a pond can be silver foil stuck on to the layout, seats formed from corrugated paper and roundabouts made from cheese boxes.

Characters in stories

Show the child how to use toys to act out a story with different characters. Provide relevant miniature figures and materials alongside small world equipment to enable this. Look out for commercial sets that accompany familiar tales like *The Three Billy Goats Gruff*, *Jack and the Beanstalk* and *Goldilocks and the Three Bears*. This is a great way for children to take on different roles and act out a sequence.

Object-miniature matching

Augment small word play with activities that encourage comparisons of real-size objects, large toys and miniature items. Make active comparisons and demonstrate the similarities between the two, starting with very familiar objects, such as a chair, a table and a shoe. The difference in size between the real object and the miniature should be great, but not so great that the child ceases to perceive the visual likeness.

- Point to a real object and ask the child to find a matching object in a selection of miniature versions. Increase the complexity by introducing a memory factor and figure-ground discrimination skills; for example, place the miniatures in a toy box so that the child has to remember their object as they search through the box.
- Put two miniature toys into a feely box or bag, point to a real object and have the child find a duplicate copy by feel. Gradually increase the choices.
- Think up new and interesting ways to present the miniatures; for example, put them in a series of boxes so the child must open the boxes to find the correct toy: hide them around the room or wrap them up in parcels.

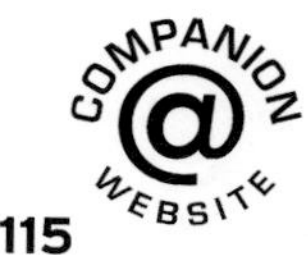

Language around size and comparison can be introduced alongside these activities.

2D to 3D

Have activities running alongside small world play that encourage the child to link the 3D components of the miniature figures with 2D representations.

- Make a home-made picture-board from stiff card. The child can make up their own picture using junk materials to illustrate a small world scene. A relief effect can be achieved using empty boxes, cartons, crumpled paper and foil.
- Use *Fuzzy Felt* to recreate similar themes to play with figures. There are a whole range of scenes, including a farm, house, sea, space, pet parlours and builders.

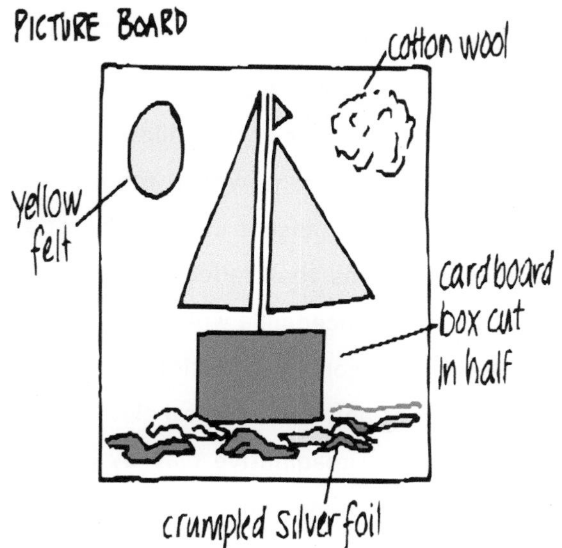

Activities for older children

- Help children match and sort items into categories by shape, size and colour, for example, sorting vehicles into cars, lorries and vans. Introduce counting.
- Make small world materials using junk and improvised materials, so furnishings for a dolls house, buildings for a farm.
- Provide paper or card in the shape of an animal, rocket or dinosaur depending on the theme that children can draw or write on.
- Show the children a composite picture of a street scene. Help them cooperate in planning and organising materials to set this up.

Role play

Early role play will centre around experiences in the home, but later, children learn to experiment by taking on new and unfamiliar roles. This leads to a greater understanding of others and an ability to make sense of novel situations they come across in real life.

Aims

To help the child represent their everyday experiences in play and act out familiar roles.
To help the child carry out a sequence of two or three actions as part of a role play.

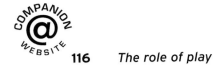

Outcomes

- Acts out roles related to their own routine and/or everyday experiences.
- Carries out a sequence of actions.
- Acts out novel or unusual roles.

Strategies

- Set up a role play space with toy furniture and different materials that reflect the daily lives and routines of the children and their families.
- Help set the scene with a range of props like toys, dolls and everyday objects, for example, pans, dishes and cutlery for a kitchen.
- Include items that reflect a range of culturally diverse experiences, so pans might include a saucepan, a wok and a chapati pan with a range of multicultural foods.
- Have an assortment of clothes for dressing up that include some traditional national costumes and multicultural clothing.
- Encourage imaginative play by providing junk material (cardboard boxes and tubes, plastic trays and odd bits of cloth), which can be used as substitution for a real object.
- Model appropriate behaviours, for example, feeding dolly and wiping dolly's face with a flannel.
- Join the child in simple turn taking routines like a tea party.
- Introduce vocabulary by commenting on your actions and the actions of the child.

Suitable materials and resources

A range of props that reflect the varied everyday experience and daily routines of the children. A collection of commercially produced dressing-up clothes, or some old clothes, especially accessories like hats, scarves, bags and jewellery. Dolls, teddies and puppets. Junk material.

Activities to encourage role play

Nursery rhymes or familiar stories

The child carries out actions with a doll, teddy or puppet described in a story or nursery rhyme. Start with those requiring simple actions that include the child's favourite characters. *Where's Spot?* has its own soft toy to use along with the story book.

Puppets

Puppets can be used in a similar way to dolls. They can wave goodbye, eat dinner and wash hands and faces.

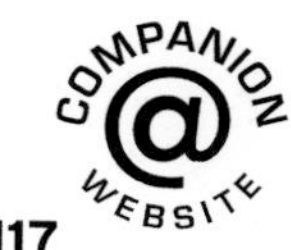

Guess 'who' mime

One child acts out a mime and the other children have to guess 'Who am I?' They might be a firefighter or a tree. Giving the children pictures of people or objects may help to stimulate their imagination.

Beep beep

Children can pretend to drive toy cars and learn to stop and go at a signal. Vocabulary might include 'stop', 'go', 'bye', 'hello', 'car' and sounds like 'beep beep' and 'toot toot'.

Acting out

Let the child act out their recent experiences using dolls, for example, a visit to the hairdressers or an outing to the park.

Pretend workers

Children can be doctors, nurses, teachers, bus drivers, police officers, carpenters, astronauts, hairdressers and so on. Encourage children to explore the language used in different roles and link this to vocabulary development.

Acting out, not acting up

Children can be helped to act out a forthcoming event that they may find worrying, for example, a visit to the dentist or hospital, starting school, or performing in front of the class. Children can take turns at acting out different roles. Such role play may help children to understand difficult situations and lessen their fear.

Activities for older children

- Children can design and make their own props and resources for role play.
- Use different scenarios to provide opportunities that target and extend specific vocabulary; for example, a post office will elicit different language to a travel agent's office. Link the role play with other curriculum areas, so a post office would provide opportunities to work on money and maths, whereas a travel agent might encourage understanding of the world.

Social play

Social play offers a natural situation in which the child's communication and social interaction skills can be practised and extended. These types of activities provide the child with an opportunity to observe and imitate others, which are basic prerequisites for

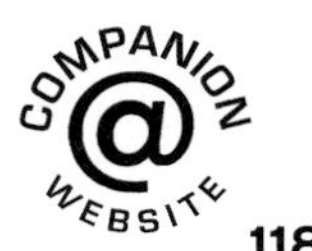

language learning (Bloom and Lahey, 1978). Play can be a solitary act or a shared activity with an adult or other child. Interaction is a key concept in social play and refers to the two-way process of give and take between the children. The child needs to understand the ideas of sharing and turn taking.

Functions

- To allow the child to develop new skills from observing and imitating their playfellows.
- To allow the child to practise old skills in novel situations.
- To provide an opportunity for the child to develop and expand their communication skills.
- To encourage the child, through shared play, to become more sociable and make friendships, thus increasing their communicative confidence.

Parallel play

Children are happy to play alongside each other but are not yet ready to play together.

Aims

To encourage the child to tolerate an adult or child playing alongside.

Outcomes

- Engages in parallel play with an adult.
- Engages in parallel play with another child.

Strategies

- Children will benefit from seeing adults around them modelling parallel play.
- Provide activities where children can play alongside each other in similar activities.
- Allow the child to play with an activity of their own choosing.
- Help the child to start participating in simple turn-taking play like peek-a-boo.
- Choose activities where it is fun to share, like blowing bubbles.

Suitable materials and resources

Puzzles; lacing and threading toys; construction toys; outdoor play equipment; bubbles; balls; balloons; foam frisbees; and toy vehicles.

Activities to encourage parallel play

Table activities

Many activities can be played by two children alongside each other at the same table, including drawing, Play-Doh, puzzles, lacing and threading toys, Lego and other construction activities.

Outdoor races

Large outdoor play items like go-karts and pedal-cars allow children to play alone or to join in the fun. Children can take turns to push each other or have races.

Push me next

As children get used to playing alongside other children on outdoor equipment, they can be gradually encouraged to cooperate with one other child. They can push or be pushed on a swing or share a see-saw.

Ball games

Children can kick, throw or roll a ball back and forth to each other.

Wheeling vehicles

Cars and toys on wheels can also be used to pass between two children.

Simon Says

'Simon says' and other similar games allow children to engage with the activity as part of a group. They are not required to interact with the other children, but they can take a turn to be leader and give commands to the rest of the group.

Activities for older children

- Provide resources like Lego or building blocks that encourage sharing of materials, but also allow the child to play on their own. The use of a personal tray, bucket or bag allows the child to select items to play with from a shared pile to then use in solitary play.
- Provide resources for children to work together like floor jigsaws, construction kits, sand and water play.
- Provide musical instruments so children can make music together but still be autonomous.

Turn taking and shared play

Turn taking is an important prerequisite to the development of shared play with other children. It is also an essential skill for social interaction, especially conversation, where speakers take turns at listening and speaking.

Aims

To encourage turn taking in simple games and social interactions and encourage carry-over into larger group activities.

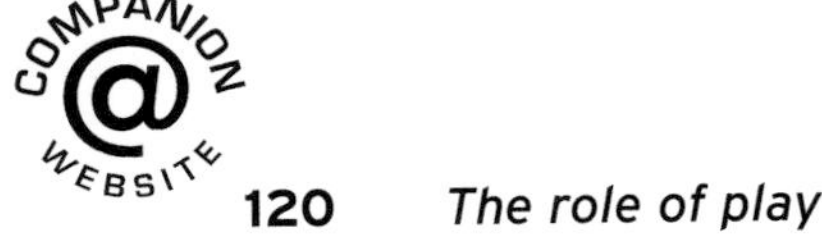

Outcomes

- Takes turns in simple games and social interactions with an adult or another child.
- Takes turns in simple games and social interactions in small group activities.

Strategies

- Follow the child's lead in play wherever possible.
- Focus on establishing a turn-taking routine, and don't worry too much if the child is not playing the 'right way'.
- Try to keep a balance of turns between you and the child. Avoid trying to lead the child; instead aim for a balance of turns.
- Use gestures and visual cues to help the child to identify who has a turn, for example, pointing or handing the child an item.
- Avoid having too many toys out at once. The focus should be on turn taking within one activity.

Suitable materials and resources

Toys for playing peek-a-boo; bubbles; toy cars; balls; balloons; inset puzzles; toy bricks; stacking cups; shape sorters; pictures and objects with a posting box.

Activities to encourage turn taking

Social games

Play social games where turn taking is a natural part of the interaction, for example, peek-a-boo.

Bubbles

Bubbles are great fun. Children may find it difficult relinquishing a bubble blower but might be encouraged to take turns at popping the bubbles.

Musical instruments

Take turns in making sounds on different instruments. Banging on a drum or tapping a chime bar is a good one for this game. Can the child copy a simple rhythm?

Tabletop games

Take turns with the child in simple tabletop games. Keep pieces in a bag or box and bring one out at a time.

- Building a brick tower.
- Piling up stacking cups.

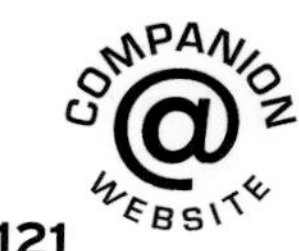

- Replacing pieces in an inset puzzle.
- Putting a shape into a shape posting box or on a shape sorter.
- Posting objects or pictures into a posting box.
- Placing a car or marble on a ramp.

Simple to and fro games

- Rolling a ball between you and the child.
- Pushing a car or train back and forth.
- Batting a balloon between you and the child.

Puppets

Play games with puppets who can model turn taking in general as well as in 'conversations'.

Books

Looking at books together offers lots of opportunities for turn taking, from simply turning pages to responding to the child's pointing, sound making and spoken language. So when the child points at a dog and says "woof-woof", you can join in and copy them. Remember to leave pauses for them to respond.

Feely bag

Let the children take turns in selecting an object from a bag and guessing what it is before taking it out. There are a number of games that could be played, including a guessing game of identifying objects by size, shape and texture, or from a spoken description.

Circle activities

Sit in a circle and pass an action around the circle, for example, passing a clap or hand squeeze around the group. This can be accompanied by language about turn taking like "Now it's Ryan's *turn*". In group games, keep activities simple with quick turns.

Activities for older children

- Be consistent in how you signal a turn, whether this is in a small group or with the whole class.
- Encourage pairs of children to share and take turns with card games like snap, matching pairs and lotto; board games like *Monopoly*; or games of strategy and skill like *Four in a Row/Connect 4* or *Jenga*.
- Let the child take a turn at being the leader in a game. 'Simon Says' is a good starter for this.
- In circle time activities use a visual or physical cue to indicate turns; for example, pass a microphone, special toy or hat around the group to signal turns.

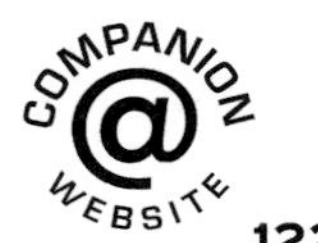

Cooperative play

Cooperative play helps the child learn how to build relationships with others as they develop abilities in turn taking and sharing. It also provides practice with nonverbal and verbal social interaction skills like eye contact, gesture and social phrases that are essential for later conversational skills.

Aims

To encourage the child to cooperate and collaborate with other children in a small group activity.

Outcomes

- Plays cooperatively with one other child or the adult, turn taking and sharing.
- Plays cooperatively with a small group of children, turn taking and sharing.

Strategies

- Children will benefit from seeing adults around them modelling turn taking and sharing during everyday routines and activities.
- Some games can be taught and practised initially between the adult and the child, and later played with one other or a small group of children at a similar developmental level.
- Early group activities need to keep all the children involved. As the children learn to share and take turns, they will find it difficult to wait during the game.
- Sing songs to help children learn each other's names and become familiar with different children in the group.
- Ensure that all the children have a chance to have a turn in a game. Do not allow one child to dominate the group.
- Provide some sort of prop that the children can pass around to indicate who has a 'turn'. This might be a special hat or cap, toy, medallion or a microphone.
- Use activities to practice social skills like eye contact, gestures and social phrases.
- Acknowledge the use of these social communication behaviours and provide positive reinforcement.

Suitable materials and resources

Ball or other toy for catching and throwing; activities and games that require collaboration like parachute games, *Twister*; construction toys; and random toys for pass the parcel games.

Activities to promote cooperative play

Pass the parcel

This can be made more interesting by wrapping a small toy inside each layer. This way the child has something to keep and something to pass on.

Hide and seek

Divide children into two teams of hiders and seekers.

Ball games

There are many different games that help turn taking and sharing. Here are just a few suggestions:

- Two children have a large beach ball that they can pass to each other.
- Children stand in a circle. One calls another child's name and throws them the ball. This child does the same and so on.
- 'Piggy in the middle': one child stands between two players and tries to catch the ball as they throw it to each other. If they succeed in catching the ball, they swap places with the thrower, who takes over as 'piggy'. Encourage different ways of avoiding the 'piggy' by throwing the ball to the side, rolling or bouncing it. You can also try this with a small group of children.
- Children stand in a circle and throw a ball to each other. If the ball is dropped, that child is out. Winner is the last one in.

Giant human knot

A group of children join hands. The aim is to tie a giant human knot. The children twist and duck under each other's arms and legs but keep holding hands. Other children can be enlisted to break the knot by picking out people to free their hands and move away.

Play Twister

This is a classic game in which two or more children get into a fine muddle as they twist between each other's legs and arms. There is a blindfold version where the players have tactile symbols.

Circle games

- Pass the gesture: Children form a circle and begin to move in one direction holding hands. At a given signal they change direction and place their hands on each other's shoulders.

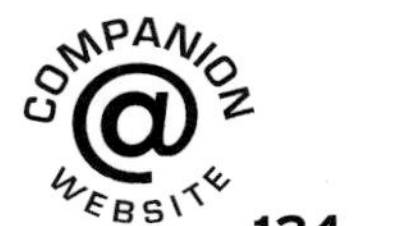

- 'Whispers': Children sit in a circle, including the adult. They take turns to send a whispered word or phrase round the circle. Is it the same word or phrase at the end?
- Squeeze: Children stand in a circle, holding hands. The adult or a child squeezes their neighbour's hand. Everyone has to pass the 'squeeze' round the circle and back to the beginning.
- Each child is given a picture of an object or someone carrying out an action with an object, for example, hammering in a nail or sawing a piece of wood. Each child has a turn at miming the action for the others to guess.

Activities for older children

- Introduce language tasks:
  - Categories – children stand in a circle and throw a ball or a quoit to each other. The thrower shouts out 'Animal, Vegetable or Mineral', and the catcher must name something from the category like a dog, a carrot or a stone. Players lose a chance to throw the ball if they fail to catch the ball or name an item.
  - Choose a theme and a trigger phrase. Each child takes a turn to complete the phrase, for example, "I like eating ...".
  - Build a story – The adult or a child gives a starter sentence, and each subsequent child must add another phrase to it and help build a story, for example, "I went to the beach".
- Play parachute games:
  - 'Merry-go-round' – children stand sideways to the parachute holding on to it with one hand. As they walk around in a circle, the chute will start to look like a merry-go-round – can they change direction when you give a signal?
  - 'Make waves' – children hold onto the edge of the parachute and raise their arms up and down. Change the tempo from slow to fast and back again.
  - 'Parachute tag' – ask the children to hold the edge of the parachute and lift it up so it fills with air in a mushroom shape. Call the names of two children who must swap places, running under the parachute before it comes down again and 'tags' them.

Sociodramatic play

At this stage of play the child is able to communicate what they want, and they know how to collaborate with other children towards a common goal. Each child will have a distinct role to play in a complex make-believe scenario where there is an elaborate recreation of real-life or imaginary situations.

Aims

To develop children's abilities to cooperate in creating complex dramatic play scenes.

Outcomes

- Builds a role play activity with other children in which each one takes on a new or different role.
- Uses language to plan and create a dramatic scenario.

Strategies

- Rather than expensive, detailed shop-bought items, use simple home-made toys or provide improvised materials, as these encourage the child to be more imaginative.
- Provide books, picture materials and other resources related to key sociodramatic themes.
- Record events using a digital camera. Post up pictures on the wall for children to refer back to and discuss.
- Help the children think about the language used by different characters.
- Guide the players when necessary but provide time for them to play without adult engagement.

Suitable materials and resources

A range of dressing up clothes and imaginative play props. However, the best resources are ones that encourage children to improvise and develop their creativity and imagination.

Activities for sociodramatic play

Social situations

Children can act out different social situations, for example, a birthday party or a visit to a fast food restaurant. Help the children share experiences and decide on roles.

Puzzles

Use puzzles that depict children and adults doing familiar things, for example, people at work, families in the park or shopping scenes. Encourage children to talk about them and then make up stories where the children can take on different roles.

Dramatic scenarios

Provide resources and play spaces for children to act out a number of dramatic scenarios:

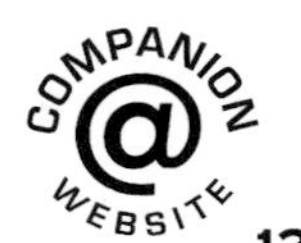

- Café – lots of opportunities to practise social language like greetings, requests and holding conversations. There is also scope for introducing money, counting and use of equipment like a till, calculator, oven and so on.
- Vets – create a dramatic play area based on children's stories about pets and visits to the vet. Provide bandages, stethoscopes, weighing scales, medicines, food and water. Toy animals can be kept in pet carriers (you may want to improvise with cardboard boxes). Opens up opportunities to talk about emotions and care for others.
- Hairdressers – provide toy hairdryers, brushes, combs, shampoos, rollers and other hair accessories. Have a mirror with seating. Children can practise asking questions, explaining, offering advice and compliments.

Fantasy world

Help children explore a fantasy world of their own creation. Use characters from films and fairy and folk tales to stir their imaginations. Build up a plot – who are the characters? Where do they live? How do they dress? What personalities do they have? Provide a cue to stimulate the development of a plot, for example, a strange creature has been found living in a nearby wood. Here one of the children can take on this role and, guided by the adult, carry out different actions that might evoke reactions from the other children (like quietly crying or rubbing their tummy).

Activities for older children

- Introduce experience of other cultures and traditions by using stories and songs that illustrate different lifestyles and roles to stimulate play.
- Provide materials that link pretend play with literacy. So a shop might have a written menu with pictures, bill slips for payment and pictures of food for sale with prices.
- Focus on social skills. Set up an audition – look at soaps on television and discuss how changes in facial expression, and in particular eye contact, express subtle meanings. Ask children to audition for different parts in a play or soap story line, using one phrase or sentence expressed in different ways.

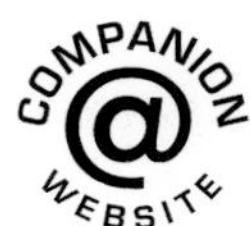

RECORD SHEET

Play skills

Name: **Review date:**

Outcomes	Comments

THE DEVELOPMENT OF VERBAL COMPREHENSION

DOI: 10.4324/9781003031109-5

Introduction

This chapter deals with the understanding of spoken language or verbal comprehension, which emerges during the first year of life and continues to develop throughout infancy and into early childhood. These language skills are foundational to the child's development as they have a significant impact on later literacy (Dickinson et al., 2010; Ouellette, 2006) and academic success (Morgan et al., 2015). Verbal comprehension refers here to the development of receptive vocabulary, including how words are related to each other, and an understanding of sentence structure. Traditionally, it has been thought that verbal comprehension precedes expressive language (Reynell, 1980), and this seems to be borne out by studies that show comprehension occurs before word production (Bates et al., 1995; Fagan, 2009). However, it may not be so straightforward, as there are many contextual and pragmatic cues like gesture and eye gaze that support comprehension (Dockrell, 2019) that may mask the child's true level of understanding. So it may be misleading to consider language understanding and language production as separate linear entities - a viewpoint expressed by Bloom and Lahey when they stated "knowing a word, knowing a grammar, and understanding structured speech apparently represent different mental capacities: it may be misleading to consider such capacities develop in linear temporal relationships, with comprehension simply preceding production" (1978, pp. 243-244).

Factors affecting verbal comprehension

There are many factors that might affect the development of a child's understanding of spoken language, including:

- **A sensory impairment:** A sensory impairment affecting hearing or vision is likely to impact a child's verbal comprehension.
  Examples include:
  - *Hearing loss:*
    - Children with significant hearing impairment show a delay in their language development (Borg et al., 2002). A study by Wie et al. (2020) found that children with a congenital profound hearing loss continued to have difficulties with receptive vocabulary post-cochlear implant.
- **An underlying neurodevelopmental disorder:** Delayed or impaired development of verbal comprehension is associated with a number of neurodevelopmental disorders:
  - *Developmental Language Disorder* (DLD): Children with DLD often have delayed receptive vocabulary (Rice and Hoffman, 2015); and have difficulty learning new words (Jackson et al., 2019).

  - *Autistic Spectrum Disorder (ASD):* Children with ASD usually present with significant impairments in language development and social communication with more pronounced difficulties in receptive language (Hudry et al., 2010).
- **Socio-economic status:** A slower rate of growth in receptive vocabulary has been found to be associated with areas of social and economic disadvantages such as 'low income, low educational attainment and high levels of unemployment' (Taylor et al., 2013).
- **Psychosocial deprivation:** Psychosocial deprivation or neglect is associated with poorer receptive language outcomes, which may be linked to less opportunities for child-directed speech and communicative interactions (Humphreys et al., 2020).
- **Type of language input:** The child learns their first words from their caregivers, who can provide them with an environment which stimulates and facilitates language learning (McDade, 1981). It is essential that these interactions are 'language rich' in both quantity and quality for the optimum development of language and cognitive abilities (Zauche et al., 2016).

Always seek professional advice where there are concerns regarding delayed or atypical development.

What is verbal comprehension?

In early development the child may only understand a word or phrase when spoken in a particular context and accompanied by gesture. True verbal comprehension begins when a child can relate a verbal concept to a meaningful object in any form it may occur (Reynell, 1977) and in any context (Bloom and Lahey, 1978).

A single verbal label has several different meanings which vary with context. Bloom and Lahey (1978) have detailed the different levels of perceptual and linguistic knowledge required by the child in the reception and understanding of spoken language.

1 Recognition of a word's sound pattern /k-a-t/.
2 Ability to recall the pattern from memory for the production of a word.
3 Knowing the word's specific referent – what object, action or event the word refers to, for example, 'cat'. This is called 'referential meaning'.
4 Knowing its full range of referents – knowing the word in relation to that object, action or event in any context, for example, all cats. This is called 'extended meaning'.
5 Knowing the relations it encodes – its meaning in regard to other words, for example, object of an action ('the boy stroked the cat') or the agent of an action ('the cat chased the mouse'). This is called 'relational meaning'.

6 Knowing the word's semantic category, for example, cat = animal. This is called 'categorical meaning'.
7 Recognising that the sound pattern is a word and that a word can consist of sounds, spoken and written. This is called 'metalinguistic sense'.

Until the child is able to show they understand all these meanings in all contexts, without cues, they do not really 'know' a word (Bloom and Lahey, 1978). This knowledge is acquired over a period of time.

The development of comprehension

First verbal labels

Common names for familiar objects first begin to have some meaning for the child at around 6 to 9 months (Bergelson and Swingley, 2015), which coincides with the emerging use by the infant of deictic gestures like 'giving', 'showing' and 'pointing' (Bates and Dick, 2002). Initially the child may rely on contextual and nonverbal cues, such as the direction of the adult's gaze, gesture or pointing, to understand the meaning of a spoken word. They may, for example, respond correctly to a request to fetch their cup as their mother brings out the orange juice but fail to select the cup from a number of objects during play when requested. The child is merely responding to the situation and has not learnt the word 'cup' as a symbol for that object. As true verbal comprehension develops, children start to recognise and understand the spoken word.

The child first learns the names of those objects that they have experienced in their everyday environment; therefore, children will differ in which words they learn first. Early vocabulary reflects the categories found in the parents' language input, which includes people, food, body parts, clothes, vehicles, animal, toys, everyday objects, routines and activities of states in the child's daily routines (Clark, 2017).

It is not until 15 to 18 months that the child begins to demonstrate true verbal comprehension (Reynell, 1977) and is able to recognise familiar objects by name even when these objects are not in their familiar surroundings. At this stage the child is able to understand several verbal concepts (Reynell, 1977) but is unable to assimilate these same concepts in a complex phrase. Although the child may respond appropriately to phrases such as 'Where's the ball?' they can only understand the word 'ball'.

Noun-noun combinations

Between the ages of 18 months and 24 months the child begins to relate two verbal concepts in an instruction, for example, 'Put the *biscuit* in the *tin*'. These concepts are nouns, as the child does not yet understand verbs, prepositions or adjectives.

Verbs

The child first learns to understand action verbs describing what is happening at around 24 months, and they are able to select pictures in response to questions like "Which one is eating?" (Sharma and Cockerill, 2014). Early verbs reflect actions the child can carry out themselves, for example, 'run', 'sleep', 'walk'; actions upon objects, for example, 'hit', 'ride', 'push'; and actions that produce changes in the child's environment, for example, 'break', 'cut' (Cole, 1982; Fenson et al., 2007).

Verbs are perceptually more abstract than nouns and therefore are more difficult for the child to learn (Roseberry et al., 2009). A noun represents an object that can be seen and manipulated, whereas a verb is without meaning unless there is a subject or object present to demonstrate its action.

Attribute and spatial relationships

Between the years 2 ½ and 4 the child's comprehension rapidly expands, so they are able to understand sentences of increasing complexity that include adjectives and prepositions (Sharma and Cockerill, 2014).

Attributes

Adjectives are words that refer to the properties and qualities of objects, and are acquired later than nouns. The child needs to appreciate that attribute represents something that is not bound to any particular object or context (Clark, 2016). They need to be able to recognise and distinguish different dimensions as a separate concept from that of the object. This conceptual development is helped by activities that involve matching and sorting of objects by different dimensions, for example, colour, shape, size. When they are able to perceive these differences, they are ready to learn the word. Some children with language delay may not learn attribute from everyday living and play, and they will need to be taught the relevant language alongside sorting and matching activities so that the association is made clear (Reynell, 1977).

As each child's experience is different, it is not possible to give a precise age by which different attribute terms are acquired, but understanding of descriptive concepts starts around three years. General terms, for example, 'big'/'little' are learnt before more specific terms such as 'tall'/'short', 'wide'/'narrow' and 'thick'/'thin'. By 3 years old the child should know several colours, and by 4 years nearly all of them (Weiss and Lillywhite, 1981). More abstract terms such as 'long', 'short', 'hard', 'soft', 'rough', 'smooth' are not learnt until 4 ½ years.

At 2 and 3 years the child perceives attributes as absolutes relative to themself, for example, 'a big elephant' and 'a small mouse'. It is not until 4 years that they can appreciate that the attributes are not fixed but are determined by context, that is, a mouse can be big as well as small.

Prepositions

It is important that children learn the concept of position before being taught the word, for example, activities where they are putting things 'in' a box or a bag, and physical games where they go 'under' or 'on' equipment. This way the child's understanding of the verbal concept does not become attached to a particular situation. The spatial terms of 'in', 'on' and 'under' are usually acquired first between 2–3 years with more complex terms learnt later. The child knows 'in front of' and 'behind' with objects where there is a logical front and back by 3 to 4 years, and 'between', 'above', 'below', 'top' and 'bottom' by 4–4 ½ years.

Question forms

Infants may respond to simple questions used by parents and caregivers in the first 18m, like "Where's mummy?" but they are using situational cues rather than showing any real understanding of the question word. It is not until 2 ½ to 3 years of age that children start to understand simple 'What?' and 'Where?' questions used directly about an object; for example, the adult says, "What's this?" pointing at an apple They can also identify items by function, for example, pointing at a picture when asked "Which one is eating?" By 3 years the child is able to understand 'Wh' questions like 'Who?' 'What?' 'Where?' and 'Why?' that ask for more specific information. By 5 they are able to understand and respond appropriately to 'How?' and 'Why?' with explanations.

Tense

It is generally agreed that the past tense is understood before the future (Cromer, 1974). As the immediate past forms part of the child's experience, it is more easily learnt. Between

4–6 years the child will start to understand talk about past and future events (Sharma and Cockerill, 2014). They will be able to understand language for sequential ordering and time like 'first', 'after', 'before' and 'last'.

Language input

The child's level of understanding cannot always be inferred from their expressive language and needs to be thoroughly assessed by formal and informal methods. It is essential that everybody involved with the child is aware of the child's comprehension ability so that they can modify their language accordingly. It is very important to monitor your language input to the child.

The level of complexity is affected by a variety of different factors.

- Introducing new vocabulary or abstract concepts, for example, size or place.
- Increasing the length of the sentence.
- The amount of information contained within a sentence:
  Sentences contain key words (or critical elements) that carry information, while some words in a sentence are redundant, as they add nothing to the message. These key words are referred to as "information carrying words" (ICW) (Knowles and Masidlover, 1982), and they will affect the complexity of a sentence and the memory load for the child (Frizelle et al., 2017).*
- The type of utterance; for example, embedded sentences require a greater level of understanding.
- The novelty of the request for the child. In the instruction "Put the doll *on* the chair" they will be able to use their own pragmatic knowledge to work out the meaning (Dockrell, 2019), whereas the instruction "Put the doll *under* the carpet" might be a little bit more difficult.

* You will not be able to find the number of information carrying words by simply counting the words in a sentence, as the words give only part of the message. The child uses other information from the situation, such as gestural cues and what they have learnt from the past, to help them to make sense of the spoken message. For example, the adult who says "Give me the *cup*" at mealtimes while holding out their hand is only requiring the child to understand one ICW – '*cup*'. The outstretched hand indicates to the child that the adult wants to be given something. If there are no other objects in the immediate vicinity of the child, then the word 'cup' becomes redundant too.

Generalisation of comprehension skills

It often happens that language skills taught do not transfer into the child's everyday communication. The child may have learnt a certain concept as specific to that situation and adult. Therefore, it is essential to make sure that learning opportunities are designed to help the child use their new skills in everyday life.

- Give the child time to consolidate their new skill through practice and reinforcement. This means ensuring that the people in their daily environment encourage them to practise their new skills and also provide the necessary feedback and repetition of language, for example, saying "Yes, that's a *ball*" when the child fetches it on request.
- Vary materials so that the child does not learn to relate a word to only one particular object or event (Gillham, 1979); for example, the word 'cup' can represent two or three non-identical cups, a toy cup, a miniature cup and a picture of a cup.
- Teach language in a variety of contexts (Gillham, 1979), for example, as the item is used at mealtimes, during a pretend tea party or while looking through a picture book.
- Teaching should normally proceed in small steps that support the consolidation and extension of learning and development.
- Present the vocabulary you want to teach in a variety of sentence structures, for example, a command, "Give me the *ball*"; a request, "*Ball*, please", or a statement, "This is a *ball*". Be careful not to increase sentence complexity, however.
- When a child first acquires a new skill, they need time to consolidate their learning with lots of practice in games and play situations.
- The home or learning environment has many distractions, and the child may find it difficult to maintain their new skills. Generalisation can be assisted in the following ways:
    - Involve the parent/caregivers where possible.
    - Carry out activities in varied environments.
    - Use cues and strategies when new skills are initially introduced into the home or general learning environment, even if these have been faded out in more structured teaching.
    - The child will continue to need praise and reinforcement for correct responses until skills become more established, even though these may have been reduced in structured teaching.
    - The general learning environment may have to be modified in order to provide the child with opportunities to practise their new skills.

Activities for developing the understanding of spoken language

These activities are designed to develop understanding of spoken language and include early vocabulary (nouns, verbs and early concepts), simple and more complex sentences.

General guidelines

- Choose activities appropriate for the child's age and stage of development.
- Use materials and resources that reflect the child's experience, interests and environment.
- Maintain the child's interest by varying materials and activities. This will also help with generalisation of learning.
- Adapt activities to suit the child's level of attention and listening skills. (See Chapter 2 for further information.)
- Adjust the amount and type of language input to suit the child's language and cognitive abilities.
- Make sure language is taught in association with its referent, so the link is clear between a particular word and the object, action or event to which it refers.
- Language activities should take place in a natural communication situation, for example, as part of a play routine, role play or game.
- Gain the child's attention before giving them a command or making a request.
- Accompany spoken language with appropriate facial expression and gesture (McNeil et al., 2000).
- Use clear speech with a varied intonation appropriate to the child's level of understanding.
- Emphasise key words but maintain a normal intonation pattern.
- Before teaching a word make sure that the child understands the relevant concept. For example, before teaching colour labels, show them how to match and sort items according to the concept.
- Shorter, less abstract words will be easier for the child to learn than longer multisyllabic words.
- Use lots of repetitions of the target language structures in daily activities.
- Gradually reduce the number of cues until the child has to rely on verbal comprehension.
- Give the child time to consolidate their new skill through practice and reinforcement. This means ensuring that the people in their daily environment encourage them to practise their new skills and also provide the necessary feedback and repetition of language, for example, saying "Yes, that's a *ball*" when the child fetches it on request.

Recording observations

Formative and ongoing assessment should help establish where the child is functioning in terms of their understanding of spoken language. Goals and strategies can then be carefully planned, although it is necessary to be flexible and adjust to the day-to-day changes in the child's needs and responsiveness. Language goals should aim to fulfil the child's immediate needs in the environment.

Observe and record the development of the child's understanding of spoken language over an extended period of time in a variety of situations within the learning environment. Observations from parents or carers are invaluable in gaining a broader understanding of the child's abilities in understanding spoken language.

Make a note of:

- the words or phrases the child is able to understand;
- the type and length of spoken instructions the child is able to follow appropriately;
- what cues the child needs in order to understand the spoken word (e.g., gestures, pictures, signs, symbols);
- how the child demonstrates this understanding, (e.g., points to an object; fetches an object; follows instructions correctly)
- the situation or context in which the child demonstrates this understanding;
- any differences in response to spoken language between formal and informal situations, (the latter may provide information on whether contextual cues are aiding understanding);
- any differences in response to spoken language between a one-to-one situation and a group activity (in the latter context, the child may watch and copy other children rather than fully comprehending the spoken word);
- responses by the child (behavioural, body language, gestures/signs or spoken language);
- consistency and frequency of responses;
- whether the child tries to copy a word or phrase;
- whether the child starts to use the word or phrase spontaneously.

First verbal labels

The first words taught to the child should reflect the objects and events that are familiar to them in their everyday environment. A vocabulary can be chosen by looking at each

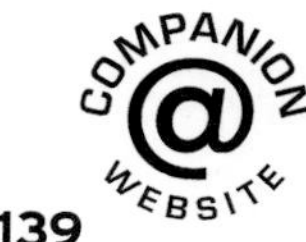

individual child's daily routines, favourite toys, food and pets. Early target words should have few syllables and be general in their reference, rather than specific – for example, 'dog' rather than 'spaniel' – as these are usually understood and remembered more easily.

Aims

To recognise and understand familiar objects by name even when these objects are not in a familiar context or routine.

Outcomes

- Identifies familiar objects by name without contextual cues.
- Identifies body parts by name without contextual cues.
- Identifies familiar animals by name without contextual cues.
- Follows simple one-part commands containing a verbal label.

Strategies

- Always link the spoken word or object name with what the child is looking at so they gradually learn to associate the word with the object.
- Use indexical gestures like pointing to help the child link the word to its reference (McNeil et al., 2000).
- Children should first be allowed to play with new objects in order to familiarise themselves with them. New objects should be introduced among familiar items, one at a time.
- A child will have a greater understanding of what a word means when they have a multisensory experience of an object; for example, as well as seeing an apple they can also hold it, smell it and see it peeled and cut into chunks, ready for them to taste.
- Talk about the function of objects to help create semantic links for the child and boost word learning (Booth, 2009).
- When teaching a new verbal concept, do not expect the child to understand it within a complex command. Activities can be modified so that the other words in the command become redundant. For example, the child is given a toy bed and a small doll and asked to "Put the doll *under* the bed". The child is not being asked to understand or remember the objects but only the word 'under'.
- Start with a small number of words and provide lots of clear models.
- At first accompany the words with lots of visual and contextual cues, gradually reducing these until the child is relying on verbal comprehension alone.

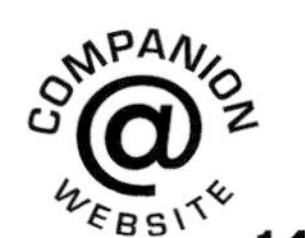

- Avoid correcting any errors the child may make when repeating or attempting to say a word. Instead provide the correct model, for example, "dup" – "cup", "dolly's cup".
- Provide lots of repetition of language targets in a variety of different contexts that include everyday routines, pretend play, picture books, activities and trips.
- Further generalise understanding by using target words in simple phrases and commands. Keep the rest of the information in the phrase redundant so the child only has to assimilate the one verbal concept.
- The key word should be at the end of the phrase and emphasised, for example, "Where's the *dog*?"
- Encourage carry-over of learning to other environments like the home by asking parents/caregivers to use the words in everyday routines.

Suitable materials and resources

Food: Real objects, empty food cans and cartons, replicas, doll-sized toys, miniature toys, pretend items made from plasticene or paper mâché, paper cut-outs, picture books, puzzles, photographs and drawings.

Clothes: Real clothing, baby clothes, doll's clothing, pictures from magazines and catalogues, cardboard cut-outs, paper dolls and cut-out clothes, picture books, puzzles, picture cards, photo cards or drawings of single items of clothing.

Toys: Teddies, dolls, puppets and stuffed animals; a range of familiar playthings like a ball, bubbles, jack-in-the-box and book; larger toy items like a kite, a rocking horse, ride-on bikes and cars; and picture cards, photo cards or drawings of toys.

Body parts: Pictures from magazines or catalogues; picture cards, photo cards and line drawings; papier-mâché models of body parts; body parts on teddies and puppets.

Everyday objects: A range of everyday objects familiar to the child. Some examples include a comb, brush, cup, plate, spoon and fork. Picture cards, photo cards or drawings of everyday objects.

Animals: Cuddly animal toys, plastic animal shapes, miniature animals, animal masks, picture books, puzzles, drawings, photographs or photo cue cards of animals.

Transport: Large toy vehicles, small toy vehicles, miniature vehicles, picture books, puzzles, picture cards, photo cards or drawings of single items of transport.

Empty food and drink containers may contain traces of allergens: for example, cereal and biscuit boxes may contain traces of nut. Avoid egg cartons, milk cartons, cereal boxes, biscuit boxes and baby food jars.

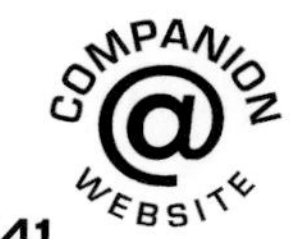

Activities to develop understanding of verbal labels

Food

Mealtimes

During mealtimes talk about the food the child is eating, drawing their attention to each item as you name it clearly. When offering them a choice of things to eat or drink, hold each item up and name it, for example, "Do you want milk?" – showing them the milk, or "Do you want orange?" – showing them the orange.

Cooking

Cooking activities give children hands on experience with food. Food names can be introduced in many different ways, from gathering items for the recipe, as part of instructions, to creating recipe picture books and story boards. Activities can focus around one food group; for example, recipes with fruit might include making a fruit salad, rainbow fruit kebabs, fruit pizza toppings, fruit rockets (melon pieces shaped like a rocket on a stick) or fruit smoothies. Follow up by finding matching items in the book *Eating the Alphabet* by Lois Elbert.

Grow a vegetable

Try growing some vegetables, preferably ones that have a fast rate of growth, so the child's interest is maintained. Let the children see the vegetables in different stages of growth. Older children can draw them and make a pictorial record of their life cycle. Get the children to draw the whole vegetable, its inside and its peel.

Printing

Look at the patterns and shapes you can create by painting and printing with different types of fruit and vegetables. Make dots by rolling corn on the cob; compare the shape of an apple cut lengthways with widthways; cut a cauliflower or broccoli head in half to make repetitive patterns; or use starfruit and melon wedges to create stars and moon crescents.

Interest table

Ask the children to bring in different foods linked with the four seasons or special festivals and celebrations. This way children get to experience a range of foods from different cultures.

Pretend food

Make pretend fruit and vegetables with the children out of plasticine, papier mâché or Play-Doh. As they make the models, they learn about the differences in colour, shape and size. Talk about what the children are doing, clearly naming the different food.

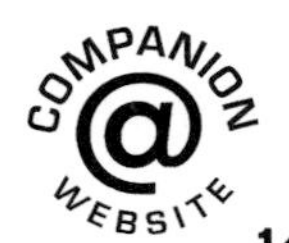

Pretend shop

Use the pretend foods in a shopping game. Set up a make-believe shop with shelves and a counter, with the children and adults taking it in turns to be the shopper and the shopkeeper. Give the child a shopping bag or basket, and tell them what to buy, for example, "Please get me an...*apple*". (Pause and emphasise the word apple using gesture or pointing, if appropriate.) Name items again when you unpack the shopping bags at the end of the game.

Café

Introduce different contexts where you might find food, like a café or restaurant. Here food names might be used with picture menus, so children can be asked to make choices and combine different food items. Children can also play at matching real or pretend food to pictures.

Going on a picnic

Use this game to introduce toy replica food in a make-believe game. The teddy bears are going on a picnic, so they need to pack a basket of things to eat and drink. Ask the child to collect together items for the picnic basket. This can be extended into a pretend tea party, with the child responding to different requests by the teddies.

Inset puzzles

Puzzles with a single inset piece provide an opportunity to reinforce a name learnt with a real food item. Inset puzzles with a food topic will help the child hear several different food names. They also help the child understand that different food items belong to the group of 'things we eat'. Categories can be general with several different foods or more specific, so all fruit or all vegetables. Ask the child to take out or put back different pieces as you name them.

Giant posting box

Make a cardboard box into a giant posting box by cutting a hole in the side. You can make the hole into the mouth of a funny face. Ask them to post different items of food through the mouth.

The Hungry Caterpillar

The Hungry Caterpillar by Eric Carle has the caterpillar eating different fruits alongside junk food and is a good starting point to talk about healthy food choices. You can also make

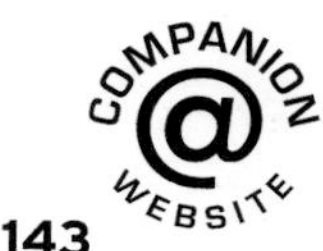

a caterpillar by painting a cardboard tube and shaping one end like a gaping mouth. Ask the child to post pictures of different foods into the mouth.

Happy families

Each child in a small group is given a card from one category, for example, fruit. This is the master card which depicts all the members of the family, for example, pear, apple, banana, orange. The adult has matching individual cards from which they take one and ask, "Who's got an *orange*?" The winner is the first to complete their family.

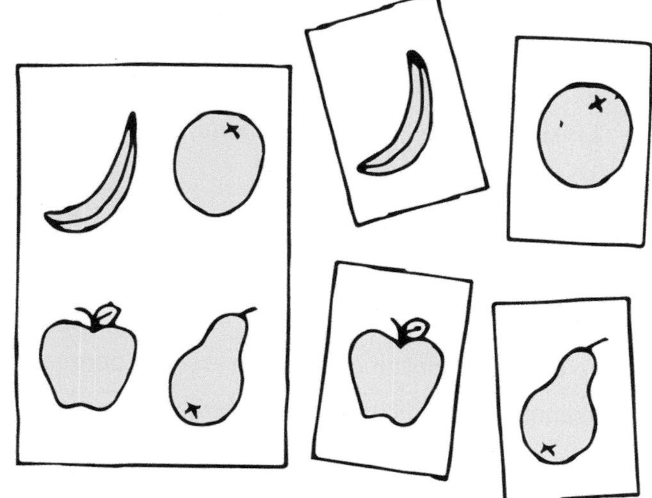

Food diary

Keep a daily diary with the child by recording the meals of the day in pictures. Meals can be photographed on a phone or tablet or drawn by the adult, or the child can look through magazines for pictures. However, there should not be too long a gap between the event and recording it.

Activities for older children

Trips to farms, allotments and markets help children understand where food comes from and how it grows. Many manufacturers are also very willing to provide information about their food-making processes and to arrange visits to see food being manufactured.

- Play a pairs game where children have to match pictures of the source food with the shop product.
- Create a food wheel to help children identify different groups of food. Ask children to talk about what they like and don't like in the food wheel. At the end children can vote for their favourite foods. Make a matrix with colour, size, taste or texture for the axes.
- Creative play – provide cut-outs of fruit and vegetables for children to create a face. Use the portraits constructed from food and other objects painted by Giuseppe Arcimboldo as inspiration!
- Use stories to introduce and explore food from different cultures. For example:

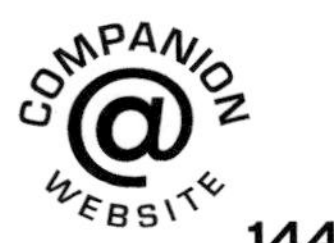

- *Handa's Surprise* by Eileen Browne tells the story of Handa and her trip to the market in Kenya. Use real examples of the fruit to re-tell the story with mischievous animal puppets that steal from Handa's basket.
- *The Ugly Vegetables* by Grace Lin introduces the reader to Chinese vegetables. Includes a glossary of Chinese characters and a soup recipe.
- *Baby Goes to Market* by Atinuke combines food names with number.

Links with on EYFS Understanding the World, Listening and Speaking, and KS1 curriculum Maths.

Clothes

Getting dressed

Name pieces of clothing as you dress and undress the child. Also name your own clothing, for example, "Look, I'm putting on my *hat*".

Dress up

Play dressing-up games using silly hats and colourful clothes. Take one item and put it on saying, "Look, I'm wearing a *hat*". Then give it to the child, again naming it – "*Hat*, Sammy's got a *hat*". Use a mirror and have lots of fun posing. Move on to giving them a choice of clothing and ask them to choose one.

Dress dolly

Dressing up dolly during pretend play is a good way to introduce and practice names of clothing. Show the child what to do with the clothes and name them as you dress the doll. Let the child join in with their own doll and clothes. Comment on what the child is doing. (Older children can put paper clothes onto cardboard cut-out figures.)

Washing day

A washing line can be hung in the play corner and washing day can be acted out by the adult.

As they peg up the clothes, they name them for the child. Clothes can be real clothes, doll's clothes, or cut-outs made from stiff card. The child can join in and perhaps be given instructions by a doll or puppet, for example, "Hang up my *sock*".

Pack my bag

Teddy is going on holiday. Have a real suitcase or travel bag with some real clothes or doll-sized ones. Ask the child to find items from a selection of two or three to pack in the

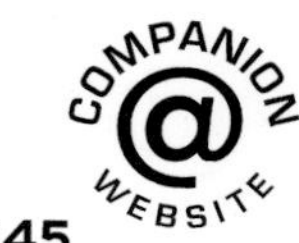

suitcase. Vary teddy's holiday destination: a warm climate versus a cold climate; a beach holiday versus a country holiday.

Clothing collage

Help the child make a collage using pictures from magazines and clothes catalogues. Cut out any articles of clothing they find in magazines and glue onto a large poster board. Hang this for them to see throughout the week. Vary the display according to the season. You can use the cut-outs to create an outline or silhouette. Can the children recognise the item of clothing?

Simon Says

Play 'Simon Says' with instructions to put on different clothing items. You will need several versions of the same item, for example, several hats, scarves and gloves. Set up team games where children compete to see who can put on the most amount of clothing the quickest. Give out instructions like "Put on a *hat*".

Story books

Look at picture books showing different clothing items. Point to the picture and name the item. Some useful books are: *We Can Get Dressed: Putting on My Clothes* by Maion Cocklico and *Let's Get Dressed!* by Caroline Jayne Church.

Activities for older children

- Help children customise old clothing or design their own fantasy clothing and put on a fashion parade. Discuss reducing, reusing and recycling and link with the fast fashion industry.
- Explore different materials. Talk about how they are made and their various uses. Use the materials in collages of colour and texture.
- Discuss the different fashions throughout history, and perhaps show the children photos of the fashions in your own youth! This should generate some interest and amusement. Finish up with a fashion show!
- Explore cultural differences in clothing. Talk about the clothes that children from different countries wear. Collect together pictures and dolls in national costume to help discussion.
    - *The Proudest Blue* by Ibtihaj Muhammad tells the story of two sisters wearing the hijab and explores faith, diversity and identity.
    - *Under My Hijab* by Hena Khan is a celebration of the hijab.

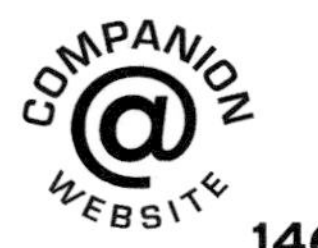

- *My Mother's Sari* by Sandhya Rao and Nina Sabnani is a fun exploration of the many uses of a sari.
- *What We Wear: Dressing Up Around the World* by Maya Ajmera and *Clothes Around the World* by Clare Lewis explore cultural differences in clothing.

Toys

Playtime

Name the child's toys you as you play with the child. Let the child have different variations of the same toy, for example, three different dollies, so they learn that the word "dolly" is not just for their favourite doll. Show them that the dolls can be used for the same things, for example, cuddling, dressing and feeding, and that they look, feel and move in the same way.

Tidy time

As you tidy toys away or get them out for play, hand them to the child and name each one. Ask the child to fetch toys from the play box. If they don't understand, find the toy for them and show it to them. Make the play box into a giant posting box by cutting a hole in the side. You can make the hole into the mouth of a funny face. Let the child tidy their toys by posting them through the hole.

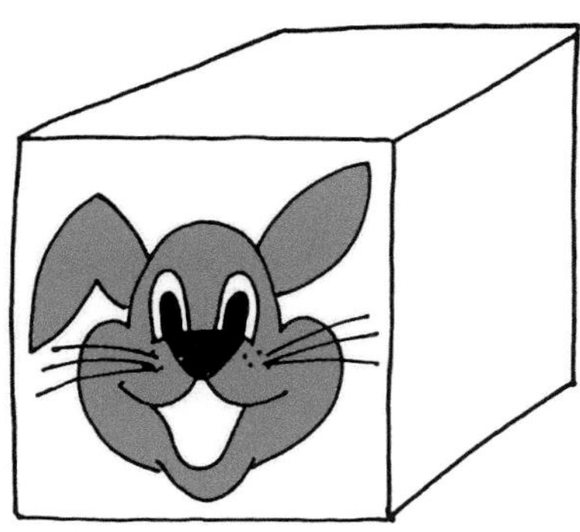

Toy shop

Set up a pretend toy shop with the children and adults taking it in turns to be the shopper and the shopkeeper. Give the child a shopping bag or basket and tell them what to buy, for example, "Please get me a... *book*". (Pause and emphasise the word book using gesture or pointing, if appropriate.) Name items again when you unpack the shopping bags at the end of the game.

'My Toys' picture book

Make a picture book of the child's favourite toys out of real photographs. Look through the book, naming each picture for the child. As the child becomes familiar with the names, see if they can find the one you name, for example, "Where's your *ball*?" Take photographs of the child using toys in different contexts, for example, playing ball on the beach, in the garden or with a sibling. This helps the child attach meaning to the verbal label in different situations.

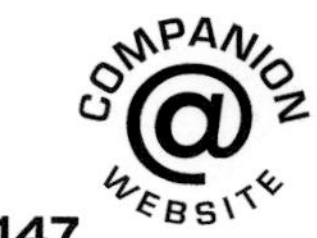

Where's my toy?

Hide a few of the child's toys around the room; name each one as you find them. Next, hide two or three toys and ask them to find one, for example, "Where's *teddy*?"

Toy sack

Place a number of different toys in an opaque bag. Let the child take turns with you in putting their hand in the bag and drawing out a toy. Name the items as they emerge from the bag. Repeat the game, but this time ask the child to find different toys. No peeking, just use the sense of touch.

Pass the parcel

Play pass the parcel with a small group of children. Wrap toys up in paper, naming items as they are revealed. Or try putting toys hidden inside each other, for example, a peg man inside a teapot or a ball inside a box.

Pairs game

Collect together several pairs of identical toys and wrap each one in paper. Help the child play a matching game where they have to find two parcels that look identical. Let the child open the parcel when they have a matching pair. Once the child is familiar with this game, they can start to have toys that are similar but not exact matches. So there may be one small ball and one big ball, or two cars the same shape and size but different colours. This will help them to generalise their learning of the verbal label to several different versions of the same toy.

Activities for older children

- Provide lots of scrap material and discarded objects for children to use in designing a toy. Find inspiration in *Toys Around the World (Adventures in Culture)* by Mary Pat Ehmann and *Toys from Around the World by* Joanna Brundle.
- Set up a toy shop with numerous examples of different miniature versions of toys. Use these to introduce counting and the concept of quantities, using terms like 'more' or 'less'.
- Have a collection of old and new toys. Discuss with the children the differences between the toys. Which toys do they like? Why have toys changed? Link with trips to toy and childhood museums.
- Explore music and songs related to toys in *The Nutcracker Suite* and *Pinocchio*.
- Create a toy hospital or repair workshop with some take apart and put together toys. Have some 'quick fixes' like plasters, string and spare wheels.

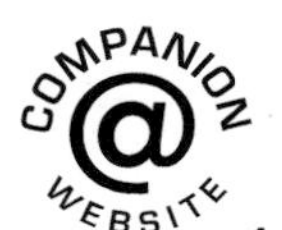

- Older children will enjoy story books with toy characters like:
  - *Toys Lost in Space* by Mini Grey. Encourage children to make up their own story inventing characters and voices for different toys.
  - *Lost in the Toy Museum* by David Lucas. Children can set up their own 'hide and seek' game with a selection of toys.
  - *Kipper's Toybox* by Mick Inkpen. Children can make their own 'Sock Thing' character using a sock and odd buttons, googly eyes and fabric bits.

Body parts

Everyday routines

When you are dressing or bathing the child, name the different parts of the body. They will learn the names of larger parts of the body first, for example, arm, leg, hand. Pretend play with dolls or teddies will reinforce this learning, so you can ask the child to "Wash dolly's face", "Wash dolly's hair". (Remember to keep the same action so the child focuses on the name of the body part.)

Puzzles

There are a number of commercially produced puzzles for learning about parts of the body. Help the child put the puzzles together, naming the pieces for them and relating them to the child's own body. Ask the child to show you different body parts on the puzzle.

Mirror play

Look in the mirror together with the child, point out different parts of their body and name them. Then point to the same parts on your body, for example, "There's your *nose*, and here's my *nose*". Talk about what you can do with different parts of the body, so the child starts to understand their function, which will help tell them apart.

Silly dressing up

Play a silly dressing-up game by putting articles of clothing on the wrong parts of the body, for example, a sock on your hand. Make comments about what you are doing and ask the child if it is right. See if they can point to the correct body part and help you put it on correctly. Give the child a piece of clothing, for example, a sock, and ask them to put it on their head or hand.

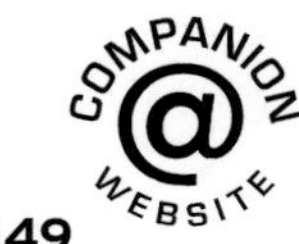

Body prints

Paint the child's hands, feet, knees and elbows so they can make prints on paper. As you paint each part, name it. A less messy activity is to draw around the child's different body parts so you can create outline drawings of a hand, foot or head.

Shadow prints

Explore the effects of light by getting children to experiment with positioning their body to create different shadows outside in the sun.

Simon Says

Play 'O'Grady' or 'Simon Says' and ask to touch different body parts, for example, "Touch your *nose*". At first point to each part of the body as you name it, but later just give the command and see if the child is correct.

Tell the child to carry out actions involving different parts of the body; for example, clap your hands, stamp your feet, wiggle your fingers or shrug your shoulders. Read and do the actions in *Ten Tiny Toes* by Caroline J Church.

Rhymes and songs

Encourage the child to copy you as you touch different body parts as you recite the nursery rhyme *Head, Shoulders, Knees and Toes*. Sing songs that focus on body parts and actions like *If You're Happy and You Know It*; or combine music and movement in *Hokey Cokey*. Children can take turns to choose an object for the song *This is the Way We Brush Our Hair* so each child has an opportunity to combine an action with an object and relate it to a body part.

Drawing

Draw a picture of a boy or a girl and ask the child to colour in the different parts. Have ready mixed skin tone paint or different coloured pencils to match different skin tones.

Activities for older children

- Older children will enjoy exploring body anatomy puzzles which provide accurate illustrations of skeletal, muscular, respiratory and digestive systems.
- Sorting matrix.

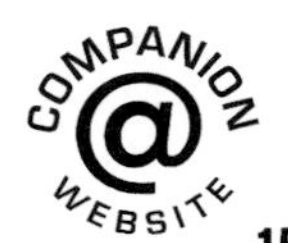

Ask children to create a matrix which compares similarities between different members of the group. Children can look in a mirror so that the children can compare parts of their bodies that are the same, for example, the same-coloured eyes, and the same length of hair.

For example: One axis could be hair length and the other eye colour.

	long	medium	short
brown	Hasan		Stefan
blue		Jack	
green	Zhen	Mary	

- Help children express their sense of identity through painting self-portraits. They will learn about how to mix paints to achieve different skin tones, eye and hair colour. Encourage the children to explore the front, back and side views of body parts.

Everyday objects

Everyday routines

During the day talk about the objects you or the child are using in everyday routines. Choose those objects that are very familiar to the child, for example, a spoon or a cup. Say the name of it, repeating the word a few times in different ways – "*cup*", "Here's your *cup*".

Pretend games

Play pretend games that involve real objects or toy replicas. Spoons, cups and plates can be used in make-believe tea parties; and brushes, combs, soap and flannels can be used to give dolly and teddy a 'wash and brush-up'. Talk about the objects as you play with them and ask the child to give you different ones.

Mystery feely bag

Put a few familiar items in an opaque bag. Put your hand in the bag and say, "I'm going to find a ... *cup*". Put your hand into the bag, draw out the cup and exclaim with great surprise, "Look, I found a *cup*". Let the child play with the cup, showing them how to take a pretend drink.

Hand the bag to the child and ask them to find a named object by feeling inside the bag. If they find it difficult, then let them go through all the objects in the bag, naming them as the child pulls each one out. When you've finished, put the items back into the bag and let the child try again. Start with two or three objects and gradually increase the number.

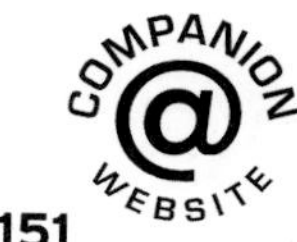

Find the hidden object

Place some objects in a Tuff Tray and cover them over with sand. Ask the child to run their hands through the sand to find the objects you name. Can they discover the objects by touch alone before they them pull out of the sand?

Pegboard puzzles

Early inset pegboard puzzles have pieces showing different objects. Name the object clearly as the child takes the pieces out. When all the pieces have been removed, ask the child to find an object and replace it in the puzzle.

Two-piece puzzles

Play a simpler version of Pelmanism with two-piece puzzles depicting everyday objects. Place two or three of the puzzles face up on the table, showing the child each picture and naming it for them. Then break up the pieces and mix them up, keeping the pictures in view. Ask the child to find an object. If they don't respond then match up the pieces for them, and when you find the right combination exclaim, "Look, a *comb*". Ask the child to find another object.

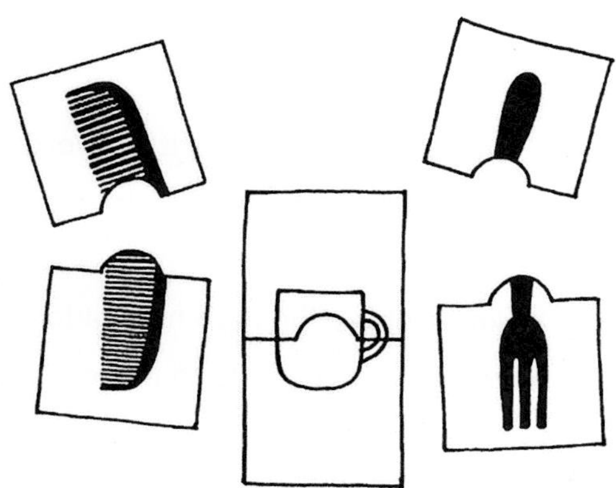

Treasure hunt

Set up a treasure hunt for a small group of children. Ask the children to search for a 'hidden' treasure object in the room. Treasure might consist of items like a small fancy 'silver' spoon, a gold-coloured pen, a decorative book, a sparkly handheld mirror and so on. Found items can be placed in a basket and at the end of the game pulled out for naming, for example, "*spoon*", who found the *spoon*?"

Once children are familiar with this activity, start to place items in unexpected places or presented at unfamiliar angles, for example, an upside-down cup or a scrunched-up scarf. These games can also be played outside where there is scope to have a lot of fun with a treasure island, pirate's boat and sunken chest in a large water tray or table.

Matching objects to pictures

Look at pictures of everyday objects using photocards or flash cards. Start with two or three images, naming the object clearly for the child. Introduce and name some real objects that

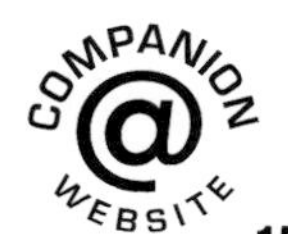

match the pictures. Show the child an object and ask, "Where's the *comb*?" or "Find the *comb*". Let the child place it on the correct picture. Gradually increase the number of photo or flash cards. Try making your own photographs of important objects in the learning environment.

Find the object

Look through picture books that show everyday objects in the home and environment. Share books like *Very First Book of Things to Spot: At Home* by Fiona Watt or *My First Words: Let's Get Talking* by DK. As the child becomes familiar with the objects and their labels, see if they can find the one you name, for example, "Where's the *ball*?" Follow the child's lead by naming items they show an interest in. Can they find an object you name? An alternative read is *Find the Duck* by Claudia Zeff, where the child has to find the little duck hidden amongst everyday items you can name as you go along.

Activities for older children

- Use photographs and written words to label drawers containing everyday items for the classroom, for example, scissors, paper and pencils, so the children start to link the spoken word with the written label.
- Make an object book to help older SEND learners link the object name with the written word. Use real objects to make a large book with cardboard pages in a ring binder. Glue or Velcro items to the pages or slip them into a plastic zip-up bag. Object names and symbols can be added to the pages.

Animals

Inset puzzles

Animals are a favourite theme for early puzzles. Name the animals as the child takes the pieces out. Have fun making the different animal sounds together with the child. As the child becomes familiar with the puzzle, ask them to take out or put back different pieces as you name them.

My pet

Encourage the children to bring in pictures or photographs of their pets to share in circle time. There will be plenty of opportunities to repeat the names of common animals. Ask questions like "Who has a cat?" or "What animal makes this sound...?" Children not yet ready to say a name can hold up a picture or make the animal sound. (Remember children with EAL may have different sounds for animals.)

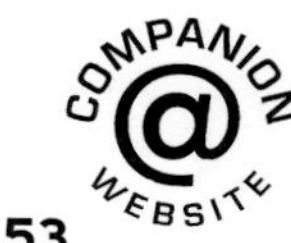

Interest table

Expand on the 'My Pet' circle activity (see previous activity) by asking children to talk about how they look after their pets and what food they like to eat. Set up an interest table or Tuff Tray around the topic of caring for pets. Children can help set this up using items from home like food or unused bedding material. Follow up with reading stories about pets. *Oh, the Pets You Can Get!* by Trish Rabe has lots of pet names to learn. Other more unsuitable pets are introduced in the funny story books *I Want a Pet* by Lauren Child and *Dear Zoo* by Rod Campbell.

Pretend pet shop

Set up a pretend pet shop using soft toys and animal replicas housed in cages, cardboard boxes, sand or water trays. Include some extra props like a pet carry box, food bowls, brushes, pet toys and leads. Children take it in turns to play the shopkeeper to find a pet for you. You can also ask for items for a specific pet, for example "I need some food for my *dog*". Allow the children time to engage in pretend play exploring different aspects of pet care, like how to hold and play with pets.

Farm

Arrange an outing to see animals at a farm. There are many 'city farms' now, so even the urban child is able to see country animals. They can help feed some of the tame animals and perhaps stroke or even ride on them! Once the child has met the real animals, help them find pictures of them in books like *Old MacDonald Had a Farm* or *I Love Animals* by Flora McDonnell. Create a group book from drawings of the farm animals seen on the farm visit.

Animal puppets

Use animal finger puppets to encourage children to imitate animal sounds. Name the animals and encourage the children to hold up the appropriate puppet and make the sounds.

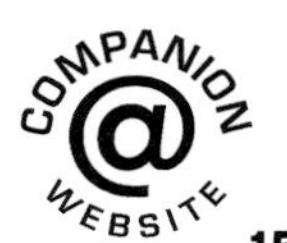

Fishpond

Make a toy fishpond by folding a long strip of card three times to form a box. A fishing rod can be made from a short stick and a piece of string with a magnet attached. Fish can be cut from cardboard with object pictures pasted on, or just use picture cards. Slip a paper clip on each one to attract the magnet. Ask the child to "catch" different animals.

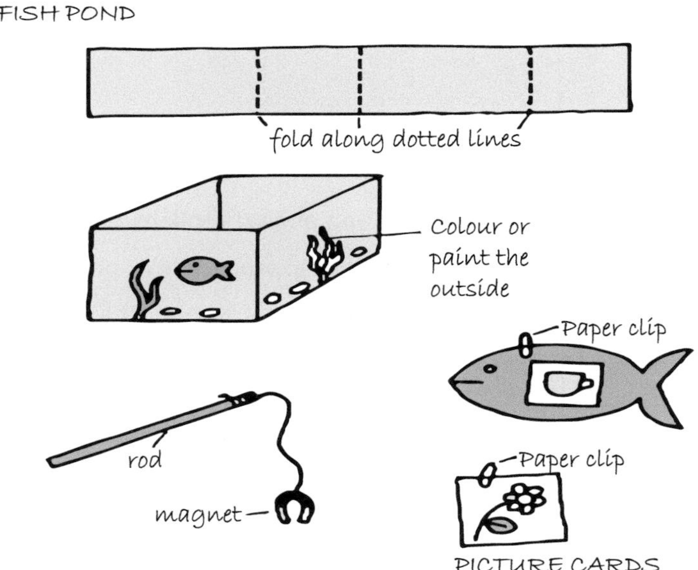

Sticker books

Use sticker books like *First 100 Stickers: Animal by* Roger Priddy to help children focus on the different animal shapes. Name an animal for the child to find and place the sticker.

Draw an animal template

Draw the child pictures of animals you have seen on outings and then ask them to draw one for you. They can choose from some animal templates to draw round or to trace over, and then you choose one for them.

Find the matching picture

You will need three or four animal pictures with matching miniature animals. Place the pictures on a table with the miniatures to one side. Ask the child to place the miniature animal on the matching picture when they hear you say its name.

Activities for older children

Create projects on the theme of animals that link with the maths and science curriculum:

- Create a pictogram to illustrate the children's pets or favourite animals.
- Use a variety of small world play resources to set up different scenarios involving animals. These might include a farm scene; parks and ponds; a zoo; and marine environments

like a river or sea. The children can learn about the animal habitats by helping to make the land or seascape complete with vegetation.

- Discuss differences in the colour and skin pattern of animals, and link this to different environmental topics like habitat and climate. Explore spots and stripes in animal patterns using a range of art materials. Provide different materials for gluing and sticking or printing, for example, paper strips, pasta shapes, sequins and buttons. Discuss the colour, shape and patterns found on different animals. Use the lines and dots for counting.

Transport

Ride and name

Point out different vehicles to the child. Use simple names like bus, car or train. On trips, the excitement of a ride in a bus or a train will help them to remember these words.

Garages

Play with different toy vehicles like cars, buses and trucks in pretend garages or along cardboard roadways. Push the toys along, naming them and making the appropriate noises; for example, "Look at my *train* – ch-ch-ch-ch".

Inset puzzles

Use a transport-themed early puzzle. Name the vehicles as the child takes the pieces out. As the child becomes familiar with the puzzle, ask them to take out or put back different pieces as you name them.

Lotto games

Give the child a lotto card and keep the pack of matching individual cards. Name the pictures, for example, "Have you got a *car*?" If the child has the picture and recognises its name, they get the card. This game is more exciting in a group, as the children can see who is first to complete their lotto card.

Rhymes and songs

Introduce transport names to the child through rhymes and songs. Try *Row, Row, Row Your Boat* and *The Wheels on the Bus*. Both these songs encourage children to carry out actions and sing along.

Story books

Look at picture books showing different modes of transport. Point to the picture and name the vehicle. Some useful books are: *Listen to the Things That Go* by Marion Billet and *We All Go Traveling* by Sheena Roberts.

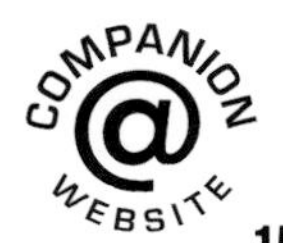

Find the matching picture

You will need three or four vehicle pictures, like a car, bus and train, with matching toy vehicles. Place the pictures on a table with the toys to one side. Ask the child to place the toy on the matching picture when they hear you say its name.

Small world play

Use a variety of small world play resources to set up different scenarios involving vehicles. These might include a farm scene; street scene; and marine environments like a river or sea.

Mark making

Explore mark making with toy vehicles like cars, trains and trucks. Roll the toys through paint so children learn about different tyre marks and mixing colours. Tape a pen or marker to the back of a toy car and roll across or down a sheet of paper. Help the children collaborate on creating a giant picture.

Activities for older children

- Have a collection of pictures or miniatures of old and new modes of transport. Discuss how transport has changed through the ages, and the inventions that have brought about these changes.
- Create transport pictograms using pictures drawn or cut out by the children – themes might include road, rail, sea and air transport. Discuss the differences between categories of vehicles and how these impact on their design.
- Make simple models of different vehicles using junk materials like cardboard boxes, plates and tubes; plastic cartons, trays, lids and bottle tops; foil trays; lollipop sticks; assorted papers and textiles; and small car tyres. Encourage the creation of vehicles for different purposes, like a car for people and a truck for carrying bricks or sand.

Relating two verbal concepts (noun-noun)

Once the child is understanding a variety of verbal labels, they can be encouraged to follow simple commands containing two of these verbal labels. These activities encourage the child to relate two named objects to each other. Note this is not about fetching two items: it is about the child making a connection between the two items.

Aims

To develop the ability to relate two verbal concepts (noun-noun) and respond appropriately to simple two-part commands.

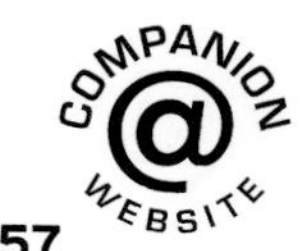

Outcomes

- Looks back and forth between two objects.
- Relates two verbal concepts (noun-noun).
- Follows a simple a two-part command (noun-noun).

Strategies

- Show the child how you want them to relate the objects by demonstrating the task.
- Make sure the child is familiar with the vocabulary. The task is to help the child relate two verbal concepts rather than the learning of new vocabulary.
- Use phrases that only contain two information-carrying words or two verbal labels. A child may be able to respond appropriately to the command "*sit* dolly on the *chair*" at this stage, but they do not understand the words 'sit' and 'on'. They are merely relating the two objects in the most usual way (contextual understanding), and the child would probably make the same response to the command, "sit dolly under the chair".
- Alternatively, you can allow them to use their prior knowledge and contextual information in making sense of the instruction, for example, a doll usually sits on a chair or lies in a bed.

Suitable materials and resources

Assorted objects like a ball, toy car, brick; pretend play items like a brush, sponge, cup, plate and spoon; dolls, teddies and other stuffed toys.

Activities to develop understanding of noun-noun combinations

Roll a ball

Roll a ball gently to teddy, telling the child what you are doing; for example, "Look, I'm rolling the *ball* to *teddy*". Draw their attention to the objects as you name them. Replace teddy with a second toy, for example, a dolly, and repeat the activity. Then, using both the teddy and the doll, roll the ball to one or the other, again commenting on what you are doing. Give the ball to the child and ask them to roll it to either teddy or dolly, for example, "Roll the *ball* to *teddy*". Point to the right toy if they need help.

Replace the ball with a car and play the game again, commenting. Give both the toys to the child and ask them to roll one of them to either dolly or teddy. Again, help them if necessary. At this point the child needs to understand both nouns in order to follow the command. As the child becomes more confident, you can gradually increase the choice of toys.

Posting boxes

Make several posting boxes with different painted faces, for example, a clown, a dog and a cat, and give the child an assortment of objects to post like a ball, large brick, toy cars and

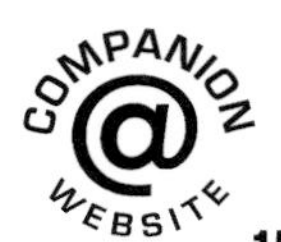

small teddy. Give the command, for example, "Post the *ball* in the *clown*!" and "Post the *car* in the *dog*!" Start with one posting box and one object and gradually increase the choices.

Water play

Put some toys in a water-tray like a boat, fish and frog and ask the children to push them to each other, for example, "Push the *boat* to *John*".

Tea party

Set out the child's favourite dolls and teddies for a tea party, and give the child instructions about handing out cutlery, plates, cups and pretend food; for example, "*Dolly* wants *cake*" and "Give *teddy* his *cup*".

Hide and seek

A group of children can play hide and seek with a selection of objects and containers like a box, basket and bag. One child leaves the room or closes their eyes while another is told where to hide an object, for example, "Hide the *ball* in the *box*".

Dress up

Collect some old clothes for the children to play a dressing-up game. The adult gives instructions, for example, "Mary, give the *scarf* to *Paul*".

Miniature figures

Children love playing with miniature figures like people, animals and toy furniture. Use the miniature items with a dolls house or a toy farm, parks and zoos. Remember to give unusual instructions to avoid the child using contextual cues, so instead of a "Put the *duck* in the *pond*", use "Put the *cow* in the *pond*". Alternatively, peg people can be put into cars, fire engines and trucks, or onto merry-go-rounds, swings and see-saws.

Activities for older children

- Older children may still benefit from the use of strategies to help follow these two-part commands:
  - Get the child's attention before giving an instruction.
  - Break complex spoken instructions into manageable chunks of information.
  - Use a gesture or sign along with the spoken command, or additional cues like a symbol or picture card showing the item.

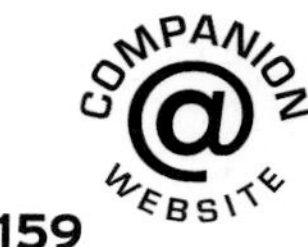

- Use everyday activities in the classroom as an opportunity to give practise in following two-part commands; for example, "Put the *peg-boards* in the *box*". In a group, ask each child to give something to another child; for example, "Give the *book* to *Michael*".
- Drawing – use preprepared sheets for children to colour in or mark. Instructions might include "Put a *cross* on the *house*" and "Draw a *circle* round the *bird*".

Verbs

Action verbs might also be known as 'action words' or 'doing words'.

Aims

To recognise and understand the meaning of a range of simple verbs including action verbs, action on object verbs and attribute verbs.

Outcomes

- Recognises and understands a range of simple verbs.
- Follows simple one-part commands containing a verb.

Strategies

- Talk about actions as they occur, so that the association between the action and the word is made clear.
- Consolidate learning by providing practise with language targets in a variety of different contexts that include everyday routines, pretend play, picture books, physical activities and play.
- Further generalise understanding by using target verbs in simple phrases and commands. Children are more likely to be able to identify the verb in sentences that require less processing (Xiaoxue He et al., 2020).
- Avoid correcting any errors the child may make when repeating or attempting to say a word. Instead provide the correct model, for example, child says "ump" – model back "jumping", "Ben's jumping".

Suitable materials and resources

Dolls and teddies with movable parts; action picture cards, picture books, photographs and photocards; action songs and nursery rhymes; physical play equipment; and construction toys.

Action verbs

These verbs describe an action (doing words) such as running, sleeping and jumping. Start with action verbs which the child can carry out themselves, like running or jumping.

Physical play

During physical play, talk about what you or the child is doing, for example, "Look, I'm *jumping*". Carry out an action and ask the child to join in, saying "Let's *jump*. We're *jumping*", emphasising the action word. Ask the child to do the action; if they hesitate or make a wrong response, repeat the action and the word again.

Action songs

Sing nursery rhymes or action songs while carrying out the actions with the child. Try *This Is the Way We...*; *If You're Happy and You Know It*; and *Wind the Bobbin Up*. See if the child can do the actions when you cue them with the action verb, for example, "If you are happy and you know it... *clap your hands*".

Action photographs

Create a photo album by taking photographs of the child carrying out different actions. Or use the Book Creator app on your tablet or iPad to capture photographs and video of the child in action. The app allows images and text to be added straight into a personalised book that might also include links to spoken stories and action songs.

Simon Says

Play 'Simon Says' using commands about actions, for example, "Simon says... *jump*". At first do the actions with the child, and later just give them the commands.

Obstacle course

Set up an obstacle course and talk about what the child is doing as they make their way through the course. Next time, ask them to carry out specific commands as they come to each obstacle; for example, "*Climb* over the boxes"; "*Hop* round the table".

Act out with dolly

Describe the child's actions as they play with dolls and say, "Look, dolly's *running*". Ask the child to show you different actions with the doll.

Action word picture cards

In a group, give each child several action word picture cards. Ask each child to mime one of the actions and see if the other children can identify the right picture. Hold up the correct picture and say, "Yes, Leo is *jumping*".

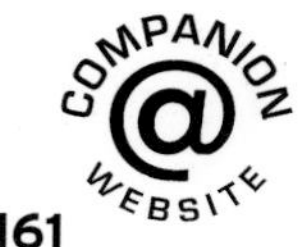

Puzzles

Collect together puzzles that have lift-out pieces, showing people carrying out actions. Show the child the different actions, describing each one; for example, "The boy's *running*". Ask the child to take out the pieces as you name the action, so "Find *running*".

Picture books

Look through picture books and talk about the different actions of the characters. Ask the child to find certain actions, so "Let's find someone *jumping*"

Ball games

Use sponge balls, beanbags or soft toys in physical play to teach verbs such as 'throw', 'catch', 'kick', 'roll', 'bounce' and 'chase'.

Activities for older children

- Introduce children to similar words, for example, 'walk', 'jog' and 'run', and discuss the similarities and differences in meaning.
- Play the 'odd one out' game with words. Can the children spot the word with a different meaning in 'wash, clean, sing'?
- Play the parachute game 'merry-go-round'. Children stand sideways to the parachute holding on to it with one hand. As they walk around in a circle, the chute will start to look like a merry-go-round. Ask the children to carry out different actions like 'running', 'skipping', 'hopping' and 'jumping'. Switch directions every now and then.
- Alternatively play 'parachute tag'. Ask the children to hold the edge of the parachute and lift it up so it fills with air in a mushroom shape. Call the names of two children who must swap places, running under the parachute before it comes down again and 'tags' them. Again, give instructions to use different actions like 'hopping', 'walking' and 'jumping'.

Action-upon-object verbs

These are verbs that describe an action on an object, for example, hitting (a ball) and pushing (the door).

Pop-up toys

During play activities, show the child different actions with pop-up toys, talking about what is happening. Give the toy to the child and describe their play. There are a number of toys that are good for teaching specific verbs.

- Jack-in-the-box (and similar pop-up toys): when the lever is touched, out pops jack. This is useful for teaching 'push', 'go' and 'press'.

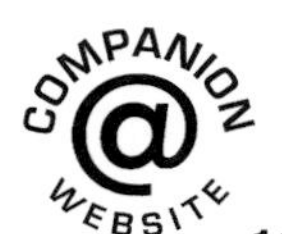

- Pop up characters in a ball: balls can be rolled along the ground, and when a button is pressed, out pops the character, so words like 'press', 'push' and 'roll' can be taught.
- Tin spinning tops: 'push' or 'press' down on the metal handle to make it spin round.

Push- and pull-along toys

Push- and pull-along toys, large toy cars and trucks also provide lots of opportunities to model the verbs 'push' and 'pull'.

Roll along...

Place several different toys and objects in front of the child, for example, a ball, a wooden sphere, a toy tyre, a cardboard tube, a coin, a lid or a bottle top. Choose one action and carry it out on all the toys, describing what you are doing; for example, "I'm *rolling* the tyre; now I'm *rolling* the ball". This teaches the child that an action is not specific to any one object. After lots of similar examples, use the toys in a game. A group of children could play at passing toys to each other, using the method chosen by the adult; for example, "*Roll* the ball to Daniel".

Large play equipment

Playground and park equipment provide a medium for such actions; for example, the child can be pushed on the swing, lifted on to the see-saw and caught off the slide. Tell the child what you are doing; for example, "I'm *pushing* you", "I'll *catch* you!"

Pretend play

Use pretend play to introduce different actions with everyday objects on dolls, teddies and other stuffed toys. So hair can be brushed and combed, faces wiped and dried.

Junk material

Gather together lots of junk materials, for example, sponges, elastic, plasticine, dough and cardboard boxes. Explore the different actions you can perform on one object; for example, plasticine can be rolled into a sausage or a ball, pulled into a long snake, squeezed and cut into shapes. Talk about what you are doing. Give the child some material and ask them to perform different actions.

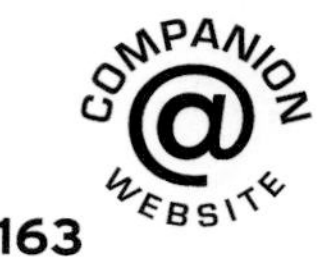

Action flip book

SEQUENCE OF ACTIONS

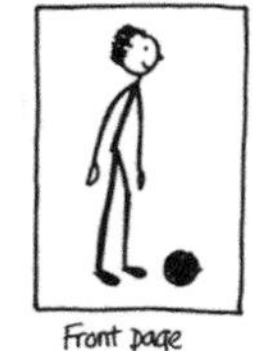

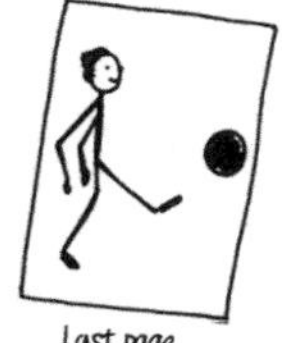

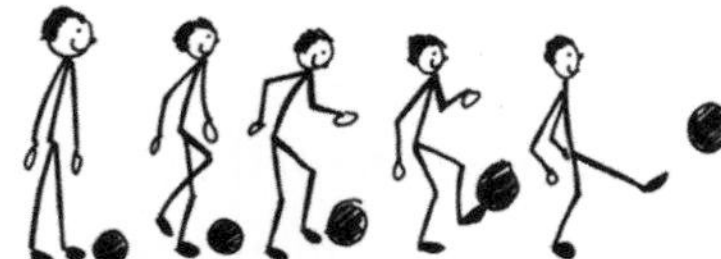

Make up several picture books of separate actions in the following way. On each page draw a picture of a person carrying out an action, for example, kicking a ball, varying the drawing slightly so that as the pages are flicked through the figure appears to move. (Note: the pages should be flicked from back to front.)

Activities for older children

- Use science projects to explore verbs that describe a change in state, for example, 'melt', 'freeze' and 'evaporate'. The child needs to have first-hand experience of these concepts and plenty of repetition of the related language.

Example: 'Melting':

  - Cooking – in cooking, show the child how different foods melt when heated, for example, butter, chocolate, jelly.
  - Snow – during winter bring in a cup of snow and let the children watch as it melts.
  - Ice cubes – place an ice cube on top of a radiator, on a table or outside on the windowsill. Let the children compare how long each one takes to melt in the different conditions.
  - Build a snowman – in winter help the children build a snowman. Each day they can check to see how much of it has melted.

- Provide clay, dough or plasticine for children to explore the effects of actions on different materials. Create different shapes with plasticine by squeezing, rolling, stretching, twisting and cutting. Push and press clay through graters, garlic pressers, colanders and sieves. Use rolling pins, scissors, cookie cutters, and potato mashers to flatten, squash and cut dough.
- Cooking provides lots of opportunities to talk about the child's actions on food, for example, stirring, beating and cutting. Some easy recipes are making sandwiches, toppings for pizza and fruit salad.

Object functions

Give the child lots of experience of seeing how different objects are used, and help them to use the objects themself. Talk about what you are doing with objects during play and everyday activities, for example, "Look, the *scissors* are *cutting* the paper".

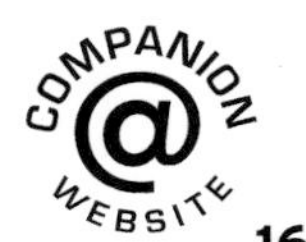

Mime an action

Put a selection of objects on the table. Pick up one of them, for example, soap, and mime its use. Say, "Look, some *soap*. You *wash* with soap". Then choose another object, and this time encourage the child to do the mime with you, saying, "Yes, that's right. You *eat* with *a fork*". When you have done this with all the objects, see if the child can mime their functions on their own.

Ask them for one of the objects, for example, "Find me something you *drink* with", emphasising the word and miming the function. If they have difficulty, show them the correct item, again miming and naming its function. When they are able to do this, ask them the same things without using gestures.

Once the child can identify objects by use, generalise with the following activities

Puzzles

Puzzles that have clear lift-out pieces of objects can be used to practice understanding of function words. Ask the child to take out or put back objects as you name the function, so "Find something you *eat* with".

Lotto games

Each child in a small group is given a lotto card, and the adult has the matching individual cards. They take one card at a time and name the functions of the object, for example, "something you *cut* with". The winner is the first to complete their card.

Spinning arrow

Place object pictures around a circular board that has a spinning arrow in its centre. Ask the child to point the arrow at different objects that you have identified by use.

Find the picture

Hide object-picture cards around the room. Ask the child to find them, for example, "Find me something you *cook* with".

Scrapbook

Make a scrapbook with the child and ask them to find pictures in magazines or catalogues, identifying them only by use, for example, "'Find something you *draw* with".

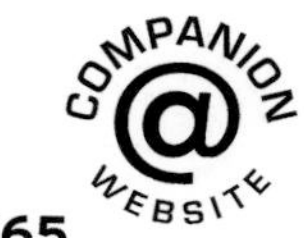

Making choices

Introduce the use of function words into activities where you need to make choices about a tool. For example, when exploring making with dough, you can ask, "Find be something to *cut* with" or "Find me something to *roll* with".

Question forms

Introduce the use of question forms to ask about function, for example, "Which one do you use to cut with?"

Activities for older children

- Create a pictogram to help children explore items that have similar functions; for example, scissors and a knife are both things you cut with.
- Introduce a range of verbs with similar meanings to express object functions. For example, for a kitchen knife you might have 'cut', 'slice, 'chop', 'spread', 'pierce' and 'carve'. Talk about and demonstrate the different actions to ensure the child understands the word.
- Play the 'how many uses' game with an object. Choose an object and ask the children to think of how many things you can do with it (functions) and also to it (action on objects).

  Examples include:
  - Book – read, look, open, shut, carry, write, draw.
  - Phone – talk, play games, hold, read, take photographs.

Extend the activity by discussing less obvious uses or more complex vocabulary. A book might be used to 'prop open' a door, as a paper weight or to help draw a straight line. A luxury phone might be used as a fashion statement or a symbol of wealth.

Prepositions

Not all prepositions are learnt at the same age, so the child's general comprehension abilities should be established before deciding on which ones to teach first. The words 'on', 'under' and 'in' tend to be understood early on. Chapter 5 also has some activities for eliciting specific prepositions, for example, 'on', 'off' and 'in', and these can be adapted for aiding comprehension.

Aims

To understand the meaning of a range of simple prepositions describing spatial positions.

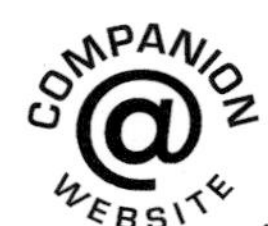

Outcomes

- Understands a range of simple prepositions describing spatial positions.
- Follows simple one-part command containing a preposition describing spatial positions.

Strategies

- Start with activities that involve the child in physical play where they experience different spatial positions.
- Talk about the position of the child using the target prepositions.
- At first accompany the prepositions with gesture and pointing, gradually reducing these until the child is relying on verbal comprehension alone.
- Some children may benefit from the use of signs and symbols.
- Provide lots of repetition of language targets in a variety of different contexts that include everyday routines, physical activities, pretend play, picture books, songs and stories.
- Further generalise understanding by using target prepositions in simple phrases and commands. Keep the rest of the words in the phrase redundant so the child focuses on the preposition.

Suitable materials and resources

Physical play equipment; construction toys; small world toys; nursery rhymes and songs; picture books and stories.

Activities to develop understanding of prepositions

Hide teddy

Demonstrate the meaning of two contrasting prepositions like ‘on’ and ‘under’ using a teddy or other prop. Talk about what you are doing and emphasise the key word, for example, "Look, Teddy's *under* the table". Help the child to carry out actions with the teddy that demonstrate the same two prepositions and describe what they do. At first accompany words with gesture to help the child understand. Keep the location constant so they have to understand only the preposition. Gradually reduce the cues until the child is relying on their verbal comprehension.

Active play

Use physical play with different equipment for the child to explore different special positions. Talk about the position of the child, emphasising the prepositions.

- climbing frames: up/down/off/on top of/under
- slide: up/down
- see-saw: up/down/on

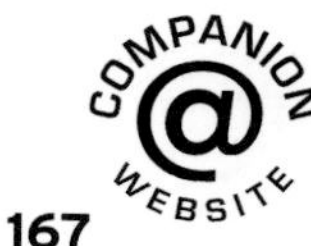

Obstacle course

Set up an obstacle course using a variety of equipment and furniture. As the children move through the course, talk about what the children are doing. Gradually introduce simple instructions for the children to follow. Suitable outdoor equipment includes:

- chairs and tables: on/under/over/next to
- large boxes: in/inside/through/behind/in front of/beside
- play tunnels: through/in
- benches: along/over/on/off/behind
- balancing planks: on/along
- bridge: over
- ladders: up/down
- hoops: in/over

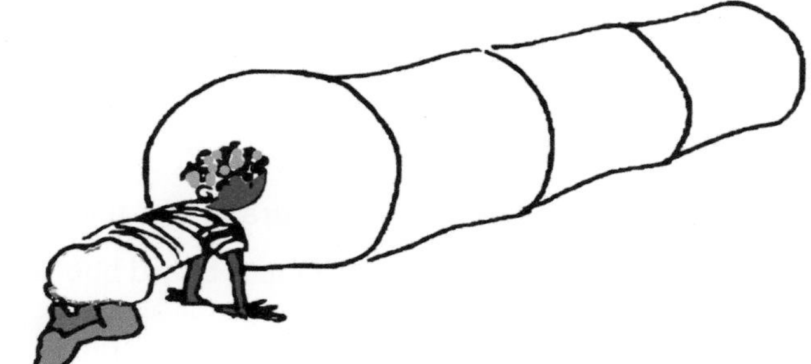

Follow the trail

Help the children to create a trail using chalk on the ground. Give instructions using prepositions like "go *round* the tree" and "*through* the tunnel" for the children to follow the trail. Lay out surprises for the children to find along the way, like a coloured balloon or a hooter.

Tidy up

During the day, try to incorporate prepositions into what you say to the child; for instance, while tidying up, ask the child to put toys in specified places, for example, "*under* the table", "*in* the cupboard". If they do not understand, take the toy and the child to the right place and say "Look, *under* the bed".

Songs

Recite nursery rhymes or sing songs that involve prepositions, for example, *Ring-a-Ring-O'-Roses* – "we all fall *down*". Do the actions with the child at first, but later see if they can do them by themself at the right verbal cue.

- On/under – *Humpty Dumpty; Little Miss Muffet; Three Billy Goats Gruff*
- Down – *Ring a Ring o' Roses; London Bridge Is Falling Down.*
- Up/down – *Hickory Dickory Dock; Jack and Jill; Incy Wincy Spider; Grand Old Duke of York; Wheels on the Bus.*
- Over/under – *Jack Be Nimble; Hey Diddle; Three Little Billy Goats.*
- In/out – *There Was an Old Woman Who Lived in a Shoe; Hokey Cokey.*
- Round – *Round and Round the Garden; Here We Go Round the Mulberry Bush.*
- Beside – *Little Miss Muffet.*

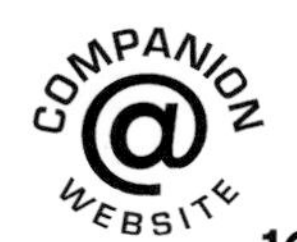

Adapt rhymes and songs to include several position words:

- *Little Miss Muffet* – the spider can sit beside, behind, above and on.
- *Hickory Dickory Dock* – the mouse can run down, under, over and behind.

Hide and seek

Play hide and seek with a group of children. One is sent out of the room while another is told to hide a toy, for example, "*under* the flowerpot". Can the child find the toy on their return?

Picture books

Look at picture books that encourage the understanding of positional words. Try *Where's Spot?* by Eric Hill and Usborne *Find It* board books with their pictorial hide and seek themes.

Small world play

Use small world play like a toy playground or park to introduce and practice a variety of prepositions. Playmobil City Life Children's Playground with swings, slides, roundabouts and a climbing frame will provide follow up practice to active play experience with 'on', 'in', 'up', 'down' and 'round'. City Life Playground includes benches and tables with several useful receptacles, like a waste bin, basket, storage crate and barbecue, where the small picnic and play items can be placed 'in', 'on', 'under' and 'next to'.

Playmobil parts are very small, so not for use by children under 3. Needs adult supervision at all times.

Trains and tracks

Train sets with tracks, tunnels, bridges and stations are great for 'in', 'on', 'round', 'across', 'under' and 'through'.

Act out a story

Tell a story around a picture scene, for example, a small mouse hiding from a big, bad cat. The child has a cardboard mouse which they move around the board as the story is told, for example, "The little mouse hid *under* the table". It will help the child if you perhaps tell the story first, moving the mouse for them, before asking them to join in (adapted from the Derbyshire Language Programme). Familiar stories can also be modified in the same way to give lots of practice of one preposition, for example, "Snow White hid *under* the table"; "*under* the bed"; "*under* the chair".

Activities for older children

- During construction play there are lots of opportunities to introduce prepositions. Talk about what the child is going to do, and then what they have done. Use giant foam blocks, Lego, wooden building bricks or junk materials. There is scope to focus on simple prepositions like 'on' and 'under' or introduce more difficult position words like 'in front of', 'on top of', 'middle', 'below', 'inside' and 'between'; and directional words like 'forwards' and 'backwards'.
- Play a parachute game – while holding the parachute aloft, give different children instructions to move under the parachute and position themselves near other children. For example, ask the child to stand "next to", "behind" or "in front of" another child.
- The books *We're Going on a Bear Hunt* by Michael Rosen, *Rosie's Walk* by Pat Hutchins and *Bears in the Night* by Stan Berenstain all have a great focus on a variety of prepositions. Children can recreate the journeys through story boards, drawing a map or acting out the story with puppets.

Attribute terms

Attribute terms are words that describe the properties of an object or material that can be observed with the senses and include adjectives about shape, colour, size and texture. These attributes help to define the characteristics of a specific object or material, so a ball is 'round' or 'spherical' and comes in many different colours and sizes. Activities for attribute terms are divided into colour, shape, size (including measures of length, height and weight), and texture. They encourage the child to explore the characteristics of everyday objects and materials and start to understand early concept words and mathematical language used to describe attributes.

Shape

Aims

To encourage the child to explore the shape of everyday objects and materials.
To understand the meaning of a range of simple and mathematical language to describe shape.

Outcomes

- Recognises common 2D and 3D shapes and knows their properties.
- Understands names of simple shapes ('round', 'square', 'triangle').
- Understands some common mathematical language ('sphere', 'cube', 'cone').

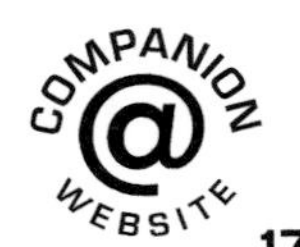

Strategies

- Children will benefit from activities that involve matching and sorting objects by shape.
- Some children may benefit from activities that focus on a contrasting pair of items, but this can be adapted for individual children's needs.
- Initially give the child materials that have very obvious perceptual differences along the dimension you are teaching; for example, a circle and an oval shape are harder to discriminate than a circle and a square.
- Draw the child's attention to the properties of different shapes, so round ones tend to roll, triangular ones have three sides.
- At first, accompany the spoken word with showing and pointing, gradually reducing these cues until the child is relying on verbal comprehension alone.
- Provide lots of repetition of shape names in a variety of different contexts.
- Further generalise understanding by using the shape name in simple phrases and commands. Keep the rest of the words in the phrase redundant so the child focuses on the shape name.

Suitable materials and resources

Shape stacking toys; shape sorter posting boxes; shape form boards; shape hammer bench; geometric 2D and 3D shapes; different shaped containers and moulds for sand play; construction toys like blocks, geometric shapes; different shaped cutters for plasticine, Play-Doh or clay; shape dominoes; shape matching games like Colorama; magnetic shape boards; threading laces and different shaped beads; attribute blocks; Hammer and Nail Pattern Boards; Mosaics; and BelleStyle Wooden Pattern Blocks for flat patterns; Pyramis 144 Primary; Constructostraws; and Polydron sets.

Activities to develop understanding of shape

Flat 2D shapes

Matching and sorting by shape

Geometric shape puzzles and shape stacking toys help develop the child's awareness and recognition of these shapes through looking and touching as they handle the different shaped pieces. Name the shapes clearly as the child manipulates the pieces, so they learn the word alongside the concept. Give them a choice of two or three shape pieces. Can they find the shape you name?

Trace a shape

Encourage lots of matching activities with cardboard, plastic and plasticine shape templates. Show the child how to feel around the shapes to discover their contours and use them to

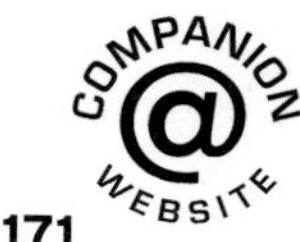

draw around the shape. Introduce everyday objects for the child to explore tracing similar shapes; for example, the bottom of a cup is round, and a box might be round, square, oval or rectangular. Help the child to copy shapes, first by demonstration, then from memory. (Practice in tracing or drawing shapes develops skills that later support the writing of letters and numbers.)

Printing

Help the child explore shape, line and colour through printing. Use a variety of household objects, fruits and vegetables as printing blocks; for example, round shapes can be made from a cotton reel, a square from a building block. Choose one item and create a repeat pattern moving left to right across the paper; then add two items to make a simple sequence. Gradually increase the number of shapes and complexity of the sequence.

Pack a bag

Cut out pictures of items with different shapes from a catalogue, for example, a square travel clock, a rectangular book, a round hat. Next, draw a large suitcase containing outlines of various shapes. The child has to pack the items in the suitcase by matching up the shapes. Once the child is confident in matching up the shapes, start to ask for items: "Find me something *round*".

Craft

Make different shapes with plasticine and dough using ready-made cutters in all sorts of shapes and sizes. Describe the shapes, drawing attention to characteristics like a circle is round and has no corners, whereas a square has four corners and a triangle three. Older children can count and sort the different shapes. Alternatively, children can cut shapes from sandpaper and other materials, though this will require more hand–eye coordination.

Baking

Make cream biscuits or jam tarts with different-shaped pastry cutters, and before eating, see if the child can match them back together. Or use plasticene or Play-Doh to create buns and cakes in imaginative play; for example, role play as a baker.

Solid 3D shapes

Posting boxes

Early play with shape posting boxes helps develop the child's awareness of three-dimensional shapes. Simple labels like 'round' and 'square' might be used, or mathematical labels like sphere and cube might be introduced. Help children examine the properties of shapes – whether they roll, stand up or have points or straight edges.

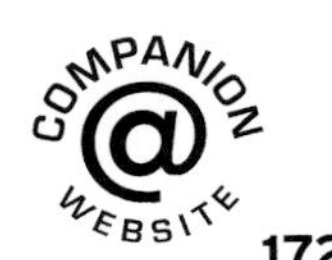

Matching and sorting by shape

Wooden beads can be matched and sorted by shape for threading on a lace or matched to a pattern card. Accompany play with talk about shape, for example, "Let's find a *round* bead".

Feeling by shape

Place objects with different shapes, like a box, ball, and a book, in an opaque bag. Can the child recognise what they are by feeling their shape? Show the child an object and/or describe its shape. Can they find its duplicate in the bag?

Interest table

Choose a shape and ask children to find objects to place on the table; for example, 'round' might have a ball, orange, drawing of a circle, bead, a ring and so on. Draw attention to the properties of the object. Most round objects will roll, as they have no corners or sides.

Sand play

Provide different shaped buckets, containers and moulds for children to fill up with sand and make sand sculptures. Comment on the different shape of containers – round, square, straight sides or curved sides. After making several sculptures, ask the child to find the matching containers.

Water play

Add several objects of the same shape to the water tray; for example, explore a sphere shape with a selection of balls – plastic, sponge, ping pong balls, table tennis and jumbo Orbeez water beads. Talk about how the round shape helps them spin around in the water.

Activities for older children

- Make pictures out of drawings using shapes, so a square becomes a house and a circle becomes a sun. Give the child a colour key, so squares are coloured red, and rectangles green. The child must first identify the shape and then choose the correct colour.
- Provide games that encourage the use of shapes to build different patterns and images. Try Hammer and Nail Pattern Boards, Mosaics and BelleStyle Wooden Pattern Blocks for flat patterns, and Pyramis 144 Primary, Constructostraws and Polydron Sets for building 3D shapes.
- Encourage children to compare geometric and abstract shapes such as circles, triangles, rectangles and squares with similar real-life shapes in buildings such as tents, doors and windows. Use mathematical language to describe the characteristics of the architecture.

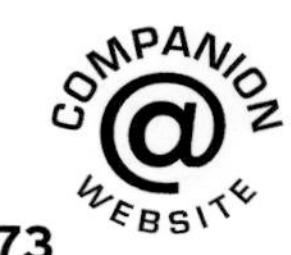

- Organise a scavenger hunt – ask the children to find natural objects like leaves, stones and fir cones on a scavenger hunt and categorise them according to shape. For example, a fir cone, as the name suggests, has a cone shape, where as a stone might be flat and round. Draw shapes on cards to help children decide on the shape of their finds.

Colour

Aims

To encourage recognition of colour as an attribute and develop understanding of several basic colour labels.

Outcomes

- Matches and sorts a range of familiar and unfamiliar items by colour.
- Recognises and understands several basic colour labels.

Strategies

- Children will benefit from activities that involve matching and sorting objects by colour.
- Initially use identical objects for matching and sorting to help the child separate the name of the object from the colour description. Later move on to using non-identical items to help generalise understanding of the concept.
- At first accompany colour labels with showing and pointing, gradually reducing these cues until the child is relying on verbal comprehension alone.
- Provide lots of repetition of colour names in a variety of different contexts that include everyday routines, physical activities, pretend play, picture books, songs and stories.
- Further generalise understanding by using colour names in simple phrases and commands. Keep the rest of the words in the phrase redundant so the child focuses on the colour name.
- Be aware of learners who may be colour blind or have colour vision deficiency. They may have difficulty distinguishing red/green or blue/yellow, or may see no colour at all. See www.colourblindawareness.org for more information.

Suitable materials and resources

Everyday objects like a blue comb, a yellow duster or a red brick; a colour set of pretend play plates, cups and cutlery; containers, beakers, bowls and boxes in primary and secondary colours; items of clothing; multicoloured physical play equipment like hoops, mats and balls; construction toys like Lego, Duplo, building blocks, Stickle Bricks, interlocking discs and geometric shapes in various colours; threading laces and coloured beads; colour dominoes; counting bears and other sets of coloured miniature figures; and a range of mark-making materials like pencils, crayons, brushes and paint.

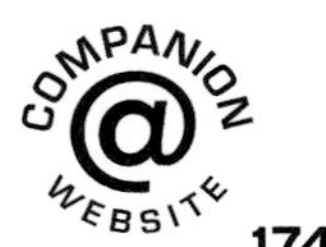

Activities to develop understanding of colour

Build a colour tower

Have a box of wooden or Lego Duplo bricks in two different colours. Start to build a tower using one colour and encourage the child to add more bricks. Then start another tower in a different colour and again encourage the child to add more bricks. Once the child is following along with this, bring out a brick and see if the child can match it to the correct tower.

Sort and thread

Thread some large, coloured beads, buttons or cotton reels in two different colours on two separate threading laces. Give the child one bead at a time. Can they find the lace with the matching colour?

Post by colour

In the commercial *Post Box Game* the child must post the coloured letters in its matching postbox. Colours are red, blue, yellow and green. Alternatively, make your own posting boxes in different colours with a variety of coloured objects or pictures for posting. Start off with a couple of posting boxes and hand the child one item to match up and post. There are lots of opportunities to use the colour name as the child learns the colour concept.

Tabletop games

There are several matching tabletop activities that encourage matching by colour. These include colour dominoes; colour snap; and colour lotto.

Colour mats

Once the child is matching identical items consistently, introduce non-identical items. Choose two coloured mats. Give the child a coloured object to place on the matching mat. Use everyday objects, toys, construction blocks and clothes. Using a variety of objects in this way will help the child learn that colour is a separate attribute.

Find a matching pair

Use household items and clothing to play a matching game. Give the child one of a pair and see if they can find the other. For example, they can match a red toothbrush to a red beaker, a yellow cup to a yellow saucer, or a blue sock to a blue shoe. Extend this activity by asking the child to find non-associated matching items, for example, matching a red brick to a red car; a yellow bead to a yellow cotton reel, and so on.

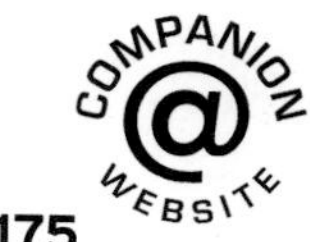

Sorting by colour

Once the child is matching by colour efficiently, they are well on the way to being able to sort by colour. Start with a few colours and use matching coloured sorting trays or bowls. Move on to sorting in plain trays and then without any prop as a cue.

Activities might include sorting out different-coloured beads for making necklaces or posting coloured pompoms down matching coloured cardboard tubes. (Have bowls to collect the pompoms at the bottom.) Children can sort almost anything. Some further ideas are coloured buttons, cotton reels, plastic animals, trees, laces, ribbons, paper, crayons and pencils.

Building blocks

Use constructional toys that have different coloured blocks, discs and tiles that can slot or clip together, for example, Lego Duplo or Slot-Together Translucent Builders. Give the child instructions about which pieces to fit together, "put the *red* one with the *blue* one".

Tidy up

Ask the child to put away items by colour, for example, "the *red* pencil", or use different-coloured tidy boxes, "pencils in the *red* box".

Hoops

In physical play place different coloured hoops on the floor. Ask the child to "hop to the *blue* hoop", or "Hop to the *red* hoop".

Obstacle course

Set up an obstacle course with mats, chairs, tables, benches, etc and put large, coloured paper on each of the obstacles. Give the child directions that involve understanding colour, for example, "Run round the *blue* table", "Run round the *red* table".

Collect an object

Ask the children to go round the room collecting objects in one target colour and help them set up an interest table.

Dress up

Put a pile of clothes in different colours on the floor. Two children can compete to put on clothes that the adult has described, for example, "a blue hat". Follow up with reading *Blue Hat, Green Hat* by Sandra Boynton whose characters try on different coloured clothing.

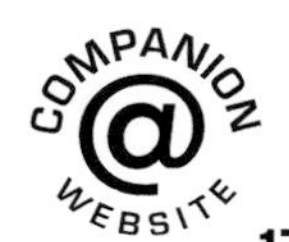

Activities for older children

- Discuss how colour can be a visual cue, for example, red for danger. Explore the different associations of colour with the children. Collect examples like traffic lights; colour of brands; and as a symbol of emotions.
- Introduce the colour wheel– Encourage the children to mix two different primary colours to produce secondary colours. Provide a giant template for the children to paint.
- Help the children make a rainbow. All you need is a glass of water, some paper and a sunny windowsill. Hold the glass over the paper, as the sun shines through the glass you should see a rainbow.

Size

Aims

To understand the meaning of a range of simple mathematical language to describe size, length and weight.

Outcomes

- Matches and sorts items according to size, length or weight
- Developing understanding of simple mathematical language (big/small; long/short; heavy/light).

Strategies

- Children will benefit from activities that involve matching and sorting objects by size.
- Some children may benefit from activities that focus on a contrasting pair of items, but this can be adapted for individual children's needs.
- Initially give the child materials that have very obvious perceptual differences along the dimension you are teaching, for example, a circle and an oval shape are harder to discriminate than a circle and a square.
- At first accompany the spoken word with showing, pointing, and gesture, gradually reducing these cues until the child is relying on verbal comprehension alone.
- Provide lots of repetition of size words in a variety of different contexts that include everyday routines, physical activities, pretend play, picture books, songs and stories;
- Further generalise understanding by referring to size in simple phrases and commands. Keep the rest of the words in the phrase redundant so the child focuses on the attribute of size.

Suitable materials and resources

Large and small boxes, containers, trays and baskets; different sized dolls, teddies, and stuffed toys; pretend play plates, cups and cutlery that vary only in size; construction toys

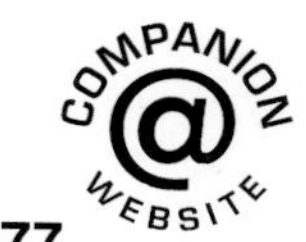

like Lego, Duplo, bricks, and blocks; buckets, spades, beakers and jugs in a range of sizes for water and sand play; doll's clothes, child and adult clothing in various sizes; pairs of large and small sized everyday objects, for example, shampoo in a travel size container with a large family bottle.

Activities to develop understanding of size

Big/small or little

Tidy up boxes

Have two boxes, one big and one small. When tidying up toys with the child, say "Look, I'm putting teddy in the... *big* box", as you drop it in the box. Give a toy to the child and say, "Put it in the *big* box", pointing to the appropriate one. Later, see if the child can put it in the right box without cues.

Water play

Provide different sized beakers, jugs, and containers for water play. Talk about the different sizes as the child explores how much water they hold, "Here is the *big* jug". Help them explore pouring from a little container into a big container and vice versa. Join in with the child's play and start to ask for "a *small* beaker" or "a *big* jug" pointing if necessary.

Sand play

Play similar games with different sized spades and buckets in the sand tray. Talk about the best size of spade to fill the bucket. So, a big spade will fill a big bucket quickly, and a small spade will fit into a little bucket avoiding spills. Make sandcastles of different sizes.

Pretend tea party

Use two different-sized teddies in a pretend tea party. Take a cup and say to the child "I'm giving the cup to... *big* teddy", putting the cup in front of the big teddy. After lots of examples, give an item to the child and ask them to give it to the "*big* teddy". Continue with different objects and pretend food but keep to one item at a time.

Dressing up

Play a dressing-up game with different-sized articles of clothing. Name the items as you put them on, "Look at my *big* hat", before you try them on the child. Ask the child to put on different-sized clothing, helping them if they still don't understand. When the child is able to follow verbal instructions without cues, they can compete with another child in a dressing up race. The adult or another child gives instructions, for example, "Put on a *big* shoe".

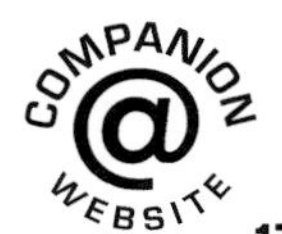

Dress dolly

Give the child two dolls of different sizes and have a variety of doll's clothes. Help the child to find an item of clothing like a hat and ask her to "Put the hat on the *big* doll".

Feely bag

Allow the child to explore through touch a large and small version of a hairbrush. Place brushes in an opaque bag and ask the child to "Find the *big* brush". Gradually build up to several pairs of different-sized objects.

Construction play

Introduce size into construction play by having different sized materials. Ask the children to put similar sized bricks together in a structure.

Hide the animal

Cut out different-sized animals like a lion, monkey, and giraffe from stiff card. Create a simple jungle scene cage (see image below). Stick the jungle scene on to a backing card, leaving one side unstuck to form a pocket. Ask the child to slip one of the animals into the jungle, for example, "Put the *big* lion in the jungle".

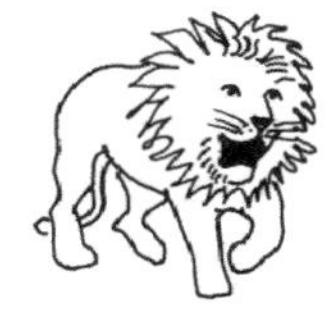

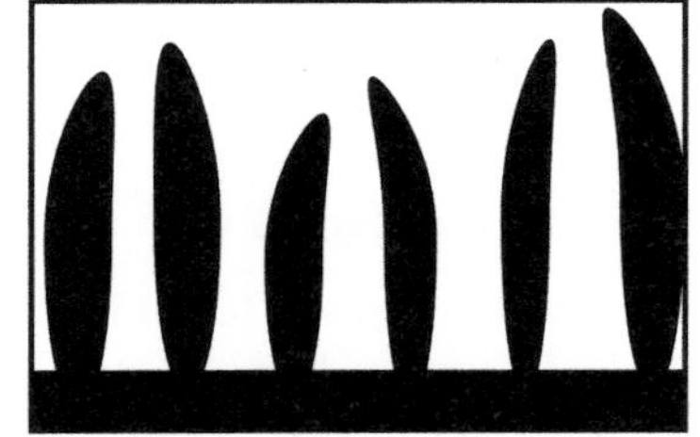

Other ideas are dog and kennel; fish and pond; car and garage; cake and oven; children and a bed. (Adapted from an idea in the Derbyshire Language Programme).

Activities for older children

- Ask the child to draw or colour big or small objects. At first, they may need to have one example, so they have something to compare their drawing against.
- The Three Bears – Read the story of the three bears with their different sized bowls, chairs and beds. Provide three different sizes of construction material (bricks, blocks) for the children to make a house for each of the bears. Children will need to estimate the size of brick needed for each house, compare different bricks in order to make choices about suitably sized items.

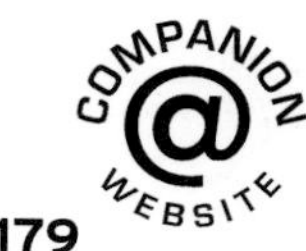

Children may also benefit from specific work on other language to describe measurement like length and weight.

Length

Long/short

Sort by length

Collect together pairs of everyday objects that vary in length like pencils, ribbons, necklaces, and natural materials like grasses. Show the child each object, describing it to them, for example, "Look, a *long* pencil", and putting it with the other long or short objects as appropriate. Ask the child to find an object by length saying "Now, the *short* ribbon", pointing to it if necessary.

Make a snake

During construction or creative play, talk about what the child has made, for example, "Well done, that's a *long* snake". Copy the child's snake, making it shorter. Compare your model with theirs, for example, "I've made a *short* snake; you've made a *long* snake", drawing their attention to the difference in length with your finger. You can also make long and short trains, cars, and buses.

Doll play

During doll-play, talk about articles of clothing that are different lengths, for example, "Look at dolly's *long* ribbon", holding it up for the child to see. Tell the child to dress dolly in different clothing, for example, "Put on her *long* scarf. (Make sure there are paired items of clothing that differ in length, so that the child needs to make a choice. Some useful garments are scarves, socks, belts, ties, and shoelaces of different lengths).

Colour by length

Provide pre-prepared sheets with drawings of pairs of items in different lengths. Ask the child to colour in the longer or smaller items, for example, "Colour the *long* snake".

Activities for older children

- Ask the child to draw a long train, a short snake. At first, they may need to have one example, so they have something to compare their drawing against.

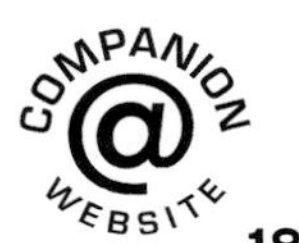

- Introduce different ways of measuring using the body, for example, a hand span; foot length; or a cubit (the length of the arm from the elbow to the tip of the middle finger). Help the children to take measurements of the room, furniture and equipment.
- Introduce different tools for measuring length, for example, ruler, tape measure, metre stick, metre wheel. Take different measurements both inside and outside and discuss which tool is the most practical for the task.

Weight

(Light/heavy)

Collection

Collect together similar objects of different weights; for instance, let the children hold a piece of paper and then a very heavy book. Say "This paper is *light*. This book is *heavy*". Repeat this with lots of pairs of different objects. Light objects might include feathers, sponges, cotton wool, small pebbles and stones. Heavy objects might include a door stop, brick, and a bag of coins or marbles. Ask the children to find something "heavy" or something "light". Help them if they hesitate or make the wrong response. Place the collection on an interest table along with some weighing scales.

Compare weights

Let the children explore similar objects with different weights, for example, two books. Talk about why one might be heavier, for example, a heavy book is likely to be bigger in size, thicker, with more pages, and have a hard cover. Compare the book with one sheet of paper and discuss how as you add more sheets the weight increases.

Cooking

Measuring out quantities is a fundamental part of successful cooking. Let the child compare different foods by first weighing them in their hands. Talk about the different weights of the food items as they hold them. Use digital or mechanical scales for the child to help weigh out quantities as per the recipe. Cooking ingredients that need to be weighed out include flour, butter, caster sugar, cheese, chocolate; and liquids like water, milk and stock.

'Moon rocks'

Wrap objects of different weights and sizes in silver foil to make moon rocks. Set up a trail for the children to follow. One team must find *light* 'moon rocks' and the other *heavy* ones.

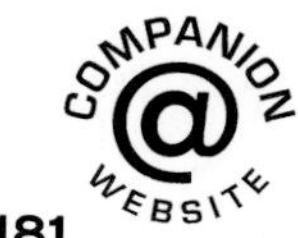

Provide examples of how being large in size doesn't mean it will be heavy, for example, a foil balloon or a large sponge compared with a small heavy rock or a small bag of sand.

Activities for older children

- Provide lots of different types of weighing equipment like kitchen scales, bathroom scales, digital and mechanical scales, spring scales, and balance scales. Children can carry out experiments with different materials, objects and even themselves.
- Use a balance scale for comparing weights:
  - Comparing the weight of two different items, for example, a sponge and a pebble;
  - Comparing the weight of two similar items, for example, two books;
  - Finding two items that weigh the same, either identical like two wooden blocks or different as in a pebble and a metal key;
  - Choosing one item and finding other items that are lighter or heavier (weigh more or less);
  - Increasing the quantity of a material to see how its weight changes, for example, a few grains of light fine sand get very heavy as you add more and more.
- Set up role play areas for topics that encourage weighing and measuring, for example, weighing out different fruit and vegetables at a market; parcels at a post office; pet food in a pet shop; or babies at the health clinic.

Texture

Aims

To encourage visual and tactile awareness of different textures in a range of materials through sensory exploration; and to introduce language to describe these tactile experiences.

Outcomes

- Notices different textures common to a range of objects and materials.
- Understands several simple words that describe these textures.

Strategies

- Children will benefit from activities that involve matching and sorting objects by texture.
- Initially give the child materials that have very obvious perceptual differences along the dimension you are teaching, for example, silk and nylon are harder to discriminate between than silk and hessian.
- Provide lots of experience of different textures using a wide range of familiar and unfamiliar objects and materials, so the child learns to generalise their understanding.

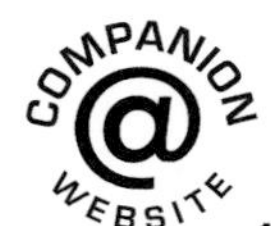

- Some children may benefit from activities that focus on a contrasting pair of textures, for example, rough versus smooth, while others may be able to assimilate a number of different textures and their names.

Suitable materials and resources

Fabrics with a range of surfaces and finishes (felt, denim, silk, satin, velvet, nylon, hessian, wool); a range of play sand, (silver or fine sand, coloured sand, slinky and smooshy sand from Hope Education); paint; glue; washing-up liquid; sequins, beads, glitter, seeds, rice, lentils, sand, grit, and sawdust.

Activities to develop understanding of attribute labels for texture

Feely bag

Choose two or three fabrics of different textures like silk, net, and denim cut into identical small squares. Allow the child to explore the different tactile sensations of feeling the material with their fingers, holding it in the palm of their hand or against their cheeks. Talk about how the different fabrics feel. Place the squares into a feely bag and give the child a matching fabric square. Can they find its matching pair in the bag just by touch?

Feely box

Alternatively make a feely box by simply cutting a hole in the side of a large box and making a loose cover for the child to slip their hand through. A box is more versatile, as you can place larger items inside or more numerous quantities of a single material. Try a variety of items that have 'wet', 'dry', 'furry', 'rough' or 'smooth' textures.

Sand play

Explore the properties of different types of sand through visual and tactile experimentation. Compare the fine granules of silver sand; get creative with coloured sand; or encourage different actions with slinky and smooshy sand (available from Hope Education).

Mix sand and water

Provide watering cans and funnels for the children to experiment with adding water to dry sand. Talk about how it changes the texture of the sand, and how dry and wet sand respond in different ways. Use a range of descriptive words like 'rough', 'smooth', 'soft', 'sticky', 'lumpy', 'dry', and 'wet'.

Touch table

Ask the children to collect items of a certain texture, for example, "Find me things that feel *soft*". Talk about the objects with the children, letting them feel them, and explore

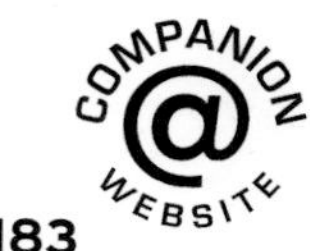

their physical properties. For example, a soft acrylic scarf can be folded, scrunched up, and wafted in the air. Put the items on a touch table or tuff tray for children to explore independently.

Creating texture

Salt dough or air dry clay is the ideal base for children to experiment with different ways to add texture. Help the children to roll the clay into smooth, flat tiles or discs or have these pre-prepared ready for use. Children can create texture by using various clay stamps, and tools like patterned rolling pins and paddles. Alternatively make use of everyday or found objects like building bricks with embossed patterns, different fabrics, buttons or shells to make an imprint in the clay. Dry materials like sequins, beads, glitter, seeds, rice and other grains, lentils, sand, grit, and sawdust can also be pressed into the clay.

Allow dough or clay with added materials to dry naturally. Not suitable for kiln firing.

Sensory tabletop games

There are several commercial tabletop activities that encourage attention to the sensory experience of touch, prompting the child to match and sort by feeling for similar textures. These include *TickiT® Touch & Match Board* with tactile counters; *Goki Memo* game 'Feel a Pair' (pairs of tactile counters in a bag); *Tactile Dominoes*; and *Tactile Memory Cards* (photographs with textured surfaces) by Winslow Resources. Make your own games using card and different textured material like felt, satin, velvet, hessian, corduroy, embossed wallpaper and different grades of sandpaper.

Sensory walks

TickiT® SiliShapes® Sensory Circle Set provides a tactile experience for the feet as the child walks on the different textured surfaces of the silicone discs.

Touch walks

Take the children on a "touch walk" to collect different kinds of natural items. Talk about how things feel, so a leaf might be *smooth* compared to a *spiky* conker shell. Can the children group the found items by texture?

Baking

Bake sweets, cakes, bread and biscuits, using different flours and dough mixtures. Let the child compare them before and after cooking. Use language to describe how they look and feel – 'soft', 'hard', 'wet', 'dry', 'cold' and 'warm'.

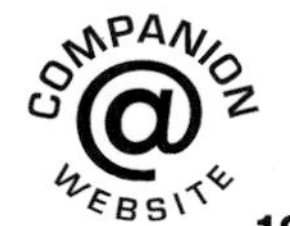

Collage

Ask the children to collect items for a large group collage. Materials might follow a theme, for example, different textured papers – craft, scrap, newspaper, magazines and sandpaper. These can be easily glued onto cardboard and used to create abstract patterns or a representative image, for example, sandpaper for a beach, blue craft paper for the sea. Other themes might be different fabrics, seaside discoveries or natural materials collected on a walk. Talk about the different textures and how they feel. Avoid being too descriptive and have fun with words invented by children to describe the different sensations.

Activities for older children

- Provide experience of different colours, patterns and texture in clay items from a range of cultures. Look for clay artefacts like tiles, bowls, vessels and pots from Egypt, the Middle East, Greece, China, Asia and Japan.
- Creative arts – talk to the children about what happens when they mix different dry and wet materials together to create textured pictures; for example, adding sand to paint makes it thick and grainy. Mix foods like flour, salt and oats directly into paints and brush on the paper. Or try combining PVA glue with various organic materials like soil, straw, sawdust and sand and apply over paintings. Introduce words like 'lumpy', 'rough', 'thick', 'shiny' and 'gloopy'. What words do the children use? Look at the work of artists who use different media in their paintings, for example, Richard Long and Anselm Kiefer, who use found organic matter like soil and straw in their artwork.
- Print a texture – create different textures in printing by using textured tools like patterned rollers, textured palm printers and printing stamps. Alternatively, explore using a variety of household objects as printing blocks to create unusual and abstract patterns. Try dipping combs, toothbrushes, nail brushes, potato mashers, bubble wrap and sponges in paint and press onto paper or cardboard.
- Create a collagraph – cut out a small square of strong cardboard as the base for a collagraph. Stick various items onto the collagraph like wool, string, beads, shells, rice, pasta, grains and various seeds. Aim for a level surface, so when you add paint to the collagraph and print an image, all of the pieces make a mark on the paper.
- Children search out different textures in the environment and take rubbings using a range of media.

Links with art and design curriculum.

Avoid uncooked raw beans and other legumes, as they contain harmful lectins.

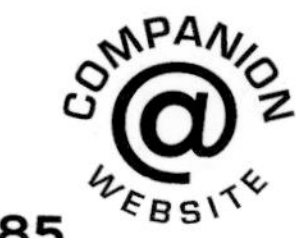

Time

The child first needs to understand that actions and events occur in a sequential order before they can begin to understand the concept of time (Cole, 1982).

Aims

To help children develop a sense of time and start to understand simple time-related language constructs.

Outcomes

- Sequences pictures of actions and events in the correct sequential order.
- Understands simple time-related language.

Strategies

- Represent the passage of time visually, as this will be easier for the child to understand.
- Provide practice with sequencing pictures so that the child understands that things happen in a particular order.
- Encourage the child to talk about things that have happened, or what they are about to do, even if they haven't mastered the correct grammatical forms for tense.
- Model the correct tense forms for the child.

Suitable materials and resources

Sequencing pictures; visual diary; visual timetables; weather charts; sand timers; sundials; different clocks, watches and timers; picture books and story books illustrating time.

Activities to encourage understanding of time

Sequence pictures

Use commercial sequencing picture sets, or make your own using drawings or photographs. Start off with a simple sequence of two cards showing a before-and-after scenario, for example, a tree upright and a tree cut down, or a whole biscuit and a half-eaten biscuit.

Set routines

Provide the child with set routines and talk about what the child is doing, what they have done and what they are going to do. Help them recreate their routine with a sequence of pictures, for example, washing, having breakfast and leaving for nursery. Introduce phrases that describe sequences, such as 'first we wash our face and hands', 'next we eat breakfast', 'after breakfast we get ready for nursery'.

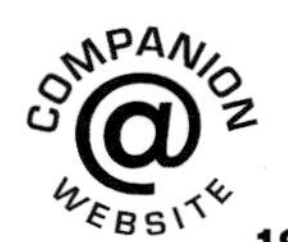

Picture books

Reinforce this learning with picture books that illustrate everyday routines indicating the structure of a typical day in relation to time, for instance, getting up and having breakfast in the morning, midday meal and bath in the evening. Introduce simple language about time, 'day', 'morning', 'evening' and so on. Try *Maisy Goes to Preschool* by Lucy Cousins and *Spot Says Goodnight* by Eric Hill.

Daily diary

Keep a daily diary with the child. Each day talk about what the child is doing, what they did yesterday and what they will do tomorrow.

Stories

Read the child a story that involves time. Ask the child questions, for example, "What did the boy do?" "What happened yesterday?"

Visualising time

Use visual methods to display the passing of time, like giant sand timers. This introduces the child to the notion that time can be measured. Introduce a variety of ways to mark the passage of time, for example, sundials and water clocks.

Counting down

Children find it difficult to grasp abstract concepts of time like days or weeks, so link the passing of time to events that are familiar to children; instead of 'five days' use 'five sleeps'.

Growth and change

Help the children explore changes over time caused by growth, for example, growing herbs, salad cress and other simple plants.

Activities for older children

- Explore old and new ways of doing things, so the children develop a sense of 'in the past'. Topics might include transport, occupations and communication systems.
- Celebrate key events, festivals and holidays during the year. Such events help us mark the passage of time and act as anchors to our understanding of the passage of time.
- Weather is a good marker of time, as it changes throughout the year but can also vary day by day. Help the children record the weather on a daily chart. Can they make predictions about the weather tomorrow or next week?
- Introduce the language of time and link it to actual events during the day.

These activities can be adapted to introduce the Wh-question form 'when'?

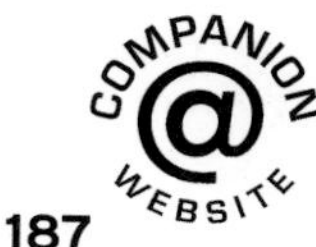

Understanding two-word phrases

When the child is able to understand a verbal label, verb or attribute word in isolation, it should be gradually introduced into simple sentences or instructions with two key words. Activities will need to be structured, so the child needs to make a choice for each of these key words.

Aims

To develop understanding of simple phrases containing two key words or elements.

Outcomes

- Follows instructions containing two key words or elements.

Strategies

- Give the child time to focus their attention before giving instructions.
- At first, accompany spoken language with lots of visual and contextual cues, gradually reducing these until the child is relying on verbal comprehension alone.
- Keep the rest of the information in the phrase redundant so the child only has to assimilate the two target verbal concepts.
- Provide lots of repetition of language targets in a variety of different contexts that include everyday routines, pretend play, picture books, activities and trips.

Suitable materials and resources

Everyday objects; picture cards; photographs; picture story sequences; toy vehicles; and small world toys.

Activities to develop understanding of two-word phrases

Noun + verb

Action pictures

Use pictures of children and animals carrying out similar actions, so a boy running and a girl running with a boy climbing and a girl climbing. Lay out a selection on the table and ask the child to point to the pictures you name, for example, "Where is the *boy running*?" It is important to have enough images so there are choices to be made between nouns and verbs.

Doll play

Give the child a doll and a teddy. Ask them to "Make *dolly jump*" or "Make *teddy run*".

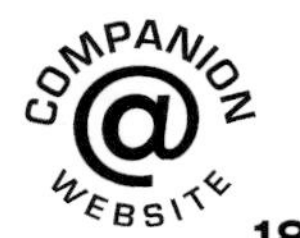

Verb + noun

Obstacle race

Ask the child to carry out different actions in relation to different obstacles. For example, "*Crawl* round the *table*"; "*Run* to the *hoop*"; "*Hop* to the *chair*".

Bath time

Have a dolly and some bath-time accessories like a flannel, soap, shampoo, cream, hairbrush and toothbrush for this game. Ask the child to "*Wash* dolly's *hands*" and "*Wash* dolly's *hair*".

Noun + noun

Tea party

Set up a pretend tea party for a selection of different dolls, teddies and soft toys. Have a variety of pretend food items. Give instructions like "*Teddy* wants some *cake*" and "*Dolly* wants some *biscuits*". The child will need to find the correct food for the right toy.

Play park

Use a miniature play park with figures and small objects along with a picture of a park scene. Give instructions about setting up the scene to the child, for example, "put the *girl* on the *bench*" and "the *dog* by the *tree*". Keep to obvious places so the child does not have to understand the position word. The child can compare their efforts with the picture once they have finished.

Attribute + noun

Vehicles

Play with toy vehicles like cars, buses and trucks in different sizes and colours. Pretend to be a customer wanting to buy a vehicle. Ask the child to "show me the *red car*", or "Show me the *small truck*".

Shopping game

This game has lots of opportunities to introduce phrases with an attribute word with a noun. Ask the child to "Buy a *big apple*". (There should be a big and a small apple amongst the food items.) As well as size, you can use 'number' and 'weight'. For example: "*two bananas*" or the "*heaviest potato*".

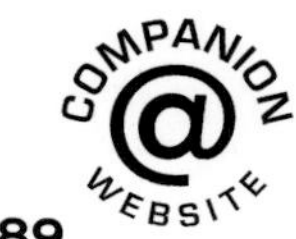

Holiday pack

Have a teddy or doll and a selection of similar clothing items that differ only in colour and size ready to pack in a bag. Ask the child to "Pack teddy's *red jumper*".

Preposition + noun

Tidy up time

Use instructions that involve prepositions, such as "Put your bag *under* the *bed*" or "Put your football *behind* the *chair*". Make sure you hand the child the object to the child first before you give the instruction.

Round up

Use miniature animals and a farm layout with buildings and fields. Ask the child to place one the animals in a part of the farm, for example, "Put the *cow* in the *field*". Start to ask the child to place the animal in an unexpected place, for example, "Put the *cow* in the *pond*". This way they will not be able to use their pragmatic knowledge.

Moving day

Play a pretend game of moving to a new house. The child or children take on the role of the removal people. Give instructions about where you want the furniture to be placed, for example, "Put the *chair* in the *living room*". Ask the child to place the furniture in unexpected places too, for example, "Put the *bath* in the *bedroom*". (You could wrap the furniture in paper or put the items in boxes!)

Drawing

Draw pictures of a chair, table and bed. Ask the child to draw "a ball *under* the table", "*on* the bed". Try to gradually introduce less obvious connections so "a ball *on* the television" or "*under* the rug". Increase the complexity by describing a simple picture to the child, who has to recreate it using Fuzzy Felt or pre-prepared pictures.

Activities for older children

- Adapt classroom instructions to give practice in understanding two-word phrases containing language targets.
- Barrier game – two children sit on either side of a screen, each with a large sheet of paper and crayons. They take it in turns to tell each other what to draw, for example, "Draw a house. Put a red roof on it. Make three windows". At the end both drawings

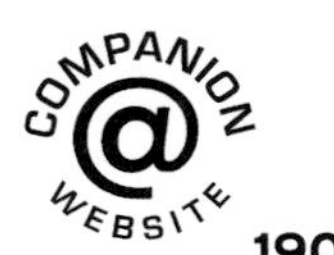

should look the same. (Only encourage children to use phrases to give instructions if their speech and language levels permit.)

Understanding complex utterances (three- to four-word phrases)

When the child is able to understand simple phrases with two key words or elements, longer and more complex sentences can be introduced. A complex sentence or instruction will have one or more of the following constituents: multiple information carrying words (ICWs), increased length of sentence, syntactic complexity and increased vocabulary demands in terms of novelty and/or abstract meaning. The activities in this section focus on sentences containing three and four key elements or ICWs.

Aims

To develop understanding of simple phrases containing three to four key words or elements.

Outcomes

- Follows instructions containing three to four key words.
- Follows a sequence of complex instructions.

Strategies

- Give the child time to focus their attention before using new and complex sentences.
- At first, accompany spoken language with lots of visual and contextual cues, gradually reducing these until the child is relying on verbal comprehension alone.
- Using supporting gestures will facilitate comprehension of complex utterances, particularly for new information (McNeil et al., 2000)
- Give instructions out sequentially or in the order in which you wish the child to carry them out.
- Provide lots of repetition of language targets in a variety of different contexts that include everyday routines, pretend play, picture books, activities and trips.

Suitable materials and resources

Everyday objects; picture cards; photographs; picture story sequences; toy vehicles; and small world toys.

Activities to encourage understanding of complex commands

Make sure there are choices for each of the elements in the sentence. Activities for two-word phrases can be adapted by adding more choice.

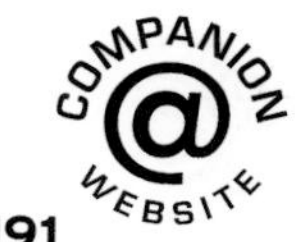

Three-word sentences

Bath time

Have a dolly and a teddy with some bath-time accessories like a flannel, soap, shampoo, cream, hairbrush and toothbrush for this game. Ask the child to "*Wash dolly's hands*" and "*Brush teddy's hair*". Introduce different action words like 'dry', 'brush' and 'clean'.

Shopping game

Set up a shop with the help of the children. Choose different items for the shop that vary in size and colour, for example, red and green peppers, a big and a small apple, and small individual cereal boxes and large family ones. Similarly, there should be a choice between a bag and another type of container, like a basket or a box. Ask the child to "Buy a *big apple* and put it in the *bag*" As well as size you can use 'number' and 'weight' – for example: "*two bananas*" or the "*heaviest potato*".

Location

Give the child a toy bed, table, chair and bed with a small doll and animal figure. Ask them to "Put the *doll under* the *table*" or "Put the *dog in* the *bed*".

Four-word sentences

Clothes pack

Have a teddy or doll and a selection of similar clothing items that differ only in colour and size ready to pack in a bag. For example, there should be a red and a blue jumper amongst the clothes items. Similarly, there should be a choice between a duffle bag and another type of luggage, like a suitcase or a backpack. Ask the child to "Pack *teddy's red jumper* in the *bag*". As well as colour you can use 'texture' or 'length' – for example: "*short scarf*" or "*woolly hat*".

Copy my world

Use miniature dolls and furniture to arrange a scene out of sight of the child, for example, a man in a bed, a cat on a chair or a boy behind a wardrobe. Give the child a duplicate set of toys and instruct them how to set it up. When they have finished, they can compare it with the adult's model.

Actions

Ask the child to carry out actions and then move to a named place. For example, "*Touch* your *nose* and *walk* to the *window*." The complexity can be increased as you include more

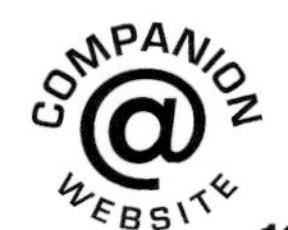

choices: "*Rub* your *nose* and *walk* to the *window*"; "*Pat* your *head* and *run* to the *door*". In this activity the child has a choice of *body part; action* on that body part; *place*; and *action to get to the place*.

Activities for older children

- Gaining the attention of the child before giving a complex instruction is even more important in a busy classroom.
- Provide practice by using more complex sentences in everyday activities.
- Reduce background noise and visual distractions so children can focus on more complex language input.
- Take photographs of actions in response to complex instructions. Place these on the wall along with a written sentence.

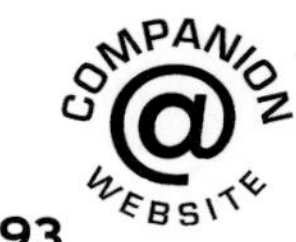

Understanding question forms

Talking together with the child and asking questions about an activity, event or story is a good way to develop their listening skills, understanding and language. Simple Wh-questions like 'what', 'where' and 'who' encourage the child to use language about objects, actions and concepts like colour and size. Higher order questions that are open ended, like 'How' and 'Why', allow the child scope to describe in detail, give reasons and explanations.

Aims

To develop understanding a range of question forms from simple to complex.

Outcomes

- Responds to simple questions like 'what', 'where' and 'who' by pointing, fetching or naming.
- Responds to more complex questions like 'why' and 'how' by giving a reason or explanation.

Strategies

- Model asking questions during everyday activities, but make this a natural part of the interaction. Avoid overwhelming the child with too many questions.
- Ensure the child is listening before asking a question by gaining their attention by calling their name and making eye contact.
- Use vocabulary that the child is familiar with so they can focus on the question form.
- Use gesture, signs and symbols to support spoken language.
- Provide a range of objects and images so children have a choice to make a nonverbal response by pointing, fetching or selecting an item.
- Model a range of spoken responses to questions from simple statements like "Here it is" to whole sentences and further questions, for example, "Where is the dog?" – "Is he in the field?" – "No, he's hiding in the barn".
- Inappropriate responses are probably an indication that the child has not understood the question.
- Most importantly, let the child know that you value their ideas by showing the child you are listening carefully to their responses.

Suitable materials and resources

Everyday objects; picture cards; photographs; picture story sequences; construction toys; small world toys; creative play materials; sand and water toys.

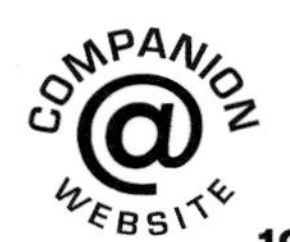

What?

What's in the bag?

Play this as a group game so there is an opportunity for repetition of the question form. Put a few familiar items in an opaque bag out of sight of the children. Ask "*What's* in the bag?" and see if the children can make a guess. Choose items that have a familiar outline or make a noise when the bag is shaken so you can give clues. Let each child take a turn to put their hand in the bag and find an object.

What do you see?

The book *Brown Bear, Brown Bear, What Do You See?* and the other three books in the series by Bill Martin have lots of simple, repetitive language that support the understanding of the question form "*What* do you see?" They provide good examples of the use of whole sentences to answer the question, although you may need to make some adaptations to some of the more complex vocabulary and American words.

What's That Noise, Spot?

What's That Noise, Spot? is a sound book by Eric Hill that links sounds to different locations like a farm or the seaside. The child can select a picture in response or name the sound. A Spot soft toy can be used to model responses.

Guessing games

Play guessing games like "*What* do you wear on your head?" Have props ready to show the child the correct answer if necessary.

What's that smell?

Put small amounts of different fragrant objects in sealed containers and cover the top with a thin piece of cloth or a piece of paper with holes in it, held on with an elastic band. Items could range from soap, lavender and fruits to herbs and spices, but they should be things the child is familiar with and is able to name, describe, select a picture or gesture about. This would be a good follow-up to a cooking session.

Where?

Hide and seek

Encourage the child to close their eyes while you hide a few of the child's toys around the room. Ask them to find one, for example, "*Where's* teddy?"

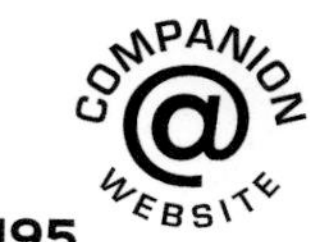

Where's Spot?

Where's Spot? by Eric Hill offers the chance of repetitive modelling of the 'where' question form. The 'lift the flap' element also allows modelling of an extension to the question: "Where's Spot? – "Is he in the wardrobe?" A cuddly Spot soft toy can also be used for games of hide and seek.

Find the picture

Share picture books with the child that show familiar everyday objects, animals or events. As the child becomes familiar with the vocabulary, see if they can find the one you name, for example, "*Where's* the ball?" or "*Where's* the boy?"

Farmer has lost his animals

Place miniature animal figures within a toy farm set up. Ask the child to help the farmer find his lost animals using 'where' questions: "Help, *where* is the cow?" "*Where* has the sheep gone?" Children can collect the figures and place them in a safe place. For older children, model further questions like "Is it in the barn?" and possible responses like "Here is the cow, it was in the barn" and "The sheep is behind the tree".

Rescue the toy

Small toys and objects will disappear in a bowl of water with some added bubble bath. With just the right amount of water, they keep peeping out for the child to find and rescue when asked "*Where* is...?"

Smash the sandcastle

Toy animals and other creatures can be partially or fully hidden in a sand tray to be dug out by hand or with a spade. Put a toy inside a cup, cover with sand, then turn it out to make a sandcastle. Make some other sandcastles without a toy. Can the child find the toy? Allow them to smash the sand towers. Gradually increase the number of toys and ask some 'where' questions.

Who?

My pets

Encourage the children to bring in pictures or photographs of their pets to share in circle time. Ask "*Who* has a cat?" and "*Who* has a dog?" Children can hold up a picture of their pet.

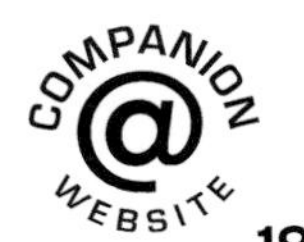

Similarities and differences

Compare similarities and differences between children. Ask questions like "*Who* has brown hair?" "*Who* has long hair?" "*Who* has blue eyes?"

Goldilocks and the Three Bears

The traditional fairy tale of *Goldilocks and the Three Bears* can be adapted to model the question 'Who?' – "*Who's* been eating my porridge?" "*Who's* been sleeping in my bed?"

Action pictures

Have several pictures or photographs of people or animals carrying out different actions. Ask children to identify "Who is running?" and "Who is jumping?" and so on.

Why? and how?

Construction

Construction tasks and building models offer an opportunity to ask questions about '*why* things happen' and '*how* things work'.

Printing

Use a range of objects to create prints. Talk to the children about which ones make the best prints and ask them 'why'.

What's wrong pictures

There are a number of commercial products available that have pictures depicting situations where things are not as we would expect them to be, for example, *What's Wrong? Colorcards*, with a woman cutting bread with a saw. Can the children spot the errors and explain why this is not right?

Busy picture scenes

Complex picture scenes are a way to introduce practice with a range of question forms. These are often themed around seasons, special activities or places and can also be used to extend vocabulary.

Activities for older children

- Carry out simple science experiments and use 'why 'questions to explore reasons or explanations for events. For example, try introducing objects into water play to explore sinking and floating, and ask questions like 'What helps you float?' and "Why?" or "What makes a boat sink?" and "Why?"

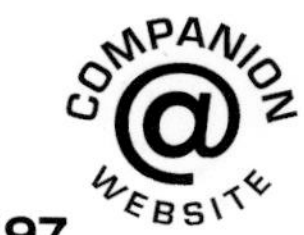

- Use a topic like minibeasts to encourage children to look for information to answer a number of different research questions like 'what', 'where', 'why' and 'how'. Encourage research using observation, textbooks, images and videos.
- The book *Ada Twist, Scientist (The Questioneers)* by Andrea Beaty is a champion of scientific enquiry, with its heroine, Ada Twist, seeking to discover answers to questions like "How does a nose know there is something to smell?"
- Help children understand how to use higher order questions that are open ended to talk through their thinking process, for example, 'What would happen if?' and 'What might happen next?' and 'Why would that happen next?' Provide alternative answers for children to make a choice. Acknowledge the value of a 'good' question that encourages children to observe and reflect on events.
- Use questions to help children with recalling and recapping the main points of a story. Remind students about the meaning of different question forms to help their understanding and to prompt recall. For example, 'Who' is about characters (people or animals) and 'What happened?' is about events and thus will have doing or action words.

See more ideas in Chapter 5, where expressive activities for questions can be modified to build comprehension.

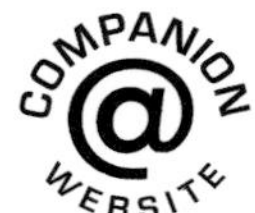

RECORD SHEET

Verbal comprehension

Name: **Review date:**

Outcomes	Comments

5

THE ACQUISITION OF EXPRESSIVE LANGUAGE

DOI: 10.4324/9781003031109-6

Introduction

This chapter sets out to describe the normal development of expressive language, starting with the child's production of their first words, to early combination of words into phrases, through to the use of complex sentences. It covers the function of language, its form in terms of syntax and morphology and its content (or semantics).

It is clear that the development of comprehension and expression are closely linked and must be considered together, and so, although for the sake of convenience this chapter is separate from the previous one on comprehension, this division is not a true reflection of normal communication.

The majority of the activities listed in this chapter presume an existing comprehension of the language involved. The reader should therefore refer to the previous chapter for ideas on the presentation of comprehension activities.

Factors affecting expressive language

There are many factors that might affect the development of a child's expressive language including:

- **A sensory impairment:**
  - *Hearing loss* - Children with a mild-to-moderate permanent hearing loss are at risk of delayed language development. For example, they produce fewer complex sentences (Koehlinger et al., 2013) and have difficulties with morphology (Tomblin et al., 2015).
- **An underlying neurodevelopmental disorder:** Delayed or impaired development of expressive language is associated with a number of neurodevelopmental disorders:
  - *Developmental Language Disorder (DLD):* There are individual differences in the way that children with DLD present in terms of understanding and spoken language difficulties. Characteristically they have reduced vocabularies and difficulties in finding the specific word to name a common object or 'word-finding difficulties' (Paul et al., 2018). Sentence structure may contain grammatical errors, for example, omitting morphemes that express tense and subject-verb agreement (Leonard, 2014).
  - *Autism (Autistic Spectrum Disorder, ASD):* There is considerable diversity in patterns of language development in children with ASD (Brignell et al., 2018). There

may be an absence or delay in language acquisition, and impairments in syntax and morphology have been noted, for example, confusion of personal pronouns (Kim et al., 2014).

- *Down's syndrome*: Studies have consistently shown that language outcomes for children with Down's syndrome is poor, with the acquisition of grammar significantly impaired (Singer Harris et al., 1997).

- **Digital device use:** Van den Heuvel et al. (2019) found that extended use of mobile media devices was associated with expressive language delay in young children between 18–36 months. A similar finding was reported by Operto et al. (2020) with longer exposure to digital devices resulting in lower language skills in this age group. They hypothesised that this might be related to the passive nature of the engagement and the lack of interaction that is common in parent-child communication.
- **Child-directed speech:** Variations in language input by caregivers/parents during early life is an important factor in predicting later expressive language outcomes for the child.
  - **Quantity of parent/caregiver language:** Infants who experience a greater amount of child-directed speech tend to learn language earlier and have larger vocabularies at 2 years of age (Hoff, 2006).
  - **Diversity of parent/caregiver language:** Along with quantity, the lexical diversity and sentence complexity of language input has a positive influence on the child learning new words and acquiring a range of linguistic structures (Jones and Rowland, 2017; Hadley et al., 2016).

Always seek professional advice where there are concerns regarding delayed or atypical development.

The functions of language

Language serves many functions, which the child learns to express in various ways in the first few years of life. Even the newborn baby soon realises that they can influence their environment by making sounds, smiles and movements. Later they develop more effective skills through the use of gestures, actions and language.

Halliday (2004) distinguishes between the pragmatic function, which refers to the use of language for communication, and the mathetic function, which refers to the use of language to explore and learn about the world. For the very young child these functions are served by the same utterances, but as language becomes more sophisticated, they learn new ways of expressing them.

Bloom and Lahey (1978) suggest that for any utterance, four elements can be described:

1. The propositional meaning, that is, the content of the utterance.
2. The locutionary act, that is, the act of uttering.
3. The illocutionary act, that is, the speaker's intentions.
4. The perlocutionary act, that is, the effect on the listener.

The illocutionary act has to do with the functions of language, and the perlocutionary act concerns how the speaker adapts their language according to the listener, the context and the situation.

Types of speech act

There are many kinds of speech act serving many different functions. They include the following:

- to ask questions;
- to make statements;
- to give information;
- to request and refuse objects and actions;
- to give orders and make suggestions;
- to solve problems;
- to describe events;
- to form concepts;
- to make threats and promises;
- to initiate and maintain conversation.

There are no exact correlations between kinds of speech act and types of syntactic structure; for instance, the same basic request can be made in the form of a question, "Can I have a biscuit?"; a declarative, "I'm hungry"; or an imperative, "Make me some tea".

It is important that children with a language delay have the opportunity to practise all the types of speech act appropriate to their stage of development.

Communication

The child must learn rules for initiating and maintaining conversation as well as how to modify what they say according to the listener and the situation.

Initiating conversation

Before the age of 2 to 2½ years, children tend to address themselves to the listener without first attempting to engage their attention. Two and a half to 3-year-olds will say the person's name before starting to speak (Bloom and Lahey, 1978), but they often do not wait for them to respond with their full attention.

Maintaining conversation

One of the basic rules of maintaining a conversation is 'turn taking'. The child is already fairly skilled at this before they begin to talk, as they have engaged in reciprocal smiling and similar games since they were tiny (see also Chapter 1).

Another foundation stone of satisfactory conversation is the 'shared topic'. The 2-year-old has a short memory and concentration span and tends to switch topics of conversation frequently. Between 2 and 3 years, children's ability to keep to the subject improves, although they can rarely sustain it for more than two consecutive responses (Cole, 1982). The child's response is usually related to a preceding adult utterance by containing either alternative or additional information, although there may be a phase when echoing is normal/

At 3years, the child's responses begin to reflect the syntax as well as the content of the adult's preceding utterance, which helps to make the conversation flow and misunderstandings less likely (Bloom and Lahey, 1978). However, although the 3-year-old is a reasonably competent conversationalist, a study of conversational patterns by Umiker-Sebeok (1979) showed that the 3-year-old often fails to attract a listener's attention and indulges in monologues which require no response, whereas the 4- to 5-year-old tends to converse more and to allow the listener an opportunity to respond to and discuss the message.

Appreciation of the listener

De Villiers and de Villiers (1978) propose four skills that are needed in order to modify one's speech according to the demands of the listener and the situation. These are:

1 Enough grammar and vocabulary to be able to choose amongst different language forms.

2 Recognition that different listeners need different amounts of information.
3 Knowledge of polite forms.
4 Recognition of which listeners require polite forms.

At 2 to 3 years old, the child is deficient in these skills, and so they tend to talk about what is already apparent to their listener (Bloom and Lahey, 1978), and to address all listeners similarly. Sometimes small children, and those with poor communication skills, are considered 'rude' by adults who do not realise that an appreciation of other people is an acquired skill. However, although young children tend to be egocentric (Piaget, 1929), there is sufficient evidence to suggest that they can adopt another person's point of view to a limited extent.

The intellectual use of language

One of the major functions of language is its intellectual use. We use language to martial our thoughts. The relationship between language and thought is very intricate and fascinating, and the subject of much research and literature.

The very young child cannot integrate the language they are hearing when they are engaged with their own activities; for example, they cannot simultaneously build a tower of bricks and listen to an adult's instructions (Reynell, 1980).

Between 2 and 2½ years, the child begins to relate language to their actions and can follow instructions; at 3½ they can direct themselves out loud to coordinate their actions and thoughts, saying such things as, "That goes there!" By 4, this private speech is used more specifically for goal-directed tasks (Winsler et al., 2000) and lays the foundation for the development of later skills in executive function. Sometime around 7 years, the child can begin to think silently, as language becomes internalised.

The language-performance link is forged, and the child can now start to plan ahead and to think through a sequence of events to its outcome rather than proceed, as hitherto, on a trial-and-error basis. (See Chapter 2 for more information on levels of attention.)

The meanings of language

Word meanings

Words stand for objects, people, actions, events, ideas and so on. The child must learn which words stand for which things in order to use language effectively. Through their sensorimotor experience children may have quite a lot of knowledge sorted into categories before spoken language develops (Clark, 2016). For instance, they know that some things move by themselves and others must be moved; that some things make sounds and others do not. The child does not at first understand and produce words as an adult would. They make a hypothesis about the new word based on the context in which they hear it used, and this may or may not coincide with its full meaning. The hypotheses are:

1 That the word has a greater meaning than it does for an adult; for example, the child hears 'dog' and thinks it refers to all four-legged, furry animals. They thus 'overextend' the word 'dog' to sheep, cats and cows etc.
2 That the word has a narrower meaning than it does for an adult; for example, they use 'dog' only to refer to their neighbour's dog; thus they 'underextend' the word.
3 That the word has a different meaning than it does for an adult; for example, the child hears 'dog' whilst looking at a dog's bowl and uses 'dog' to refer to bowls and dishes.
4 That the word has the same meaning as it does for an adult.

Overextensions are very common up to 2½ years. Clark states that the child gradually narrows down the range of objects covered by one word as they learn both new vocabulary and the essential differences between objects. They need feedback from adults to confirm or refute their hypotheses (Brown, 1973). It is probable that for a while the child may use 'dog' for other animals, although they understand that they are different, because they are unable to access the right word.

Two to 3-year-olds learn words first at an intermediate level, for example, 'dog'. At the age of 4 to 5 they acquire the superordinate terms, for example, 'animal', and specific terms, such as 'Alsatian'. The awareness of size follows a similar pattern; that is, children use the general terms 'big' and 'little' at first, and as they develop both cognitively and linguistically, they learn more and more specific terms, generally in the order 'tall/short', 'wide/narrow' and 'thick/thin' (de Villiers and de Villiers, 1978).

Sentence meanings

Children talk mostly about what they are doing, what they are about to do or what they are trying to do, and what they want other people to do (Bloom and Lahey, 1978). In other words, their talk revolves around actions and how objects affect actions or are affected by them.

Children's early rules for sentence construction appear to be based on words functioning in semantic roles such as agent, action and object, and not as syntactic constituents such as subject, verb and predicate, which are learnt much later. Young children express a limited set of semantic relations based on concepts that they acquire in the sensorimotor period (Brown, 1973). These relations develop in a relatively consistent order according to (Bloom et al., 1975) who describe them thus:

1 Existence – "there ball"; non-existence – "all gone"; recurrence – "more milk".
2 Action – "Run Mummy".
3 Locative action – "Put dolly there".
4 Locative state – "Box", in reply to "Where's teddy?"
5 Possession – "Daddy sock"; attribute – "Dirty".
6 Other categories, which occur only rarely before MLU 2.5 are: instrument – "bang (with) hammer"; intention – "want go park"; dative – "Give Mummy soap"; place of action – "swim bath".

Although action relations appear after existence, its relative frequency soon surpasses the other categories. Early verbs are usually very general ones which can be used in a variety of ways, for example, 'do', 'put' and 'go' (Bloom and Lahey, 1978).

Locative action refers to an object that is moving to a place and is usually expressed before locative state, which refers to objects that are stationary.

These semantic categories have very narrow definitions for the child early on; for instance, an agent of an action is nearly always animate, while the object of an action tends to be inanimate, so the 3-year-old might say, "Man hit bus", but rarely "bus hit man" (Cole, 1982). When expressing possession, the young child refers to alienable possessions, for example, "Mummy bag", before inalienable ones such as "Mummy nose". Possession and attribution are rarely used contrastively by small children, that is, they say "red sock" and "baby bottle" as part of naming and not to distinguish them from "blue sock" and "Mummy bottle" (Bloom and Lahey, 1978).

The development of language structure

First words (9 to 18 months)

The child says their first consistent and recognisable words at about 12 months, although the normal range varies from 9 to 18 months (Clark, 2016). At this stage, clear words may be embedded in long, jargon-like patterns. These first words may have a unique, idiosyncratic significance for the child (Adamson, 2019), for example, before they become aware that 'mama' stands for a particular person, they may understand it as a means of getting someone to smile and play with them. Early words are predominantly a way of initiating and maintaining interaction rather than a symbolic representation of objects and people. Such words include social expressions like 'bye-bye' as well as object names.

This early use of words is distinguishable from the first verbal labels, which appear at about 12 to 18 months, coinciding with the development of symbolic understanding. The earliest verbal labels represent familiar objects in the child's environment; people, food and drinks, toys and household items that are involved in their daily routines (Reynell, 1980; Schneider et al., 2015). These are words with a clear referent, and at 18 months expressive vocabulary is approximately 50-100 words. First words are usually very context bound; the child uses 'cup' only for their own cup at mealtimes and not for other cups or for their own cup in other situations. Later the word becomes more flexible and overextensions are common. Verbs are less common and occur later, with their use increasing sharply at the two-word stage.

Single-word utterances

There is general agreement that many single-word utterances have propositional meaning, and the child is not just naming objects. The single-word utterance may stand for one of many different functions, for example, "coat" might mean "Please take my coat off", "Where is my coat?" or "I want to go outside". The child uses context, gesture and intonation to specify the content and intention of their utterance, for example, they say "Mummy" and point to a toy that they want (Dore, 1974). The adult must do likewise in order to infer the message.

The functions of the single-word utterances include:

- Commenting: calling attention to things in the environment.
- Requesting: requests for objects, actions.
- Social interaction: gaining attention and initiating interaction.
- Refusing: protesting or rejection, use of 'no'.

From single words to two-word phrases

During the first half of the single-word stage, each communication act entails just one word. In the latter half, several different single-word utterances may be used in succession. They are still single-word utterances because they have equal stress and are separated by intonation and pause, but they refer to one event and comprise a single communication act, for example, "Tommy. Milk. Dirty" (meaning that Tommy has spilt his milk).

Children often combine two words in a fixed expression, such as 'geddown' or 'all gone' and treat them as if they were single words (Buckley, 2003). The individual words are not used flexibly in other expressions such as 'get coat' or 'all bricks'. This use continues into the two-word stage in such utterances as 'all gone soap'.

Two-word phrases (18 to 24 months)

By the age of 2, the child uses about 200 to 300 words and understands many more, again with wide normal variation (Fenson et al., 1994). Two-word phrases emerge between 18–24 months after this vocabulary spurt, distinguishable from successive single-word utterances because they are bound by a single intonation contour. At 20 months children encode similar relational meanings in different languages and include refusal, denial, requests, possession and agent-action-object (Bates et al., 2003). Early two-word combinations consist of a relational word, for example, "more", and a verbal label, for example, "biscuit", related through word order. Braine (1963) called this "Pivot Grammar". Braine postulated that the child has two classes of word: a small number of "pivots", for example, "all gone", which occur in a fixed position with any of a larger class of "open" words, for example, "teddy" and "milk". This is now seen as an over-simplification of the way children generate new utterances. Bloom (1973) calls this type of sentence, which does not create any new meaning, a pivotal combination. Later combinations, which Bloom calls hierarchical combinations, do create new meaning, for example, 'Mummy baby' expresses a relationship between Mummy and baby that is not inherent in either of the two words separately.

Reynell states that at 2 to 2½ years old, the child can assimilate and combine two operative words, usually nouns representing objects and actions, such as 'Daddy car'. At 2½ their two-word phrases also include noun-verb combinations, for example, 'Daddy wash', which are more complex, as verbs involve both an action, an agent to perform the action and, in some cases, an object to be acted upon (Reynell, 1980).

The child shows a good grasp of word order. Errors are rare; for example, if a 2½-year-old is shown a picture of a man carrying a lady, they might say "man carry", "carry lady" or "man lady" but not "carry man" or "lady man" (de Villiers and de Villiers, 1978).

Bloom (1973) suggests that if a child uses the relations agent-action, for example, 'Mummy wash', action-object, for example, 'wash baby' and agent-object, for example, 'Mummy baby', they must be able to understand the superordinate structure, agent-action-object, 'Mummy wash baby'. Therefore, if a child is producing these two-word relations consistently, they should be ready to progress to three-word phrases.

Three-word phrases

Brown (1973) and de Villiers and de Villiers (1978) have proposed two ways of moving from two- to three-word phrases.

1 By combining two previously learned constituents:
  For example:
    Agent + Action + Action + Object (Jack throw) (throw ball)
    = Agent Action Object (Jack throw ball)
2 By expanding one previously learned constituent:
  For example:
    Action + Object
    (throw + ball)

  Child is taught attribute (big)
    Attribute + Object (big ball)
    Action Attribute Object (throw big ball)

The first type tends to expand clause structure and the second type phrase structure. The level of difficulty seems about the same, and both types of expansion may co-occur.

Syntax at this stage is often called 'telegraphic' because the child's utterance contains only the most informative words, especially nouns, verbs and adjectives, and omits grammatical words such as 'the', 'of' and 'to'. The adult uses context, questioning and inference to interpret the full message.

Children still produce two-word phrases at this stage.

Bloom (1973) found that the following factors influence the length of utterance:

1 grammatical complexity (for example, noun and verb inflections, adverbs);
2 new vocabulary;
3 whether nouns or pronouns are used;
4 the conversational context.

Bloom discovered that complex and novel language produced a constraint on the length of utterance, whereas using pronouns such as 'they' and 'it' rather than noun-phrases such as 'the man' or 'the dog' made it easier for the child. It is also easier for the child to produce a three-word utterance if two of the constituents have already appeared in the conversational context. For instance, if an adult asks a child "Can you see the doggy eating?" this facilitates an answer such as "Doggy eating bone". The child's own preceding two-word phrase may likewise prompt a three-word sentence, for example, "get car", "Mummy get car".

Beyond the three-word phrase

Children can achieve goals and satisfy needs by using simple sentences in context, but they cannot divorce language from context or convey shades of meaning until they use more complex syntax, inflections and words. Between 2½ and 4-years-old there is very rapid language development, with growth in syntax (Sharma and Cockerill, 2014). The 3-year-old understands directions involving three or more operative words, including nouns, verbs, adjectives and prepositions, and produces short simple phrases (Reynell, 1980). Pronouns appear relatively late, around 3 years, with the use of subjective pronouns like 'I', 'he' and 'she' and 'it', and objective pronouns 'me' and 'you'. At 3½–4 years they start to use other pronouns consistently, although there may be frequent errors such as "me do it", which have generally disappeared by about the age of 4½ (Crystal et al., 1976).

The complexity of utterance is increased by:

- Combining and expanding constituents, as described previously.
- Adding morphological inflections, for example, '-ing', -ed' and auxiliary verbs.
- Introducing new constructions and expressions (Clark, 2016).

Increasing the complexity of utterances

Grammatical morphemes

Roger Brown described the stages of language development based on mean length of utterance (MLU). Stage I (between 12–26 months) related to MLU of 1–2 with utterances mainly single words with the beginning of sentence forms that combine two words. His model had four more stages outlining morphological development, where a morpheme is the smallest unit of meaning. Grammatical morphemes emerge between MLU 2 and 2.5 (Brown, 1973), at about 2 to 3 years of age. The rate of development varies considerably, but the order is relatively consistent.

The order of acquisition according to Brown is:
Stage II
27–30 months:

1 progressive [-ing] as in 'running'
2 the preposition 'in'

3 the preposition 'on'

4 the regular plural [-s] as in 'balls'

Stage III

31–34 months:

5 the irregular past tense, for example, 'sang'

6 possessive [-s] as in 'Mummy's coat'

7 the uncontracted copula [-is] as in 'Daddy is tired'

Stage IV

35–40 months:

8 determiners/articles 'a' and 'the'

9 the regular past tense [-ed] as in 'walked'

10 3rd-person singular, regular [-s] as in 'he walks'

Stage V

41–46+ months:

11 3rd-person singular irregular, for example, 'he catches'

12 the uncontracted auxiliary, for example, 'Are they hungry?'

13 the contracted copula [-s] as in 'Daddy's tired'

14 the contracted auxiliary [-s] as in 'she's finished'

This order was also confirmed by de Villiers and de Villiers (1978).

Children often produce common irregular forms correctly at first, but when they learn grammatical rules, they tend to apply them to everything, producing words such as 'runned' and even 'ranned', which may persist for some time. It is rare, however, to find errors across categories; the child does not inflect nouns with verb endings or precede verbs with articles.

The child may not distinguish between mass and count nouns for some time, and even a 7-year-old may produce forms such as 'a snow' and 'some spaghettis', but other noun-inflection errors usually disappear between the ages of 3½ and 4½.

Confusions between determiners are still common at 3½ to 4 years, especially between terms such as 'this' and 'that', which change their referent relative to the speaker (Crystal et al., 1976).

Auxiliary verbs

The stereotypes 'gonna', 'hafta' and 'wanna' are the first to appear, followed by the negative auxiliaries, 'do', 'can't' and 'won't'. Their positive counterparts appear much later, as they are semantically redundant elements, whereas the negative auxiliaries convey negation.

Children rarely use auxiliaries with the wrong verbs, for example, 'I am liking you'; or in the wrong constructions, 'Have get me book'. Occasionally they do use other words as if they were auxiliaries, for example, 'you better'd do it!', but this kind of error is usually gone by 4½ to 5 years.

At about 3 years, children may begin to use two auxiliaries, although they continue to make errors, for example, 'They have been crying' (Crystal et al., 1976). By MLU 3.5 at around 4 years of age, most of the auxiliaries have appeared, except complex ones involving subtle mood or tense.

Tense

Researchers are unanimous that very young children talk exclusively about the here and now, with the use of past tense in speech not emerging until around 3 years. The immediate past is part of the child's actual experience and therefore more easily understood than the future, which has yet to happen. Children initially refer to past events using the present tense, for example, 'Look at the picture I do'. Subsequently they mark the past time with an adverb, for example, 'Last night I see it', before using the appropriate inflections. Irregular past-tense verbs are learnt slightly earlier around 2½ years, and then the regular past-tense verbs appear nearer to 3 years, along with the use of 'do', 'can' and 'will' as future tense emerges.

Bloom and Lahey (1978) comments that children typically talk about what they are about to do, using the form 'I'm gonna', rather than what they have done, but many comprehension studies have found that understanding of the past is better than the future. Appropriate and consistent use of the future tense is not expected until the child is 4 to 4½, as it involves preplanning, a higher language function. The form 'I'm going to' or 'I'm gonna' is both simpler and more frequently used in everyday conversation, even between adults, than the more complex 'I will' and 'I shall', which appear later.

While children are acquiring the auxiliary system, inflections and rules for marking tense, certain types of errors are common. They frequently double-mark tenses and leave out essential words, for example, 'I did painted that picture' and 'I running very fast'.

Increasing the length of utterances

Children continue to expand their utterances by combining and expanding constituents, as previously described. Object-noun phrases are usually elaborated earlier than subject-noun phrases, as children tend to expand the ends of sentences first. In other words, a sentence such as 'I painted birds and flowers' would be produced earlier than one such as 'The boys and girls went to the seaside'.

Complex sentences begin at about 3 years of age or when they have obtained a mean length of utterance (MLU) of 3.0 (Lahey, 1988). The child begins to express two or more thoughts in a single utterance by first using coordination and, later, embedding.

Coordination is the joining together of two separate utterances or simple sentences that are related by context with a conjunction, which can be coordinating ('and', 'but', 'or') or subordinating ('because', 'when'). The former is termed a compound sentence, whereas the latter is termed a complex sentence (Steffani and Dachtyl, 2007). The conjunction 'and' appears earliest and is used in a variety of constructions whether or not it is appropriate or necessary; for example, the 3-year-old may say, "I got tummy ache and I goed to bed"; "I sit here and you sit here". A complex sentence has one or more dependent clauses joined to an independent clause, usually by a subordinating conjunction, for example, 'The boy was late because he missed his bus'. The order of appearance of the main conjunctions was found by Bloom and Lahey (1978) and Clark (1970) to be: 'and', 'because', 'what', 'when', 'but', 'that', 'if' and 'so', with the use of 'and' decreasing as the other words are learned.

Embedding refers to the process where one clause is included in or embedded in another clause in a sentence. The joining of these two interdependent clauses within one utterance results in a new meaning. For example, 'The bike, which was old, had a puncture' contains a main clause that can stand alone, whereas the embedded clause makes no sense on its own. By 4–5 years, 20 per cent of spontaneous sentences contain conjoined or embedded clauses (Paul, 1981).

Types of sentence

There are four sentence types in English:

1 Declarative sentence – most basic sentence that serves to relay information. Includes negative statements: The dog is not chasing the cat.

2 Interrogative sentence - interrogate or ask questions.*
   Yes/no questions: Is the dog chasing the cat?
   Wh- questions: Where is the cat? What is the dog chasing? Who is chasing the dog?
   Tag questions: The cat isn't here, is he?
3 Imperative sentence - tell or give instructions.
4 Exclamatory sentence - expresses emotion.

*Negative interrogative sentences are also possible.

Negatives

The child expresses various forms of negation:

1 Non-existence.
2 Disappearance.
3 Non-occurrence.
4 Cessation.
5 Rejection.
6 Denial.
7 Prohibition.

Between 2 years and 2½ years these are all expressed by 'no' or sometimes 'not' preceding the utterance, for example, 'no juice', 'no tickle', 'not play now'. The negative auxiliaries 'can't' and 'don't' emerge next, but they do not reflect knowledge of the auxiliary system, as they are used interchangeably with 'no' and 'not', and the positive auxiliaries do not occur. Initially the child omits the subject when using negatives, which reduces the length and complexity of the utterance, for example, 'can't see me', 'don't want book!' Finally, the child uses negative auxiliaries consistently as they master the auxiliary system at about MLU 3.4 to 3.9 (de Villiers and de Villiers, 1978).

Questions

From 1½ to 2 years children can discriminate between yes-no type questions and Wh- type questions but are unable to respond appropriately to the latter (Cole, 1982).

At about 2 years the child asks many stereotyped questions - for example, "What's that?" or "What's it called?" - without any real understanding, which is evident from their inability to respond to similar questioning by adults. From 2 years the child can ask yes-no questions with rising intonation but no subject-auxiliary inversion, and often omits the auxiliary altogether, for example, "That my juice?" Subject-auxiliary inversion occurs in these questions at around MLU 3.0. (35–37 months).

The child cannot use Wh- questions appropriately until they can understand them (Soderburgh, 1974). They can only do this after they have learned to express the appropriate concepts in a simpler form in their own speech. For instance, they can only understand why-questions once they are able to express causal relations (Hood, 1977).

It seems that children learn specific questions individually and not the question form as a single concept. At 2½, the most common Wh- question used is 'What?' about objects and 'What doing?' about events. At 3 it is 'Where?' 'What' and 'Who?' and by 4 years, 'Why?' predominates. The child may repeat the same questions over and over again to begin with, suggesting that they are practising and confirming the linguistic forms as well as seeking factual information (Rutter and Martin, 1972).

Until MLU 3 (35–37 months) the child typically puts the Wh- word at the beginning of the sentence and uses appropriate intonation but does not invert the subject and auxiliary, for example, 'Where you go?' 'What you are doing?' Subject-auxiliary inversion usually occurs with some Wh-questions before others.

At about 4 years, tag-questions appear. These are questions that are literally tagged on to the end of a sentence, as in, 'You did the washing-up, *didn't you*?' These are often preceded by the easier forms 'right?' and 'OK?'

Setting up a language group

Activities to develop expressive language skills are best carried out with small groups of children, as language functions primarily as a medium for communication.

Language groups:

- Create a more natural communication situation.
- Provide an opportunity for communicating and interacting with peers, so the child is able to learn social conventions and interaction skills.
- Have more opportunities for using language functionally to request, command, suggest, ask and answer questions, and so on.
- Help the child to practise and generalise skills they have learnt in individual sessions.

- Ease the pressure on individual children.
- Make healthy use of children's competitive instincts.
- Offer more flexibility for a greater range of games, play situations, projects and discussions.
- Allow a mixture of abilities so that children who have acquired certain aspects of language act as models.

Some children will still benefit from some regular one to one support, which might take part within the language group or in the child's wider learning environment.

Individual work:

- May be more suitable for shy, disruptive or highly distractible children.
- Enables more time and concentration to be given to specific tasks.
- Reduces environmental distractions and allows the child to focus on the task.
- Offers the child undivided attention.
- Allows the practitioner to make focused observations of the child.

Whenever possible, language teaching should be an integral part of the activities that the child is engaged in; for example vocabulary such as 'run', 'jump' and 'quickly' might be introduced during a physical activity. There may be times when face-to-face teaching is necessary, however, and the older child can certainly tolerate periods of working on specific aspects of vocabulary or sentence structure, as long as these are presented in an interesting manner.

The uses and functions of language should be paramount, both in planning and carrying out activities. Both general theories of function and the individual child's particular needs in their own environment are to be considered. Language should not be something that happens for a specific half-hour period; it is a tool for the child to use throughout the day. Therefore, although there are suggestions of specific ways of eliciting language, these are supplementary to the kinds of language stimulation that should be taking place during the child's everyday activities.

The child will be motivated to speak if they need to speak, and they want to speak. They will need to speak if their needs are not always anticipated and satisfied before they have to express them, so sometimes put their favourite toys out of reach and arrange things so that they have to make choices between drinks, foods and toys, and so on. They will want to speak if they are having fun or have created something that they are proud of and want to tell other people about.

Specific teaching strategies

Structure activities to provide opportunities for target vocabulary and language structures to be modelled by the adult. Use the following strategies:

- **Modelling** relies on the child actively analysing the model and reproducing it, or aspects of it, in their own spoken language. The adult has to model the language target many times, in many contexts, for example, naming fruits at mealtimes and pointing to pictures in a story book. This is useful for reinforcing and generalising learning. These differ from recasts (see more on this later) as the models are not dependent on what the child is saying in the previous turn.
- **Parallel talk** – adult commentary is focused on what the *child* is seeing, hearing, touching or doing. This should be a real-time experience as things happen, so the link between words and their referent is made clear, for example, "Milly has bought some bread and cheese", "I like cheese". Such commentary can be conversational in nature with a back-and-forth element as the adult leaves pauses for the child to respond; however, there should be no requirement or prompts for children to copy words or make any sort of response.

Both expansion and extension can also be used to provide an example of a specific language target.

- **Expansion:** the adult expands on what the child has said by filling in missing words, for example, child instructs adult "apple" as they feed a dolly, and the adult models back an expansion, "*eating* apple". (Target language here is action words.) The original meaning and intention of the child's utterance is retained. This strategy is useful for children who need to extend their sentence structure.
- **Extension:** the adult extends what the child has said by adding in more descriptive words, for example, "the car is beeping" might be extended to "the *red* car is beeping". (Target language here is colour.) Again, the original meaning and intention of the child's utterance is retained, with the additional information being optional.
- **Sentence closure (or cloze statement or procedure):** the adult models a word or structure and then elicits it by requiring the child to finish the sentence, for example, "I'm drinking milk. Mary's drinking milk. You're drinking . . .". This is good for eliciting

specific linguistic structures; for example, if you want the child to produce an action word or verb, say "Mummy is cooking; baby is...(sleeping)".

- **Role reversal** is a very useful technique. Usually, the adult models the language target first, for example, giving the child a two-part command, and then they swap roles, and the child gives the same or a similar command. In a group with each child taking a turn, there will be many repetitions of the language target.
- **Forced alternatives** is another way of covertly modelling the required vocabulary or linguistic form. For example, the adult asks the child if they would like an apple or an orange; the child then has only to imitate one or other of the words.
- **Making links** – build the child's knowledge of a word by learning language in context and helping them learn how words relate together. So food words might be used in a shopping game and a pretend play tea party, so the child starts to learn food is for eating and you buy it from a shop. The colour, shapes, insides and outsides of fruits and vegetables might be explored through printing activities. Really important is that children get to taste the food!
- **Recasting** (Cleave et al., 2015) **or reformulating** (Clark, 2018) is a way to provide the correct example following an omission or error by the child in their speech or language. The words and meaning of the child's utterance are retained, but corrections are offered by the adult. If the child mispronounces a word, for example, "dups" for 'cups', the adult models the word clearly in response – "Yes, I need *cups*". There should be no attempt to prompt imitations or repetitions from the child. Omissions and language errors can be responded to in the same way. For example, "I runned in park" might be recast as "You ran in the park" or "I want eat" might be recast as "I want to eat too". It is important that a reformulation is made within the next conversational turn by the adult, so feedback is given immediately to the child (Clark, 2018).

Motivation and rewards

Children are motivated by curiosity:

- Use lucky dips or mystery bags and boxes; unusual containers for toys, such as miniature chests of drawers.
- Collect a selection of interesting objects and miniature toys, the more curious the better, and keep them in a portable expanding craft box or toolbox.
- Introduce a hide and seek element – treasure hunts (hide items in sand, inside boxes, inside books); set up hideouts (a dark space to explore); hiding games from peek-a-boo to the traditional hide and seek.

- Engage children through surprises or the unexpected. Try wrapping or hiding toys. Read story books with unusual plot lines like *On the Way Home* by Jill Murphy.

Children are motivated by success:

- Use age-appropriate materials or those materials suitable for the child's level of functioning.
- Take into account their level of functioning in other areas, such as symbolic understanding, verbal comprehension and performance skills.
- Make rewards intrinsic to the task wherever possible. What would 'success' look like in an activity? – Completing a puzzle or shape sorting task? A correct response to the child's question or instruction? An artefact created by the child like a painting or a Lego building?
- Extrinsic rewards might include – positive reinforcement from the adult, time on a favourite activity or playing with a popular toy or game.
- Opportunities to use language in everyday real-life situations makes learning meaningful and is a great motivator.

Children are motivated by competition:

- Circle games – pass-the-parcel, fruit salad, Chinese whispers or telephone game.
- Group games like musical chairs or bumps, musical statues, dance freeze and grandma's footsteps.
- Use chance games, for example, spinners and dice, to choose an activity.

Children respond to interactive toys:

- Have a selection of toy and real telephones for the children to access during child-initiated activities.
- Puppets rarely fail to break the ice with small children and can be used in a variety of ways to develop language (see Chapter 3 for more ideas on using puppets).
- Interactive books with pop-up characters, flaps to open, pages to feel, buttons and buzzers to press for sounds.
- Games – language development board games; Who am I? guessing games, *Connect 4*.
- IPads or other tablets/smart phones – check out www.funwithspot.com; *Talking Tom/ Pierre the Parrot/Ben*; or check out various apps at www.educationalappstore.com.
- Book creator apps – children can add images, text, sound and speech to make up bespoke digital books.

Generalisation of expressive language skills

It often happens that language skills taught in a specific situation and with a specific adult do not always transfer into the child's everyday communication. Therefore, it is essential to make sure that learning opportunities are designed to help the child use their new skills in everyday situations outside of the language group (Rahn et al., 2019).

- Vary materials so that the child does not learn to relate a word to only one particular object or event (Gillham, 1979); for example, the word 'cup' can represent two or three non-identical cups, a toy cup, a miniature cup and a picture of a cup.
- Teach language in a variety of contexts (Gillham, 1979); for example, the item is used at mealtimes, during a pretend tea party or while looking through a picture book.
- When a child first acquires a new word or language structure, they need time to consolidate their learning with lots of practice in games and play situations throughout the day.
- Communicate the child's language targets to everyone involved with the child, so the child is able to practice the use of language with a variety of people both at home and in the learning environment.
- Make sure that the people in their daily environment encourage them to practise their language production and also provide the necessary feedback and modelling of language targets; for example, when the child says "cat jumping", the adult responds with "yes, I see the cat jumping".
- Encourage other people to respond to the child whenever they try to communicate in an appropriate manner. Let them know what to expect from the child. All forms of communication, like sign, gesture, pointing and spoken language, should be valued.
- Use cues and strategies to help generalise language use into the home or general learning environment, even if these have been faded out in more structured teaching.
- The general learning environment may have to be modified in order to provide the child with opportunities to practise their new language skills in varied environments. This might involve taking the child out on trips, for example, to the shops or a café in order to *use* the language that has been taught.
- The child will continue to need positive reinforcement for correct responses until language structures become more established.

Activities to facilitate expressive language

This chapter covers the acquisition of expressive language and contains a wide range of practical activities to support the development of these skills. Sections cover early vocabulary, development of two- and three-word sentences and more complex sentences involving grammatical morphemes.

General guidelines

- Materials used should be at an appropriate developmental level and of interest to the child.
- Allow enough time for the child to explore new play equipment and materials before expecting them to use it in a specified way.
- Be flexible and take the child's lead as far as possible. If the child is showing no interest in your choice of materials, adapt your planned activity to whatever they are interested in. They will learn more quickly if they are learning willingly.
- Involve key people in decisions about language targets so everyone has input, including the child, if possible, and all are aware of the words or phrases the child is learning.
- Make sure the child understands the necessary vocabulary or concept before you start to teach language production (see Chapter 4 on 'The Development of Verbal Comprehension'). Otherwise, they may learn linguistic forms parrot-fashion but be unable to use them meaningfully and creatively.
- Monitor your communication and language to ensure you provide a good model for the child. Language input should be appropriate for the child's level of comprehension.
- Always try to understand the child and encourage them to point, show you or give other clues to help you interpret the content of their message.
- Be interested in *what* the child is saying, over and above *how* they are saying it.
- Encourage different types of communicative interaction, for example, structured conversations, discussions.
- Ensure that the child gets all the repetition and practice they need to consolidate their learning.
- Be prepared for periods when children's use of linguistic forms and words fluctuates; they must test out and practise language before it becomes firmly established.

Recording observations

Formative and ongoing assessment should help establish where the child is functioning in terms of their expressive language. Goals and strategies can then be carefully planned, although it is necessary to be flexible and adjust to the day-to-day changes in the child's needs and responsiveness. Language goals should aim to fulfil the child's immediate needs in the environment.

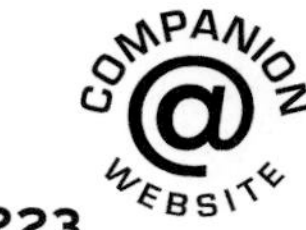

Observe and record the development of the child's expressive language over an extended period of time in a variety of situations within the learning environment. Observations from parents or carers are invaluable in gaining a broader understanding of the child's abilities in language production

Make a note of:

- the words and phrases the child is able to say and use appropriately;
- the type of sentence structure (e.g., subject-verb-object);
- the length of sentence structure; (e.g., two-word phrases, three-word phrases);
- the situation or context in which the child uses language targets;
- consistency and frequency of responses;
- any change in language use between different contexts (in a group context the child may watch and copy other children rather than having fully learnt a word or language structure);
- nonverbal responses used by the child to communicate (behavioural, body language, gestures or signs);
- whether the child tries to copy a word or phrase;
- whether the child starts to use the word or phrase spontaneously or only when elicited;
- which strategies are successful in helping the child produce language (e.g., forced alternatives, modelling).

First words

Bloom (1973) suggests some useful early words to teach children that express meanings around appearance, disappearance and recurrence. Activities focus on 'more'; 'again'; 'gone'; 'all gone'; 'go'; 'here'; 'here y'are'; 'up'; 'down'; 'on'; and 'off'. None of these words have a clear referent and might seem difficult to teach, but in fact they are among the earliest words used by the typically developing child. These are also useful words which later combine well with names of objects and actions.

Aims

To develop early expressive vocabulary with a focus on common first words.

Outcomes

- Copies words modelled by the adult.
- Uses words meaningfully to request or command.

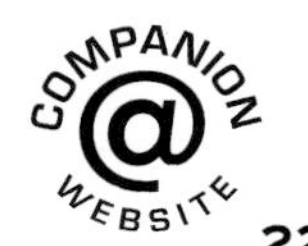

Strategies

- Start with a small number of words and provide lots of clear models in a variety of contexts.
- Vary materials and activities so that the child does not associate the use of a word with one particular object or event.
- Monitor your communication and language to ensure you provide a good model for the child.
- Language input should be appropriate for the child's level of comprehension. Introduce first words in one word or simple phrases.
- Accept all attempts at communication by the child, whether this is a sound, gesture or word.
- Avoid correcting any errors the child may make when repeating or attempting to say a word. Instead provide the correct model, for example, "or" – "more" "more juice".
- Encourage carry-over of learning to other environments like the home by asking parents/caregivers to use target words in everyday routines and to respond positively to the child's attempts.
- Make sure the child understands the necessary vocabulary or concept before you start to teach language production.
- Modelling and role reversal would be useful strategies to implement.

Suitable materials and resources

Bubbles; money box and coins; wind-up toys; music box; spinning tops; posting boxes; puppets; toy vehicles, tunnels, and garages; various balls for physical games; marble runs and helter-skelters; building bricks; remote control toys; robot toys; outdoor physical play equipment and sports day kits; toy swings, roundabouts, see-saws and ladders; dressing up clothes and accessories; torches; and board games.

Activities to elicit 'more'

Drink time

If the child shows that they want more of something, for example, they finish their juice and hold out their beaker, say "More?" with exaggerated intonation and pour some out. Use the word with a variety of drinks in different situations so they learn to generalise their understanding and use of the word. Avoid the child confusing the word 'more' with 'juice' by waiting until the child has finished before you say the word, and then bring out more juice.

Bubbles

Blow a few bubbles. When they have all burst, say "More?" as you blow some more. Next time wait until the child makes a response of some sort to indicate 'more'. Model the word

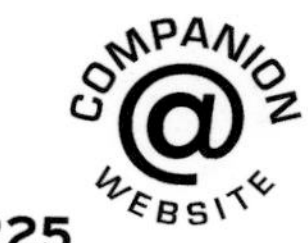

if the child uses a sound or gesture to indicate a request – for example, "You want *more?*" "*More?*"

Coins in a money box

Have some coins to pop in a money box. Give the child one at a time and wait for the child to indicate or ask for "more". Look out for money boxes with sound or movement like the Coin Stealing Monkey and Fisher Price Laugh and Learn Piggy Bank.

Snacks

Give the child some small pieces of fruit or vegetables at snack time so that they need to ask for "more".

Activities to elicit 'Again'

Rough and tumble

Any physical activity that the child enjoys can be used to elicit 'again', for example, rough and tumble, being pushed on a swing or on a roundabout.

Wind-up toys

Use a wind-up toy, music box, or spinning top, anything that the child has to ask an adult to do for them.

Nursery rhymes and songs

Choose one with fun actions that encourage interaction between you and the child like *Ring-a-Ring-O'-Roses, Zoom, Zoom Like a Rocket* and *This Is the Way the Ladies Ride*. Do once, stop, and ask "Again?" before you repeat.

Activities to elicit 'Gone'/'All Gone"

Toys away

The child puts their toys away as you say, "all gone". Make this into a game by having the child put toys into a homemade posting box.

Bubbles

Blow bubbles, and as the child bursts each one, say "all gone".

Peek-a-boo

Play peek-a-boo with puppets. Call out "gone" when the puppet hides out of sight. Similar games can be played to accompany *Two Little Dicky Birds*.

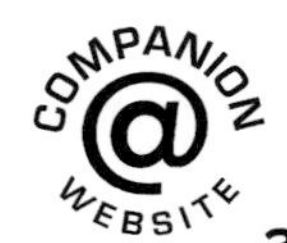

Into the tunnel

Play various hide and seek activities to elicit 'gone'; for example, when playing with a train or truck, push it into a tunnel or garage so it is out of sight.

Ball games

Create a goal using a cardboard box with one open side concealed with strips of shiny paper. Play games with the child rolling the ball into the goal. When the ball disappears inside, call out "Where's the ball? *Gone*".

Picture book

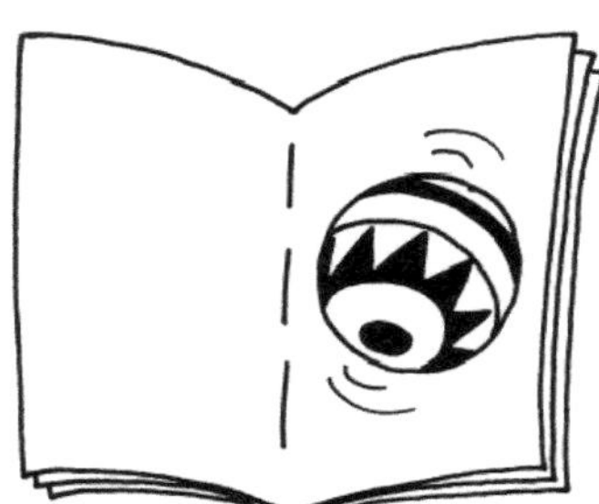

Make a picture book with clear colourful pictures. Make every other page a blank, and as the child turns to the blank page, they can say "gone".

Bye-bye games

Wave and say "bye-bye" when a person leaves the child's presence. Encourage the child to join in, and when the person has gone, say "Gone!"

Activities to elicit the word 'Go'

Starting signal

Let children take it in turns to give the signal "Go!" to start a whole range of activities. It is particular good for games involving movement, including tag, obstacles courses or skipping competitions.

Ball games

Introduce 'go' into ball games as varied as football, skittles and ping pong,

Ready, steady...

Build up the anticipation with the "Ready, steady" cue phrase. The child completes the phrase with the word "*Go*". Activities might be releasing a marble down a marble run, pushing a car down a ramp, knocking down a tower of bricks or sliding figures down a helter-skelter. Children can take turns in either giving the cue or carrying out the action.

Moving toys

Have a selection of toys that children can move when commanded with "*Go*". Try Scalextric cars and a racing track; robot toys; remote control stunt cars, planes and boats. Try role reversal so the child starts to command with the word 'go'.

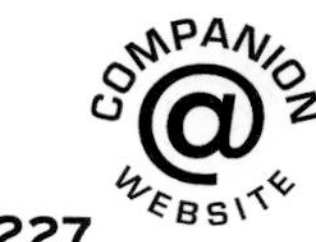

Commands

Use in activities where the command *"Go"* is used to instruct other children or adults on what to do; for example, in hide and seek the command "go" is used to instruct players to hide; or in parachute games players are instructed to start a movement or to change direction. Children can take turns in giving the command.

Activities to elicit 'Here' or 'Here y'are'

Attracting attention

The child is encouraged to attract a person's attention by saying "here" or "here y'are" while pointing to an object. They can be shown that this is more useful than silently pointing or making noises, which may be misunderstood or go unnoticed.

Handing objects

The child says "here y'are" while handing objects to the adult to put away or set out. Play give-and-take games where objects are exchanged between you and the child.

Object re-appears

The child says "here y'are" or "here it is" when an object reappears, for example, from a tunnel, a posting-box, a helter-skelter, a money-box, and so on.

Activities to elicit 'Up' and 'Down'

Physical games

Physical games provide lots of opportunities for modelling and eliciting the words 'up' and 'down' from the child. Examples include:

- as they are picked up, swung round and put down again.
- as they go up the ladder and down the slide.
- as they bounce up and down on a trampoline.
- as they go up and down on a see-saw, taking it in turns with another child to say "up" and "down".
- as they move up and down on a swing.

Action songs

Introduce 'up' and 'down' into the lyrics of different songs. For example, *Wheels on the Bus* might have "people on the bus stand up and down"; "the children in the bus jump up and down"; and "the babies on the bus bounce up and down".

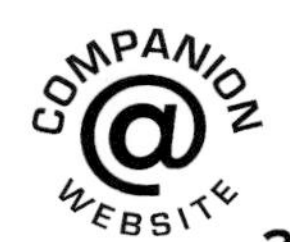

Pop-up puppets

Pop-up puppets have different figures like clowns, elves or animals that the child can push up and down.

Climbing toys

There are various toys and games where little people or animals climb up and down ladders, for example, *Penguin Dash Action Game*.

Toy swings and see-saws

Make different figures go up and down on a toy swing. Toy see-saws with their repetitive movement also give ample opportunity for the child to practise the words.

Climbing ladder

Draw or cut out a picture of a large cardboard ladder and stick it on the wall. Attach cardboard figures or climbing animals like squirrels or monkeys to the bottom of the ladder with Blu-Tack. Take turns with the child to make the figure climb up and down on command.

Activities to elicit 'On' and 'Off'

Dressing

The child says "on" as they put on their shoes, socks and coat. They say "off" as they take them off again. Extend this by playing dressing-up games with a group of children.

Dress up dolly

Have lots of clothing and accessories that dolly can put "on" and take "off".

Switches

These expressions can be used as the child switches on and off a torch or flashing light, the electric light, domestic appliances, a music-box and so on.

Funny faces

Make funny faces using a false moustache or beard, fun glasses and make-up that you can put "on" and take "off".

Activities for older children

- *More*
  - Encourage requests for "more" during creative activities when the child has to ask for more materials by keeping them out of reach or only supplying small amounts at a time.

    - Similar requests can be elicited during cooking when the child has to ask for more items, for example, pour out a little flour and wait for the child to ask for "more".
- *Go*
    - Use the word to start different sections of a relay race so the child passes a baton on to the next child, but that child must wait for the signal "go" before moving off. Add another layer of skill by having an egg and spoons rather than batons (use hard boiled eggs or a commercial set of egg and spoon games).
    - Play Hoop La- on the signal "go" children race to see who is quickest to throw their rings (or quoits) on to sticks. Alternative games might be throwing bean bags into hoops on the ground or small pebbles into an egg box.
    - Children mime movements of favourite animals as they follow an obstacle course around the room. This can be as simple as mats laid out on the floor. Children must wait at the mat until they hear the word "go" again.
- *Up and down*
    - *Snakes and Ladders* - Use a commercial game, or better still make your own visually simple board. The child pushes their counter "up" the ladders and "down" the snakes.
    - Simple board games can be devised that require the child to move up and down the board.
    - Use 'up' and 'down' as the children climb up and down from climbing-frames, climbing ropes and other outside play equipment.
- *On and off*
    - Play games where stickers are put "on" different parts of the face, hands and feet.
    - Players give instructions to each other in games, for example, in *Twister* "put your foot on red:.

Early verbal labels

A study by (Schneider etal., 2015) found that early vocabulary included words referring to animals, games and routines, and that these results were consistent for both early and late talkers.

Aims

To develop acquisition of early expressive vocabulary.

Outcomes

- Uses words to label objects, toys and animals.
- Uses object names meaningfully to:
    - direct;
    - request;

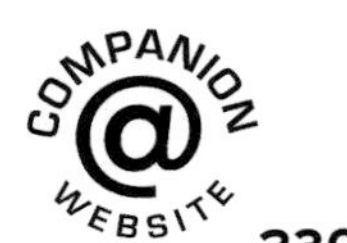

- suggest;
- command.

Strategies

- Start with a small number of words and provide lots of clear models in a variety of contexts.
- Vary materials and activities so that the child does not associate the use of a word with one particular object.
- Monitor your communication and language to ensure you provide a good model for the child.
- Language input should be appropriate for the child's level of comprehension. Introduce target verbal labels in one word or simple phrases.
- Accept all attempts at communication by the child, whether this is a sound, gesture, or word.
- Avoid correcting any errors the child may make when repeating or attempting to say a word. Instead provide the correct model, for example, "at" – "cat".
- Encourage carry-over of learning to other environments like the home by asking parents/caregivers to use target words in everyday routines and to respond positively to the child's attempts.
- Make sure the child understands the necessary vocabulary or concept before you start to teach language production.
- Modelling and role reversal would be useful strategies to implement.

Suitable materials and resources

Puppets; bean bags; posting box; mystery bag or box; feely bag or box; picture books; photographs; picture cards; magnetic picture boards; fuzzy felt; jigsaw puzzles; selection of toys and everyday objects; picture cube; croquet golf; a selection of games like dominoes, Snap, *Happy Families* and *Picture Lotto*; slide viewer; and digital camera.

Activities to elicit object names

Naming an object

Responding to questions

Child names an object in response to the adult's questions "What's that?" or "What have you got/found?" Use a puppet so the adult addresses the questions to the puppet and the child answers on the puppet's behalf. (Have a selection of objects hidden in a bag.)

Naming objects

The child names real or toy objects as they:

- Post them into a box.
- Hand them to the adult.
- Pull them out of a mystery bag or box.
- Tidy up and put them away.

Naming pictures

The child names pictures or photographs of objects as they:

- Look at a picture book.
- Post them in a postbox.
- Hand them to the adult.

Make a picture

The child names objects as they put them on to a magnetic picture boards or Fuzzy Felt layout. The adult can then tell a simple story about the pictures.

Jigsaw puzzles

The child is given jigsaw-puzzle pieces to name and complete a simple puzzle.

Hiding games

The adult hides toys around the room, and as the child finds one, they name them.

Surprise presents

The child names "presents" as they take them out of a surprise post bag. These can be wrapped so you can encourage the child to make guesses.

Picture cubes

The child names pictures on a picture-cube. This can be bought from a photographic suppliers or made at home by pasting pictures onto a large play brick.

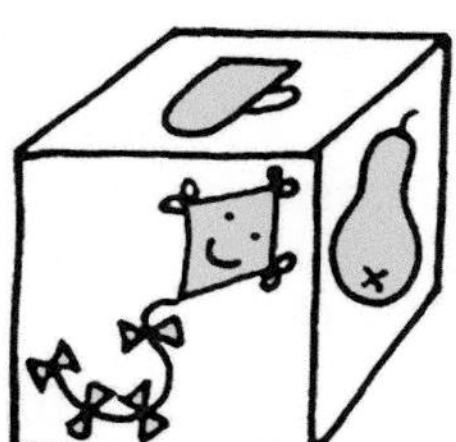

Naming as part of a game

Tiddly-wink

Make a sturdy board and mark off large squares. In each square paste a picture card. The child has to flip a tiddly-wink or shove a coin onto the board and name the picture it lands on.

Fishing-game

A large empty container or washing-up bowl can serve as the fishpond. The fish are made out of robust card and have paper clips attached to them. The fishing rod has a small magnet attached, which attracts the 'fish'. The game can be played either as a reward, for example, if the child names a picture correctly, they have 30 seconds to hook as many fish as they can, or it can incorporate the naming activity by pasting pictures onto the fish themselves. If the child names the picture, they get to keep the fish.

Spinning wheel

A spinner is attached to a board. Around the outside of the board are placed miniature objects or object pictures. To make this more natural, the children try and guess which picture the arrow will point to when it stops.

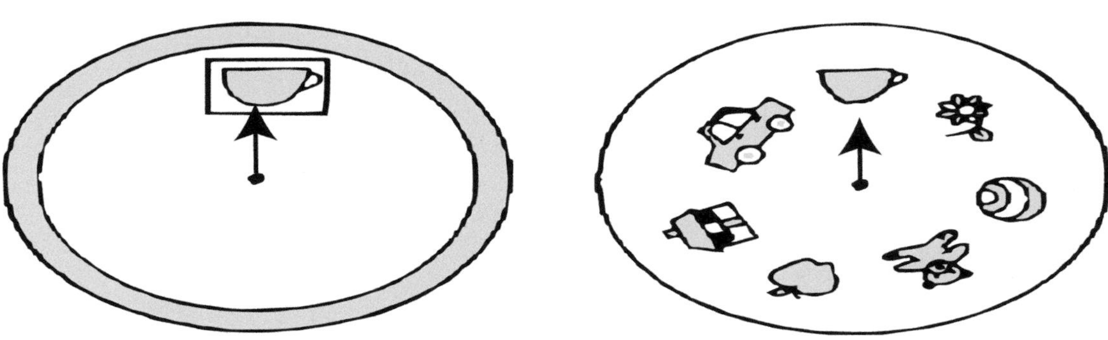

Croquet golf

Very large cardboard pictures are made that will stand up on the floor. A hole is made in them large enough for a small ball to pass through. Child-sized croquet or golf sticks are used to knock the balls through the holes. If the child can name or describe the picture, they double their score.

Games

The child names pictures as they play various games, such as dominoes, Snap, *Happy Families* and Lotto. The naming should be woven into the game as far as possible so that it does not detract from the fun.

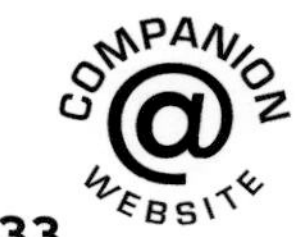

Pass the parcel

Inside each wrapper is a small toy. Prompt the child to name it with questions and cues.

Guessing games

Guessing games have an intrinsic purpose. It also gives more purpose to the act of naming if the adult cannot see what the object or picture is; the child is then giving worthwhile information.

- Feely box: a selection of objects is placed in a box with a hole cut out, large enough to place one hand through. The child manipulates the object and tries to guess what it is.
- Feely bag: used in the same way as the feely box. The child attempts to guess the objects by feeling them through the bag.
- Blindfold: the adult blindfolds themselves. They then choose an object from a tray and name it. The adult asks the children, "Am I right?" and the children either agree or tell the adult what it really is.
- Presents: wrap up some distinctively shaped objects and see if the child can guess what they are. This is only suitable for children with fairly good shape recognition.
- Lotto: the caller shuts her eyes, holds up a card and asks the children what they are holding.

Kim's game

The children have to memorise the objects on a tray and then name the one the adult has taken away.

Halves-to-wholes

Make a set of pictures displaying halves of objects that have to be matched up in a pairs game. At a simple level the child is given the halves of very dissimilar objects – for example, car, apple, cup – and they have to guess what they are. At a higher level, the pictures are perceptually more similar.

As a variation of this, you can make your own halves-to-wholes dominoes. As each piece is laid, the player guesses what the object is. Children love correcting adults, so occasionally give a wrong guess, but do not use this strategy if the child is likely to be confused or intimidated.

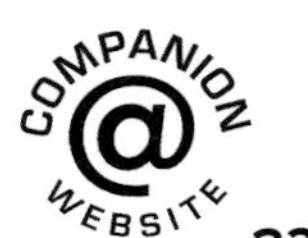

Crackers

Pull some crackers. The children name the objects that fall out. You can modify the crackers beforehand by unwrapping them and putting miniature objects or toys inside.

The child must also learn how to use words to draw attention to, comment on, and request objects:

Attention

Attracting attention

Model for the child how to attract attention to an object by holding it up, pointing at it, showing it to the person, and saying its name.

Daily environment

Encourage the child to point to objects in the environment, for example, while they are in the park or looking out of the window, and to say their names.

Request

Mealtimes

When the child shows by their gestures and intonation that they want something to eat or drink, for example, a biscuit, then show them the object and model the word before you give it to them. Gradually expect them to say the word or an approximation of it before they get their reward.

Toys

The child is given a choice of toys to play with, and to get their choice they must correctly name the toy. The younger child will need to be shown the objects, but an older child at the appropriate cognitive level may not need these visual clues.

Shopkeeper

One child acts as the shopkeeper while the other children make requests to buy certain items from them. The level of difficulty can be varied; either the adult tells the child what to buy, so they have only to imitate, or the child has to make a free choice. Names can be modelled during the set-up of the shop, and later when emptying the items out of the shopping bag.

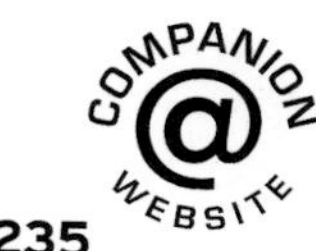

Jigsaw animals

Fold a piece of thin cardboard in half and draw an outline of an animal. Cut it out so that you have two shapes. Cut one into large jigsaw pieces and use them as stencils to make the same outlines on the other animal-shape. Then draw or paste small pictures onto each piece. The end result should look like this:

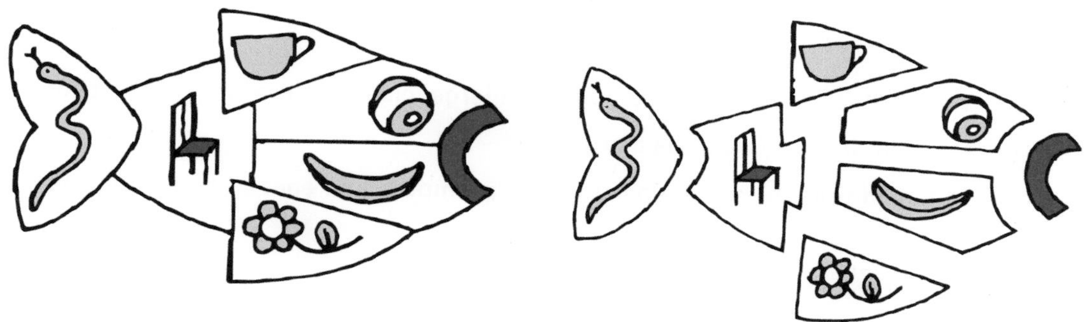

The child matches the pieces to their copy by correctly asking for the picture.

Suggestion and command

Hiding game

Play a hiding game with different objects, taking turns with the child to tell each other what to hide.

Shopper

Children take it in turns to tell each other what to buy. For children who enjoy role play, they can act as a 'parent or caregiver', teacher or even a chef telling the other children what to buy. Afterwards the child can tell the 'parent' or 'caregiver' what they have bought.

Floor map

Set up a construction, floor layout or play situation with the child, who has to tell you or the other children what they need, for example. A 'car', 'bus' or 'house'.

Creative play

If the child wants to do some painting, they ask for "paper", "paint" or "apron".

Cooking

Set out a range of items for a recipe to cook with the child. Keep this out of reach so the child has to asks for things like "eggs", "milk" and "flour". (But make sure that the items are still in view as a visual reminder for the child.)

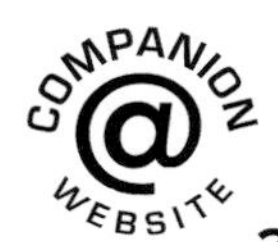

Beanbag toss

Lay out several picture cards on the floor or stick these on a box. Each child takes it in turn to name a picture for another child to aim at with their beanbag. Alternatively put the pictures on cones and use quoits for a Hoop La game.

Activities for older children

- Drawing:
  - The child is shown a picture book with large, clear line drawings. They choose one to colour in by naming the picture.
  - The child tells the adult what to draw, prompted and encouraged by another adult when necessary.
  - Jigsaw animals can be turned into a game for older children; for example, only when a six is thrown on a die can the child ask for a jigsaw piece.
- Visual perceptual tasks:
  - The adult begins a drawing from the least obvious angle, and the children guess what it is.
  - Show the child photos of objects taken from unusual angles, like the inside of an object or an upside-down or inside-out object. Can the child name the object?
  - The child looks at pictures through a toy viewer or a real slide-viewer and tells the adult what they see.
- Barrier games:
  - Children tell each other what objects to draw or paint while sitting either side of an easel. Afterwards they compare their drawings, which should be the same. The adult is on hand to prompt.

Action names

Action words or verbs are acquired later than object names or nouns, as they are perceptually more abstract (Roseberry et al., 2009) and lack a concrete referent. These activities focus on actions the child can carry out themselves, for example, running, sleeping and walking. (See Chapter 4 for ideas on developing a wider range of action words. These activities can be easily adapted to support the development of expressive vocabulary.)

Aims

To use a range of simple action words to name everyday actions.

Outcomes

- Uses a range of simple action names.

Strategies

- Start with a small number of words and provide lots of clear models in a variety of contexts.
- Monitor your communication and language to ensure you provide a good model for the child.
- Language input should be appropriate for the child's level of comprehension.
- Talk about actions as they occur so that the association between action and word is made clear.
- Accept all attempts at communication by the child, whether this is a sound, gesture or word.
- Avoid correcting any errors the child may make when repeating or attempting to say a word. Instead provide the correct model, for example, "ump" – "jumping", "Ben's jumping".
- Encourage carry-over of learning to other environments like the home by asking parents/caregivers to use target words in everyday routines and to respond positively to the child's attempts.
- Provide lots of repetition of language targets in a variety of different contexts that include everyday routines, pretend play, picture books, physical activities and play.
- Further generalise understanding by using target verbs in simple phrases and commands. Keep the rest of the words in the phrase redundant so the child focuses on the verb.
- Make sure the child understands the necessary vocabulary or concept before you start to teach language production.
- Modelling and role reversal would be useful strategies to implement.

Suitable materials and resources

Dolls, teddies and stuffed toys with movable limbs; puzzles and jigsaws illustrating actions; action picture cards, picture books, photographs and photocards; action songs and nursery rhymes; physical play equipment; and construction toys.

Activities to elicit action names

Questions

The adult asks "What are you doing?" while the child is engaged in a range of activities, for example, during mealtimes when they are "eating" and "drinking"; during physical play

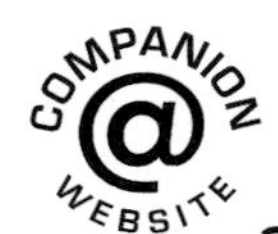

when they are "jumping" and "climbing"; during playtime when they are "playing" and "reading"; and at bath times, when they are "washing" and "splashing".

Simon Says

The children give each other and the adult instructions to carry out different actions, for example, "Skip", "Hop" and "Clap".

Doll play

Take turns with the child to carry out different actions with a doll. Comment on the actions as you play with the doll: "Dolly is *jumping*". Ask the child "What are they doing?" The child tells the adult what actions to make dolly do.

Tell teddy

Play a game where you give teddy different instructions. It may help to have one teddy for yourself and one for the child. Show the child how to manipulate its arms and legs when you give commands like "dance", "walk", "run" or "wave". Later you can say, "Now you tell Teddy what to do" and expect the child to generate their own ideas.

Paper dolls

Make paper dolls with moving arms and legs that the child can manipulate; for example, a leg can be moved so that it seems to kick a ball. Talk to the child about how different actions are carried out – "Dolly moves her leg and foot to kick the ball", "Can you make doll's leg move?" Introduce a teddy so different movements can be compared. Ask the child "What is dolly doing?" "What is teddy doing?"

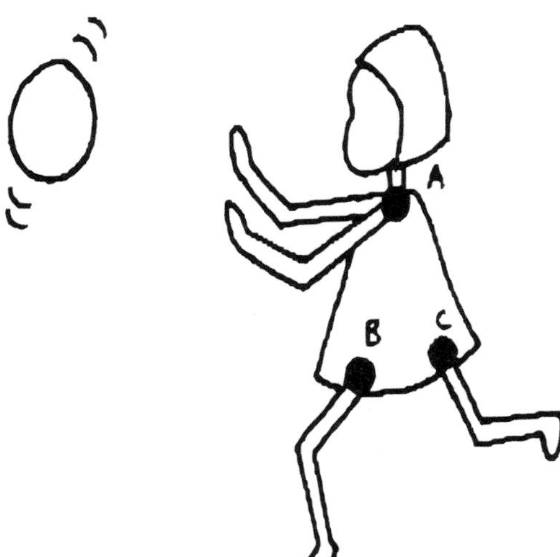

Action puzzles

The child completes a simple action-themed puzzle. Name the actions as the child takes out the pieces. Put the pieces in a bag. Take turns at naming an action and finding the appropriate piece in the bag and replacing it in the puzzle.

Picture cards

The child names the actions depicted in pictures and action cards, which can be bought or home-made. The child may enjoy capturing their own actions in images or videos that can be uploaded to a tablet and used in a book creator app.

Mime the action

Play this with a group of children. A series of action cards are placed face down. The children take turns to pick a card and mime the action, for example, "digging", "cutting", "swimming", "throwing". The others try to guess and name the action. The adult helps by giving clues and close guesses.

Book creator app

Create a digital book using a book creator app by taking photographs or, even better, making a video of the child carrying out different actions. The app allows these images to be added straight into a personalised book that might also include links to spoken stories and action songs that use the target language.

Activities for older children

- Play the 'odd one out' game with words. Can the children spot the word with a different meaning in "washing, cleaning, singing'?
- Play the parachute game 'merry-go-round'. Children stand sideways to the parachute holding on to it with one hand. As they walk around in a circle, the chute will start to look like a merry-go-round. Children take turns to shout out an action everybody has to follow like 'running', 'skipping', 'hopping' and 'jumping'. Switch directions every now and then.
- Use *Action Words on Clapper Boards* by Twinkl to play games and introduce the written word alongside the spoken name.

Two-word phrases

The early two-word utterances to teach are combinations of either a relational word plus the name of a person, object or action, for example, "look, car"; "more Mummy"; "all gone milk"; "again tickle", or a name of a person plus an object or action, for example, "Daddy coat"; "Sammy push". Each of the "pivotal" words should be used with many different objects and actions to facilitate generalisation. Many of the activities listed previously can be used for eliciting two-word utterances.

Aims

To develop two-word utterances using relational words plus the name of a person, object or action.

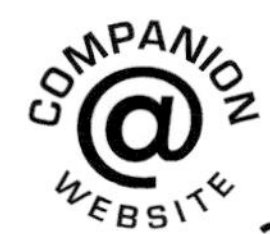

Outcomes

- Combines a relational word with a noun in a two-word phrase.

Strategies

- Monitor your communication and language to ensure you provide a good model for the child.
- Language input should be appropriate for the child's level of comprehension.
- Accept all attempts at communication by the child, whether this is a sound, gesture or word.
- Avoid correcting any errors the child may make when repeating or attempting to say a word. Instead provide the correct model, for example, "bye-bye bu" – "bye-bye ball".
- Encourage carry-over of learning to other environments like the home by asking parents/caregivers to use target phrases in everyday routines and to respond positively to the child's attempts.
- Provide lots of repetition of language targets in a variety of different contexts that include everyday routines, pretend play, picture books, physical activities and play.
- Make sure the child understands the necessary vocabulary or concepts before you start to teach language production.

Suitable materials and resources

Large dolls and teddies; pretend play items; everyday objects; puzzles; posting boxes; picture books; action pictures.

Activities to elicit two-word phrases

Early pivotal combinations

Puzzles

Graded-size inset puzzles are useful as the child can repeat the same expression many times, for example, "more dog".

Posting boxes

Encourage the child to produce a two-word utterance as they post an object in the box, for example, "Bye bye ball".

Picture book

Picture book with every other page blank for eliciting expressions like "car gone".

Other activities listed under one-word utterances can also be adapted for eliciting two-word phrases.

Later hierarchical combinations

It is quite usual for the child at this stage to express relations by combining two object names, for example, "dolly cake". This need not be discouraged in favour of the noun-verb combinations, "dolly eat" and "eat cake", although the adult should model these for the child. When introducing new object names, keep the verb constant, and vice versa, for example, "give ball, give brick, give apple"; "show cup, get cup, hide cup"; and so on.

Commentary and description

Physical play

The child is asked what they are doing while engaged in play or physical activities – "doing housework" and so on. They must answer in a two-word phrase, for example, "sweeping floor"; "dressing dolly".

Symbolic play sequences

The adult and child act out symbolic play sequences with large toys, and the child describes what is happening.

Object functions

Show the child various objects and ask, "What do we do with this?" The child answers "brush hair", "clean teeth". Hide the objects in a mystery bag to make this more fun.

Action pictures

The child is shown a picture of a person and then another picture of them performing an action. The child progresses from naming the pictures separately, "man", "digging", to a definite two-word phrase, "man digging".

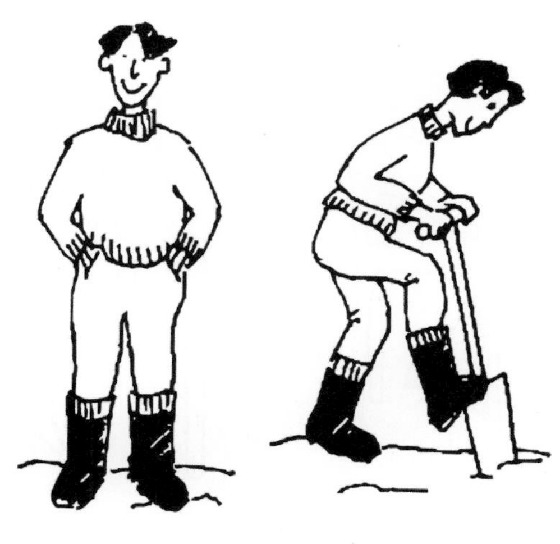

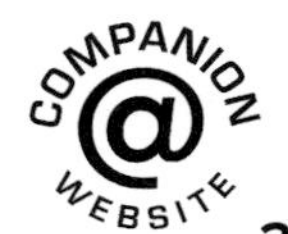

Picture pairs

Divided a book into upper and lower halves. Insert pictures of people or animals in the top section and pictures of actions in the lower section. They are encouraged to discuss which combinations can and cannot go together, for example, "man read" and "doggy read".

Picture books

Look for toddler picture books that show a picture of an object, for example, a bib, and on the opposing page a picture of somebody using the object, for example, a baby wearing the bib. The child is prompted to produce "baby bib".

Silly pictures

Make two packs of picture cards, one showing objects or people, and the other actions. Shuffle the separate packs and lay them face down. The child turns over the top cards in each pack, "reads" the sentence and judges whether it is "silly" or "proper".

Some amusing sentences can be created, for example, "eating teddy". The cards can be placed in different orders to create either agent-action relations or action-object/location relations.

Word-order games

Draw pictures to illustrate the importance of word order, for example, "fish eating" and "eating fish" have quite different meanings. The child must name them correctly (adapted from the Derbyshire Language Programme).

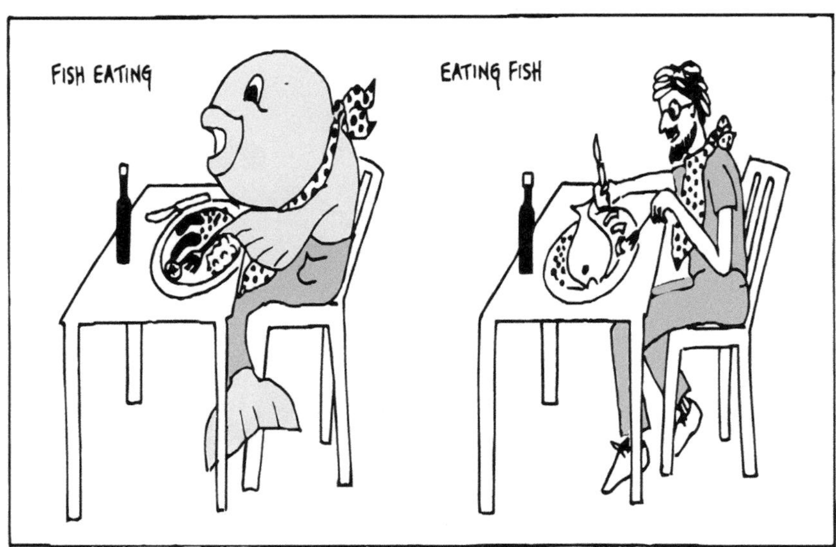

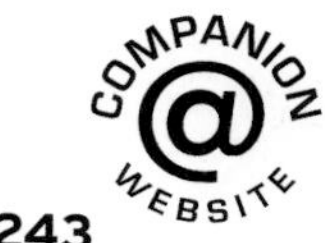

Commands and suggestions

Giving commands

The children take turns to give each other commands:

- Involving parts of the body, for example, "touch nose", "find ear".
- Involving actions, for example, "stand up", "touch wall", "sit down".
- Involving objects, for example, "cut paper", "throw ball", "open box".
- Involving musical instruments, for example, "bang the drum", "blow whistle".

Follow-my-leader

One child acts as the leader and performs lots of actions, the sillier the better, as they lead the others around the room, in and out of the furniture. They accompany their actions with verbal directions, and the other children copy them.

O'Grady says

Similar to follow-my-leader, but the children stand in a line facing the leader. Initially the child gives just the commands, "touch toes", and later adds the words "O'Grady says touch toes", which increases the length but not the complexity of their utterance. The proper rules can be introduced later for older children.

Dollies

The child gives teddy or dolly commands; using two dolls ensures that they have to use two words to specify both the action and who is to perform the action, for example, "Dolly sleep".

Tell dolly

The child gives teddy or dolly commands involving an object. This time only one toy is used so that the child can concentrate on the action-object relation, for example, "Eat lolly", "Wash car". When appropriate, another toy can be included.

Tea party

Have a tea party with the children telling each other what to do, for example, "Orange [in] glass", "Teddy [sit] chair". This can be done at mealtimes, breaks and during home-corner play.

Wizard

Take turns to be a wizard who turns everybody into animals who are in their power. "Monkeys, jump", "Lions, roar".

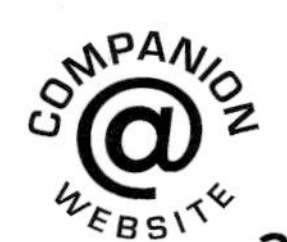

Request

Use the activities listed under the one-word utterances section to elicit two-word phrases. Teach the child several ways of expressing request, for example, "Give dolly", "Milk please", "Want play", "Need wee".

The activities given for single-word and two-word utterances can also be adapted to elicit three-word phrases.

Activities for older children

- *Leader* – each child has a chance to be "leader", telling the others what to get out for the day's activity, for example, "get pencils".
- Provide models during everyday routines and activities. Let the child have a turn at giving instructions or commenting to the group.
- Introduce activities that give an opportunity for words like action words, descriptive words and early prepositions so the child can use these to add to nouns.

Three-word phrases

The child should now be capable of commenting upon their constructional play while they are playing and using language to direct himself. They first describe what they are doing and then what they are about to do. The adult should model this for them by commenting on the things the adult is doing (commentary) or describing what the child is doing (parallel talk).

Aims

To facilitate development of simple sentence structures containing three or more words.

Outcomes

- Puts three to four words together to make a simple sentence.

Strategies

- Monitor your communication and language to ensure you provide a good model for the child.
- Avoid correcting any errors the child may make when repeating or attempting to join words in a phrase. Instead provide the correct model, for example, "bird eating" – "bird is eating a worm".

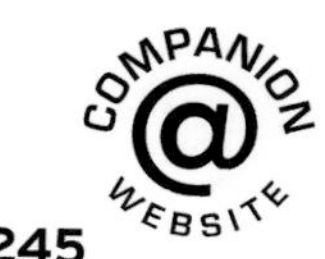

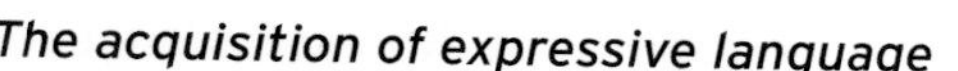

- Encourage carry-over of learning to other environments like the home by asking parents/caregivers to use target phrases in everyday routines and to respond positively to the child's attempts.
- Modelling, expansion and recasting would be useful strategies to implement.

Suitable materials and resources

Toys; teddies and dolls; doll's house furniture and figures; small world play material and floor layouts; dressing up clothes; action pictures; and picture sequencing cards.

Activities to develop three word phrases

Commands and requests

Name and instruction

To increase length without complexity, the child can give commands to other children, using their names. So instead of "touch the table" it becomes "Susan, touch the table!".

Instructions with toys

In a similar fashion the child gives commands to their toys, which can be given real names or called "horsie" and so on; for example, "Monkey drink juice".

'Give me' games

In a group game the children take turns to ask each other for toys and other objects. The phrase 'give me' remains constant, but the object changes. Later include other names, for example, "Give Hasan teddy" and "Give teddy drink".

Shopkeeper

Introduce a fantasy element; for example, three children take the roles of shopkeeper, parent and child. The parent/caregiver tells the child what to get at the shops, and the child asks the shopkeeper. This basic game can be varied by changing the role play scenario to a pet shop, restaurant and so on. The role plays can be built around themes to introduce or practise related vocabulary, such as foods, household items and vegetables. More imaginative children can play at spacemen, wizards, pirates, cops and robbers.

Moving house

Children take turns being in charge while the others are removal men, putting furniture into the house; for example, "Put oven [in] kitchen"; "Toilet goes [in] bathroom (adapted from Derbyshire Language Programme).

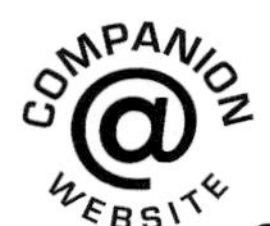

Commentary and description

Action songs

Simple action songs help the child express action relations in well-rehearsed routines.

For example,
Teddy Bear

Teddy Bear, Teddy Bear, dance on your toes

Teddy Bear, Teddy Bear, touch your nose

Teddy Bear, Teddy Bear, stand on your head

Teddy Bear, Teddy Bear, go to bed

Teddy Bear, Teddy Bear, wake up now

Teddy Bear make your bow.

Pancakes

Mix a pancake, stir a pancake

Put it in the pan,

Fry a pancake, toss a pancake,

Catch it if you can.

Large toys

The adult acts out situations with large toys while the child describes what is happening. If necessary, two elements can be held constant while the third is varied, until the child is consistent in their responses, for example, "Dolly making cakes"; "Dolly making picture"; "Dolly kicking ball"; "Teddy kicking ball"; "Teddy cuddle Dolly"; "Teddy push Dolly".

Because the child will often respond with a one- or two-word utterance, the adult must provide lots of models to give the child the idea that three words are needed. Do not correct their utterance but expand it. If the child does not produce three-word phrases after plenty of modelling, adapt the situation so that they must do so in order to make their message clear. This can be achieved by introducing a third person, a student, classroom aide or older child, who cannot see the action. The child has to describe the events to this person, who can question them if they are not being specific, for example, "But *who* is falling over?" "*What* is teddy eating?" The first adult is then free to help the child with their responses.

Miniature toys

The same activities can be carried out with miniature toys, Playmobile sets and doll's house furniture.

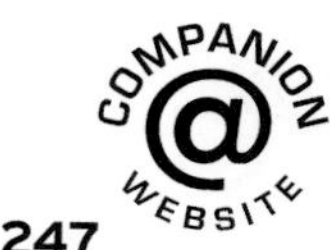

Action pictures

Clear action picture cards can be used to elicit the same constructions. Reusable sticker pads and books provide an enjoyable variation on the picture-description theme, because the child can arrange and rearrange the pictures to their own satisfaction.

Miming

The adult and children take turns to mime activities which the others try to describe.

Sequence of pictures

The adult draws a sequence of three pictures for the child to label. For example:

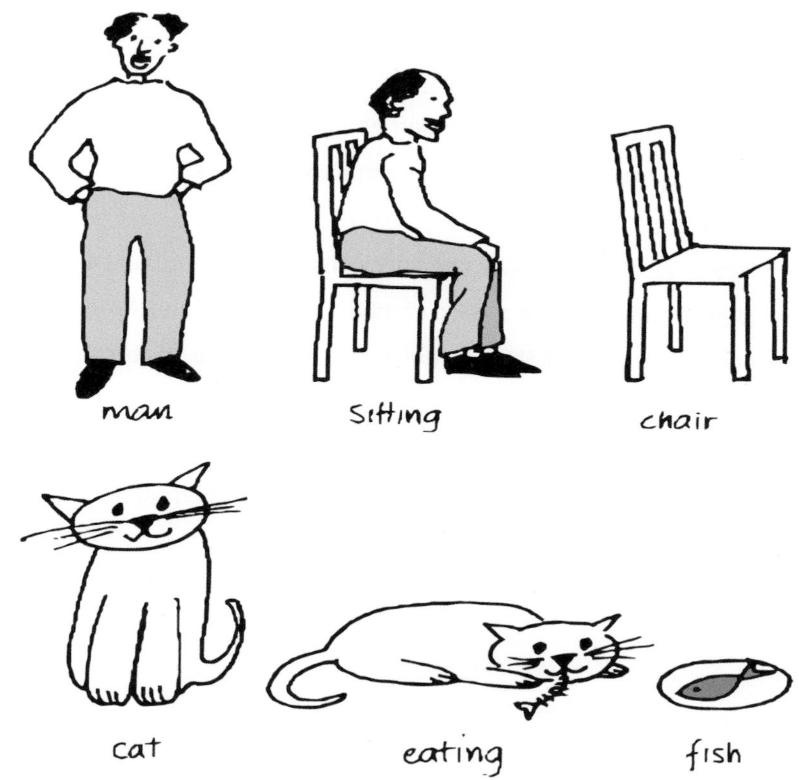

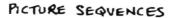

The child starts by labelling the pictures as they are drawn, producing them like successive single-word utterances, and then reads the completed strip as a whole. Each picture acts as a visual reminder.

Picture sequences

The child labels picture-sentences showing contrastive word order, for example, "lady stroking cat" and "cat stroking lady". Amusing cartoons can be made up for this purpose. You should try to discuss with the child the plausibility of each sentence.

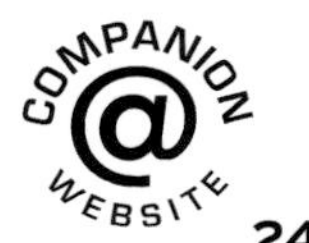

Large floor layouts

Use large floor layouts of a zoo, a farm, a house, a park or a street scene. The child moves model figures around the layout, saying "man go shop", "car drive garage".

Painting and drawing

The child tells the adult what to paint, draw or make, for example, "man kicking a ball" "man wearing brown trousers", "woman driving big car".

Activities for older children

Three-word phrases can also be produced by expanding a constituent the child already uses, for example, expanding a noun-phrase by adding a possessive or attribute: when the child says "car go", the adult can model "the blue car go".

- *Follow-my-leader:* During gross motor games like 'follow-my leader' or O'Grady Says', the child has to be more specific in their commands, for example, "Touch Sally's toes"; "Climb the big slide".
- *Dressing up:* Two piles of identical or similar clothing are placed on the floor. Two children have to race to put them on while a third child gives instructions, for example, "Put on red hat", "Put on green blouse". If they forget to say the whole sentence, they are replaced by another child. A variation of this for children who can cope with losing is to have only one pile of clothing, and the winner is the child who ends up wearing the most.
  The other children get the opportunity to practise related language such as "Come on", "Hurry up", "You're winning" etc. and to support the children by calling their names.
- *Action songs*: Action songs that involve adjectives, for example:

My Red Engine
My red engine goes Chuff Chuff Choo, Chuff Chuff Choo.
My shiny drum goes Rum Tum Tum, Rum Tum Tum.
My Teddy Bear goes Grr Grr Grr, Grr Grr Grr.
My wooden bricks go pitter patter, pitter patter, rattle, bang, CRASH!
(Make up your own lines to use the adjectives you want to practise.)

One Red Engine
One red engine
Puffing down the track.
One red engine
Puffing back.

One blue engine, etc.
One dirty engine, etc.
One wooden engine, etc.

- *Hiding games*: The adult and children take it in turns to hide a collection of objects around the room. The hider then calls out which object is to be found first, and the others race to find it. Make sure that the child needs to use a possessive or attribute to specify the object, and take care that the child is familiar with the vocabulary.
- *Hidden pictures:* Pictures are hidden around the room or stuck onto the wall. As in the previous game, the hider calls out a picture, and the first to spot it brings it to them. To give everybody a chance to find a picture, each winner can sit out the next round. Ensure that there are as many pictures or objects to find as there are children playing. An alternative is for the adult to slowly uncover a picture and the child guesses what it is. Afterwards they describe the whole picture, for example, "Man wearing red hat".

Beyond the three-word phrase

The length and complexity of utterance can be gradually increased by continued expansion of both noun and verb phrases and by combining whole utterances. To do this successfully the child needs to learn grammatical morphemes and new vocabulary, including prepositions and adverbs. Novel words and constructions should first be introduced in shorter, simpler utterances, for example, the child should be taught "Mummy in kitchen" before they are expected to say "Mummy washing up in kitchen".

'In' and 'on'

Start with the preposition 'in' and when the child can consistently express this, introduce 'on'.

Aims

To encourage the use of the prepositions 'in' and 'on' in a range of sentence structures.

Outcomes

- Uses 'in' and 'on' appropriately to express position of objects.

Strategies

- Start with activities that involve the child in physical play where they experience different spatial positions as they hear and use the prepositions.

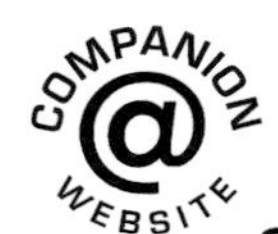

- Monitor your communication and language to ensure you provide a good model for the child.
- Provide lots of repetition of target prepositions in a variety of different contexts that include everyday routines, physical activities, pretend play, picture books, songs and stories.
- Encourage carry-over of learning to other environments like the home by asking parents/caregivers to use target prepositions in everyday routines and to respond positively to the child's attempts.
- Further generalise understanding by using target prepositions in simple phrases and commands. Keep the rest of the words in the phrase redundant so the child focuses on the preposition.

Suitable materials and resources

Toys; teddies and dolls; doll's house furniture and figures; sports day equipment for races; obstacle course equipment; small world play material; story books; and complex pictures.

Activities to elicit 'in' and 'on'

Daily activities

Be sure to emphasise the prepositions as they occur naturally during the day's activities, for example, when sticking the children's paintings *on* the wall, or mixing eggs *in* a bowl. Comment on what you are going to do and ask prompting questions, such as, "Where shall we mix the eggs?" or "What shall we put the eggs in?" This will depend upon the children's level of comprehension.

Hiding games

Gather some toys for hiding. Organise the room so that as many different hiding places as possible can be used. Early on it is best for 'in' to refer to a definite container, for example, cupboard, box, bag or barrel, and later to more abstract places such as a ring, a square marked out on the floor, or the corner. One child or more are the seekers and leave the room while the other children hide the toys in the room. The seeker/s returns and must call out where they think the toys are hidden, "in the box"; "on the cupboard".

Hide and seek

Play a traditional hide and seek game. Give the child a few minutes to find their friends, and then they must call out where they are.

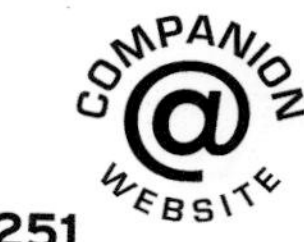

Races

Hold races that emphasise different prepositions, for example, a sack race focuses on 'in' (the sack); an egg-and-spoon race focuses on 'on' (the spoon); and so on.

Obstacle course

Set up an obstacle course that mixes up the two prepositions, for example, the child has to go *in* a hoop, on a bucket, in a bin and on a box. The others shout out the instructions in unison. This can be turned into a race against time (use an egg timer or stop watch) or a race between children.

Child gives instructions

The child tells the adult or other children where to put things away, for example, "That goes *in* the cupboard"; "Put the cups *on* the shelf".

Naughty puppet

A "naughty" puppet does all the wrong things, for example, pours the tea in the bath, puts a book in the bin and so on. The child must keep repeating the instruction until the puppet gets it right.

Hide a toy

The children take turns to hide a soft toy, for example, a Snoopy dog, and the others try to find it. If they cannot find it, the child who has hidden it has to tell them where it is.

Home corner

Setting up and rearranging the home corner or doll's house is useful for preposition work. The child and adult discuss how to arrange the furniture, and the child can direct the adult in what to do.

Miniature toys

Act out symbolic play sequences with miniature dolls or Playmobil to encourage the use of prepositions, for example, a dolly tea-party; "Pour the tea *in* the cup"; "Put plates *on* the table, Mummy". Other symbolic play themes can include:

- Shopping: putting the food *in* the bag.
- Putting baby to bed: *in* the bed; put *on* pyjamas.
- Getting dressed: put *on* your jumper.
- Doctors: medicine *in* the bottle; *in* hospital.

Reusable pictures

The child tells the adult where to stick pictures onto a reusable sticker pad or book or Fuzzy Felt board, or what to draw; for example, "Put flowers *in* the garden"; "Put roof *on* house".

Pictures with movable parts

Make special pictures with movable parts, for example, you can draw a bedroom with a cupboard that has opening doors, which reveal the clothes inside, and a duvet that comes off the bed. Ask the child questions – for example, "Where's the little cat?" "Oh he's in the bed" – as you lift up the duvet.

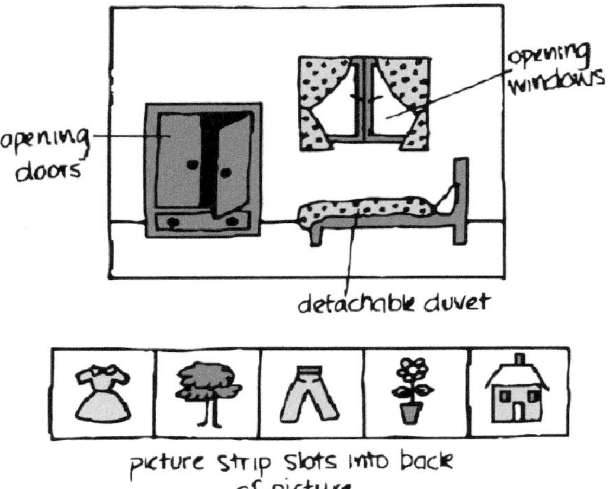

Picture description

The child describes what they see in pictures illustrating different prepositions in response to the adult's 'where' questions. Pop-up books, reusable sticker pads or books, and jigsaws make interesting variations of this.

Stories

Tell stories emphasising the prepositions and ask the child questions such as "Where was Goldilocks?" Answer – "*in* baby bear's bed". Progress from well-known stories to inventing your own.

Activities for older children

All these activities can be adapted to elicit more difficult prepositions later on. "Under" is usually the next to be understood.

- Washing day: a miniature line with doll clothes can be put up; or draw and cut out clothes to stick on to a washing line in a book, using Blu-Tack. The child gives instructions, "Hang the trousers *next to* the shirt".
- Obstacle courses: crawling *under* benches, ducking *under* ropes and other actions can be incorporated to practice the preposition. (See Chapter 4 for more ideas that could be adapted to practise using prepositions.)

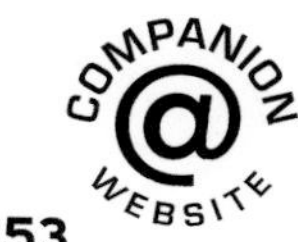

Regular plural

A plural noun indicates that there is more than one person, object, animal, toy and so on, and in English this is usually marked by adding 's' (or 'es') to the end of the noun. These words are known as regular plurals. Some nouns that do not follow this rule are known as irregular plurals where the word might remain the same, for example, 'sheep', or some letters may change or be added, as in 'man/men' and 'child/children'.

Aims

To encourage attention to and practice in the production of regular plurals.

Outcomes

- Produces simple plurals by adding 's'.

Strategies

- Make sure the child understands the concept of 'more than one' before you start to teach language production.
- Monitor your communication and language to ensure you provide a good model for the child.
- Provide feedback to the child that illustrates the importance of signalling the difference between singular and plural, for example, offering one 'shoe' when they say shoe but mean 'shoes'.
- Avoid correcting any errors the child may make instead recast or reformulate their response to include the regular plural.
- Encourage carry-over of learning to other environments like the home by asking parents/caregivers to provide opportunities to practice plurals in everyday routines and to respond positively to the child's attempts.
- Further generalise understanding by using target plurals in simple phrases and commands.
- Modelling and role reversal would be useful strategies to implement.

! Some children with a speech sound difficulty may not be able to produce the /s/ sound, and this may not be a realistic or achievable goal for them.

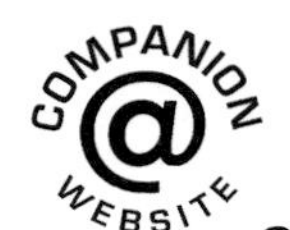

Suitable materials and resources

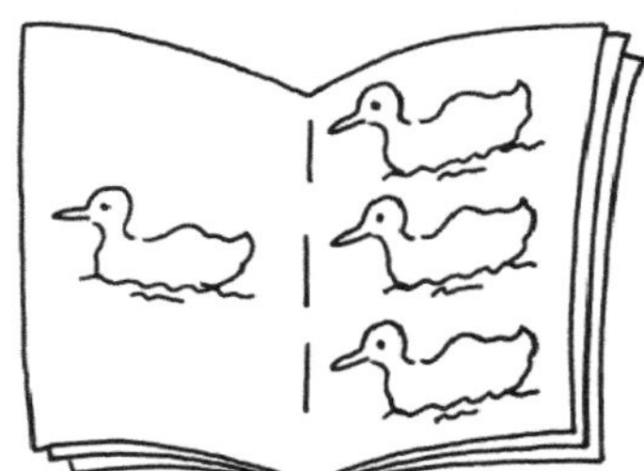

Paired items of clothing; pairs of objects (clothing); pairs of similar toys (cars, teddies); rhymes and songs that include plurals.

Activities to elicit the regular plural

Daily routines

The child can be taught the regular plural by contrasting one object with many objects. The contrast may be emphasised by making results contingent upon what the child says; for example, if they ask for "chip" at lunch-time, give them one chip. If they say, "Do shoe up", say "Just one shoe?" and do one shoe up and wait. The same goes for "Play with brick now", and so on. Be sure to model the correct structure when the child indicates that they want more than one object.

Noah's ark

Noah's ark is full of animals, which of course must always travel in pairs. The child must ask for the different animals, so give one if they ask for "cow" and two if they ask for "cows".

Rhymes

Rhymes, songs and finger plays encourage attention to and practice of plurals.

For example:
Ten Green Bottles
Ten green bottles
Hanging on the wall.
Ten green bottles
Hanging on the wall.
If one green bottle should accidentally fall,
There be nine green bottles
Hanging on the wall, and so on until there are no green bottles.
Try alternatives like "Ten fat sausages sizzling in a pan".

Five Little Frogs (a finger play)
Five little frogs sitting by a well,
One looked in and down they fell.
Four little frogs sitting by a well... and so on until all the frogs are in the well.

Dressing up

Dressing up and getting dressed or undressed are useful activities to elicit plurals because shoes, socks, tights and gloves usually come in pairs. The child can tell the adult

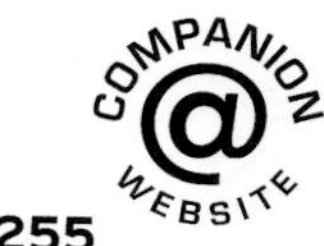

or another child what to put on. Dressing a cardboard doll with paper clothes can be used in the same way.

Books

Make a book with a picture of one object on one page, and on the facing page, many identical or similar objects. This gives the child a visual clue as they name each picture. Using a phrase such as 'lots of' helps to reinforce the plurality, for example, "a flower – lots of flowers".

Activities for older children

- Give instructions in the classroom that provide practice in listening for plurals.
- Encourage the child to request items during cooking. Use recipes that require more than one of something, like two eggs or three apples.
- Once the child has mastered the regular form of plurals, start to introduce irregular plurals.

Possessive (-s)

The possessive form expresses a relationship of belonging between one thing and another. To form the possessive (-s) is added to singular nouns preceded by an apostrophe (the apostrophe occurs after the (-s) in plural nouns).

Aims

To encourage attention to and practice in the production of possessive (-s).

Outcomes

- Marking the possessive by adding 's' to singular and plural nouns.

Strategies

- Monitor your communication and language to ensure you provide a good model for the child.
- Avoid correcting any errors the child may make; instead, recast or reformulate their response to include the regular plural.
- Encourage carry-over of learning to other environments like the home by asking parents/caregivers to provide opportunities to practice possessives in everyday routines and to respond positively to the child's attempts.
- Modelling, forced alternatives and role reversal would be useful strategies to implement.

Some children with a speech sound difficulty may not be able to produce the /s/ sound, and this may not be a realistic or achievable goal for them.

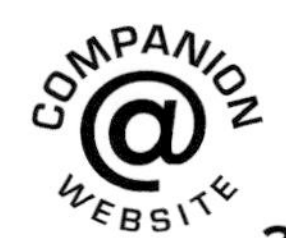

Suitable materials and resources

Picture story books; dressing-up clothes for dolls; everyday possessions of the children.

Activities to elicit possessive (-s)

Simon Says

This can be introduced into the activities already described earlier, for example, "Simon says – touch Nicky's arm". Children take it in turn to be the leader and give instructions.

Questions

Use picture book stories to model the structure for the child. Ask questions concerning possession, for example, "Whose bed is this?" Answer – "John's". Adapt stories like *Goldilocks and the Three Bears* and *The Three Little Pigs* to include phrases with possession.

Picture book

Make a picture book with a person or animal on one side and an object (acting as a possession) on the other. It is best to start with common associations, for example, a baby and a bottle; a firefighter and a hose; a dog and a bone.

Wash day

The child undresses their dolls and teddies and pretends to wash and iron their clothes. Afterwards they sort them out, saying "That's teddy's jacket; dolly's socks", and so on (adapted from the Derbyshire Language Programme).

Board game

Make a board game divided into large squares, each with a colourful picture of an unusual dwelling place. The children throw a dice to move their counters round the board and name the picture they land upon, for example, "I'm in the monster's cave". The board could be made to follow a fairy tale such as *Jack and the Beanstalk* incorporating "the giant's castle", "the old lady's room", "Jack's beanstalk" and "Jack's cottage", and so on. Rules could then be added to follow the story; for example, each player is a character from the story and must try to get home first.

Activities for older children

- Whose is this? – the children sort out possessions ready for an activity, for example, their workbooks, shoes for sport. Children can take it in turn to ask the question.
- Classroom instructions – incorporate instructions into the day that involve possession. For example, talking about "Danny's picture", "Sarah's picture".

Tense

Once the child can express a sense of time by talking about things that have happened or what they are about to do, they may be ready to learn the appropriate tense markers.

Aims

To encourage attention to and practice in the production of tense markers for past and future tense.

Outcomes

- Marking tense appropriately for past and future tense.

Strategies

- Encourage the child to talk about things that have happened or what they are about to do, even if they haven't mastered the correct grammatical forms for tense.
- Monitor your communication and language to ensure you provide a good model for the correct tense forms for the child.
- Avoid correcting any errors the child may make; instead, recast or reformulate their response to include tense markers.
- Encourage carry-over of learning to other environments like the home by asking parents/caregivers to provide opportunities to practice tense forms in everyday routines and to respond positively to the child's attempts.
- Modelling, commentary, parallel talk and role reversal would be useful strategies to implement.

Suitable materials and resources

Small world material; story books; cartoons/films; verb tense photo cards; comic strips.

Activities to elicit tense

Past tense

It is easier for the child to express the immediate past (Reynell, 1977).

Daily activities

When the child has completed an activity, talk about what they have just done, modelling the past tense form: "You painted a picture?" Send them to tell another adult or child what they have just done.

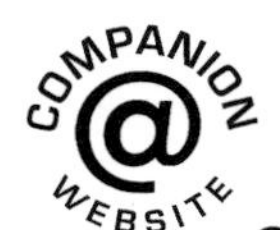

Gradually move on to the child learning to talk about things in the recent but not immediate past. Gradually increase the delay between the completion of an action and the child talking about it; for example, when the child has made a plasticine model, ask them to tidy up *before* you ask them what they have been making.

Spontaneous

Use any spontaneous incident to elicit the past tense; for example, if an aeroplane flies overhead, tell the children to listen and ask them about it afterwards.

Miniature dolls

Set up play situations with miniature dolls; for example, pretend it is dolly's birthday. Act out a sequence. Afterwards ask the child what happened using open-ended questions. Give the toys to the child to act out a role play and ask you questions.

Action pictures

Contrast past and present in action pictures. There are lots of commercial verb tense photo cards. Play a hiding game where you take turns to find pictures.

Stories and rhymes

Tell the children a simple story or nursery rhyme (using the past tense), which they then act out to help them remember the story. Afterwards they must retell the story. Start with familiar tales and rhymes.

Pick up time

When the child is collected by their parent/caregiver, help them to tell her what they have been doing. Pick out the most memorable activity.

Vary activities

Make sure that children have the opportunity to do slightly different things so that they can tell each other what they've been doing.

Story books

Share stories that use the past tense. Try *Be More Bernard* by Simon Philip and Kate Hindley.

Composite pictures

Tell the children the story happened yesterday. Ask them to describe what happened.

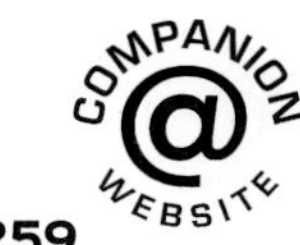

Film

Show a short children's film or cartoon if you have access to the necessary equipment and discuss it with the children afterwards. The programmes must be short and interesting. Rerun the action so the children can check how much they remembered.

Outings and visits

Let the children act out and talk about outings, visits and special occasions that have recently taken place. Pictures can be used as visual prompts to ease the load on the child's memory and allow them to concentrate more upon the linguistic forms. Use a digital camera or iPad to take images on the trip.)

Future tense

The child can be taught to use adverbials such as 'yesterday' and 'tomorrow' to express time, before the appropriate syntactic forms are used.

Asking ahead

Encourage attention to the immediate future by asking the child what they would like to play with, drink, eat, wear.

After a routine

When the child has finished an activity and discussed it, ask them what they are going to do next. Teach the forms "I'm going to" and "I want to", which are less complex than using the modals "I will" and "I shall".

Act out with small toys

Act out situations with miniature toys and ask the child "What is going to happen next?" For example, play at families with miniature dolls, setting a scenario for the child. "Baby is getting very tired – what should Mummy do?" Encourage the child to make a scenario and ask questions.

Acting out sequences

Carry out activities with the child that must follow a particular sequence, for example, "getting dressed", "making a cake or cup of tea", and at each stage ask the child "What shall I/we do now?" Do the same with other activities that the child usually carries out in a certain order. Encourage the child to use a similar structure to ask for advice.

Picture books

Picture books can be made to show people who are about to perform actions on one page and people in the process of performing them on the opposite page, for example, a footballer about to take a penalty, and taking the penalty; a plane about to take off, and flying. The child is helped to progress from expressing the present, for example, "The plane is on the ground", to the future, "The plane is going to fly".

Sequential stories

Use commercially produced packs of sequential story cards either in line drawing or photographic form, which vary from easy to very difficult. After the child has placed the pictures in the correct order, tell them the story. Once they can sequence them without error, they are ready to tell the story himself. Teach words such as "then" and "next" to help the sequence flow. Make sure the child sticks to the same tense throughout the story.

PICTURE-BOOK FOR PRESENT AND FUTURE TENSE

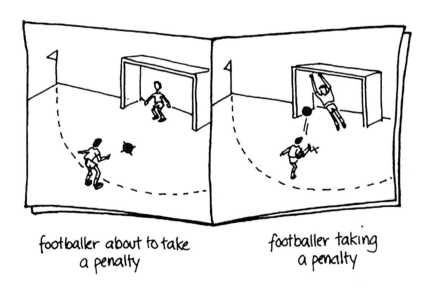

footballer about to take a penalty

footballer taking a penalty

Comic strips

Use comic strips and cartoons in a similar way to the sequential stories. They can be left in their strips or cut up for the child to sequence.

Shopkeepers

The child tells you what they are going to buy from the "shop", and this is then acted out immediately, for example, "Mischa is going to buy carrots". Food photo cards are very useful to prompt the child.

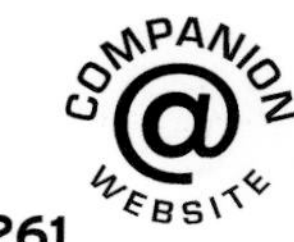

Rehearsal

Role plays can be used to rehearse a real situation, for example, going to a real sweet shop or going to the pictures. This can lead on to planning ahead using phrases with "I am going to …".

Drill games

Tomorrow: the adult and children play question-and-answer drills, turned into a game or chant.
Adult: "What will you buy tomorrow?"
Child: "I'll buy a new coat tomorrow"
Adult: "What will you eat tomorrow?"
Child: "I'll eat a nice apple tomorrow."
Adult: "Who will you visit tomorrow?"
Child: "I'll visit the queen tomorrow."
Actions can be added to the words.

Picture description

When the child can express present, past and future events, all three can be contrasted in picture form, for example, in tense photo cards or cartoon images.

Activities for older children

- Use timelines to help children understand the concept. Link this with the written word.
- Set up a time machine (This could be an arch to represent a portal). Time travellers might go forward or backward in time. They need to recount their role plays using the correct tense form.
- Children listen to a recorded story. Afterwards they can discuss the content and retell the story.

Wh- and open-ended questions

These questions help the child with conversation skills, as they are important for starting and maintaining interactions. They are also useful tools in planning and researching information about topics.

Aims

To develop understanding a range of question forms from simple to complex.

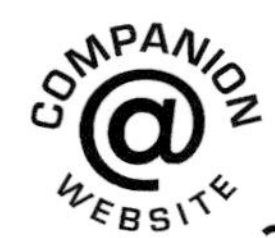

Outcomes

- Uses simple questions like 'What?' 'Where?' and 'Who?'
- Uses more complex questions like 'Why?' and 'How?'

Strategies

- Model asking and responding to questions during everyday activities, but make this a natural part of the interaction. Avoid overwhelming the child with too many questions.
- Model a range of spoken responses to questions so the child starts to make a connection between a question and what it achieves.
- Show the child you are listening carefully to their questions.
- Be flexible and allow for questions and responses to generate further questions.
- Model the use of questions that build on language already used by the child.
- If everything is always as children expect it to be and if they never have any problems, their questions can become very stereotyped and limited. Genuine questions should not be ignored, or the child may become discouraged.
- Commentary and parallel talk are useful strategies to implement.
- The linguistic form of questions may need to be modelled many times.

Suitable materials and resources

Puppets; pretend doll play material; picture cards; photographs; and picture story sequences.

Activities to elicit Wh- and open-ended questions

Mealtimes

Each child has an opportunity to be in charge at mealtimes and ask the other children what they would like to eat and drink.

Class monitor

Similarly, a child is put in charge of sharing out the toys or equipment for creative arts and asks each child what they need for an activity.

Hiding games

The adult and children take it in turns to hide around the room or in an outside play area. The seeker must ask the hiders where they are: "Where are you Sam?" Each child takes it turn to be the seeker.

Pretend doll play

The child asks teddy and dolly questions during the course of their play. The adult should answer for the toys. Themes like mealtime, bath time, and dressing will provide a stimulus for asking questions.

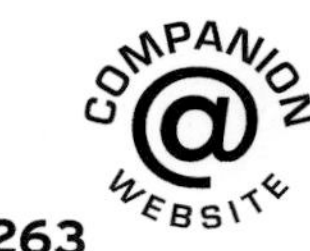

Puppets

The child asks a puppet questions while the adult takes the puppet's part in responding.

Action games and rhymes

Action games and rhymes such as *Queenie, Queenie, Who's Got the Ball? What's the Time, Mr Wolf?* and *Ding-dong Bell, Pussy's in the Well*, elicit questions as part of the game.

Show and tell

The adult and children have sessions where they ask each other questions, for example, about their family and pets, their favourite music, foods, stories and animals, what they did at the weekend or on an outing.

Role play

Help the children to set up role plays where the main characters have to ask questions. This could be a vet asking questions about a pet; a doctor asking a patient questions; or a postal worker in a post office asking about parcels.

Story books

Share books with the child that encourage repetitive use of question forms like *Brown Bear, Brown Bear, What Do You See? Where's Spot?*, '*What's That Noise, Spot?'* and *Goldilocks and the Three Bears*.

What's wrong?

There are several commercial *What's Wrong*? cards. Children usually enjoy the ridiculous pictures and can take turns to ask "What's wrong?"

Activities to elicit yes-no questions

Guessing games

- The child thinks of something in the room and the others try to guess what it is. Their guesses will usually be fairly concrete.
- 20 Questions: as in the previous suggestion, but the children have only 20 guesses between them. At a higher level, they should be encouraged to ask "Is it big?" "Is it an animal?" and so on.
- The children guess what is wrapped up in a parcel.
- The adult draws a silhouette of an object for the children to guess.
- The children try to guess what object is being mimed.
- The children listen to a recording of common everyday sounds or animal noises and try to guess what is making them.

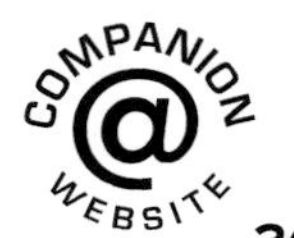

- The children are shown common objects photographed from an unusual angle and have to guess what they are.
- The children pretend to be animals, and the others ask "Are you a lion?" etc.

Activities for older children

- Why/because picture cards – use cause and effect pictures cards to help the child to express causal relations. This leads on to the appropriate use and understanding of "Why?" questions.
- Set up a problem-solving situation to prompt questions – sometimes new toys and games can be introduced and not explained in detail to the children. Children can be prompted to ask questions to find out how things work.
- Solving hypothetical situations: these must be made fairly concrete with plenty of visual clues to prompt the child. Read a story about a child who loses their money, breaks a vase, etc. and ask the children what they would do and why in the same situation. They can challenge each other's answers using questions.

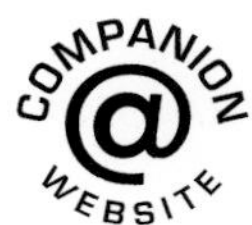

RECORD SHEET

Expressive language

Name: **Review date:**

Outcomes	Comments

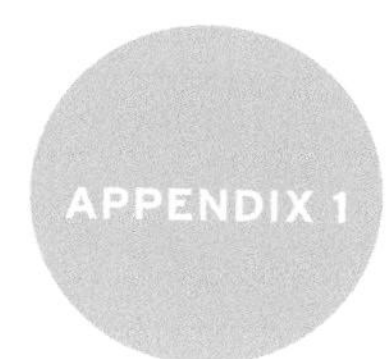

SUMMARY OF DEVELOPMENTAL STAGES

AGE RANGE	DEVELOPMENTAL MILESTONES
0-1	Pays fleeting attention to objects, people and events, and easily distracted by new stimuli **Ch1 Ch2** Turns to a familiar voice (6m) **Ch1** Enjoys social play in proto conversations with parent/caregiver **Ch1** Definition of use or functional play with objects (12m) **Ch1 Ch3** Use of deictic gestures with eye gaze to direct attention of others (8–10m) **Ch1** Development of joint attention by 12m **Ch1 Ch2** Shows understanding of 'no' and bye-bye (9m) **Ch1** Follows simple requests used in daily routines (9–12m) **Ch1 Ch4** Understanding of single words for everyday objects when used with gesture (9–18m) **Ch1 Ch4** Make sounds, cooing, gurgling and babbling, especially when spoken to (6m) **Ch1** First recognisable words (9–18m) **Ch1 Ch5**
1-2	Rigid attention to an activity of their own choosing. Concentrates intently on an activity or object for a short period of time. Needs to ignore other stimuli, especially noises or speech **Ch1 Ch2** Coordinated joint attention as child shifts attention between the object and the adult **Ch1 Ch2** Enjoys games like pat-a-cake and peek-a-boo (12m) **Ch1 Ch2 Ch3** Enjoys songs and rhymes and tries to join in with actions or vocalisations **Ch1 Ch2** Relates real objects to large doll material. Talks to a toy phone (15–18m) **Ch1 Ch3** Looks or turns when they hear their name called (12m) **Ch1 Ch2** Recognises familiar objects by name without contextual cues (15–18m) **Ch4** Understands between 200 and 300 words by 24m **Ch4**

AGE RANGE	DEVELOPMENTAL MILESTONES
	Follows simple instructions like "Show me your nose" **Ch4** Use words about familiar objects and people (12-18m) and able to say 50-100 words at 18m **Ch4**
2-3	Attention is single channelled, so they need to stop activity and listen. Prefers own choice of activity but will attend to adult choice of activity **Ch1 Ch2** Early pretend play with toys and dolls **Ch1 Ch3** Parallel play alongside other children with little concept of sharing **Ch3** Follows longer instructions with three key words or three separate pieces of information **Ch2 Ch4** Shows understanding of some simple prepositions (in, on, under) **Ch4** Understands simple What? Where? and Who? questions **Ch4** Selects pictures in response to questions like "Which one is eating?" **Ch4** Spoken vocabulary of 200-300 words (24m) **Ch5** Putting two words together, "more juice", using action words as well as nouns (18-24m) **Ch5** By 36m produces short two- and three-word phrases (36m) **Ch5** Able to have a simple conversation **Ch3 Ch4 Ch5**
3-4	Able to shift focus of attention between task and adult, but still needs to either 'listen' or 'do' **Ch2** Plays with other children, joining in play and sharing (36m) **Ch3** Understands, and able to talk about, play involving pretence, "this brick is baby's cup" **Ch3** Enjoys early make-believe play involving role play with other children **Ch3** Identifies objects by function **Ch4** Understands and often uses descriptive words for colour, basic shapes and size ('big' and 'little') **Ch4 Ch5** Knows 'in front of' and 'behind' **Ch4** Understands Who? What? Where? and Why? that ask for more specific information (36m) **Ch4** Grammatical morphemes emerge for plurals, tense, superlatives and comparatives (30m-46m) **Ch5** Use longer sentences and link sentences together with 'and' and 'because' **Ch5** Listens to simple stories with pictures, anticipating and joining in with key phrases (30-50m) **Ch4 Ch5**

AGE RANGE	DEVELOPMENTAL MILESTONES
4-5	Listens to spoken instructions without interrupting task. Concentration span is still short **Ch2** Listens to longer stories and answers questions about what they have heard **Ch2 Ch4 Ch5** Retells an event using the correct order **Ch2 Ch4 Ch5** Understand language for sequential ordering and time like 'first', 'after', 'before' and 'last' **Ch4** Knows more complex prepositions 'between', 'above', 'below', 'top' and 'bottom' by 4–4½ y **Ch4 Ch5** Understands more abstract terms ('soft', 'hard', 'rough', 'smooth') and knows nearly all colours (54m) **Ch4** Understands talk about past and future events **Ch4** Understands and responds appropriately to 'how' and 'why' questions **Ch4 Ch5** Use of conjunctions like 'when', 'so', 'if' **Ch5** Enjoys make-believe play and uses language to organise themselves **Ch3 Ch4 Ch5**
5-6	Integrated attention is well established and sustained **Ch2** Takes turns in longer more complicated conversations **Ch4 Ch5** Uses long and complex sentences that are fully formed with few if any grammatical errors **Ch5** Enjoys listening to stories and will retell a story or make up their own **Ch3 Ch4 Ch5** Enjoys imaginative play where they take on different roles and develop their own storyline **Ch3** Uses language to frame this play, take on roles and to negotiate with other children **Ch3 Ch4** Uses language to problem solve and organise thinking **Ch4 Ch5**

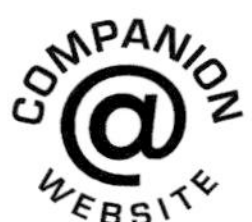
COMPANION
@
WEBSITE

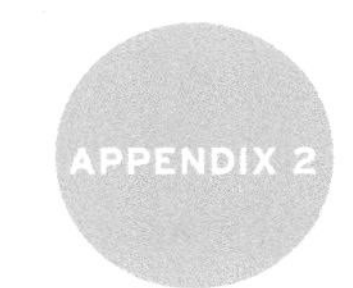
APPENDIX 2

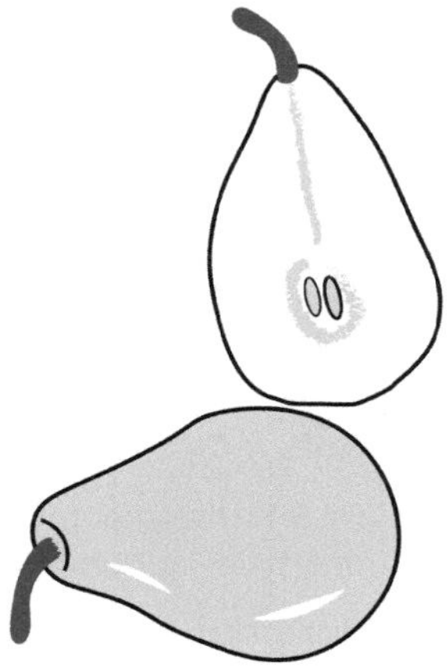

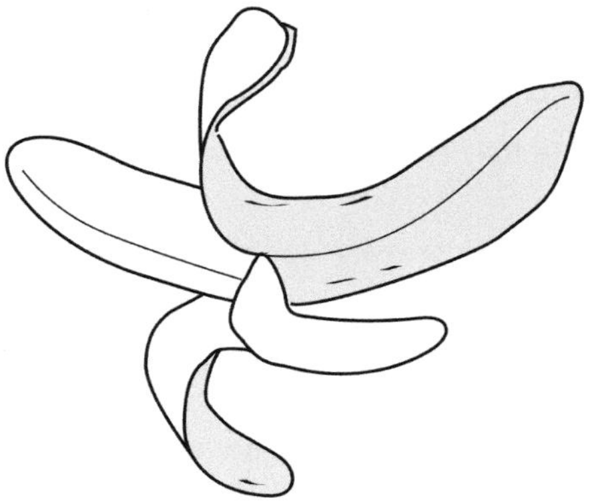

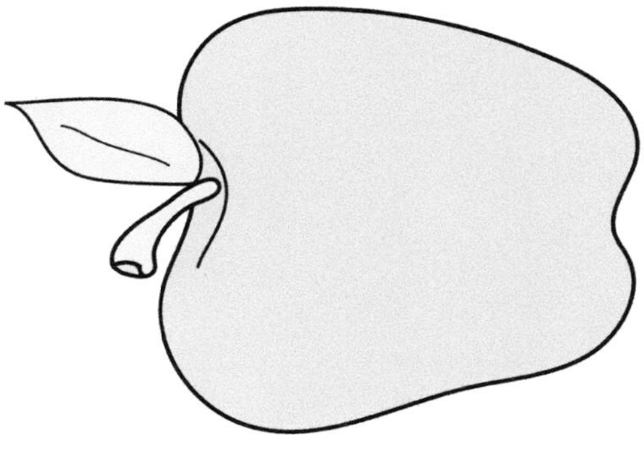

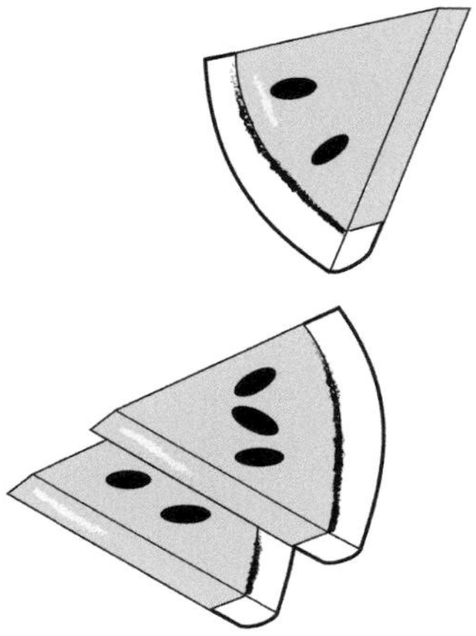

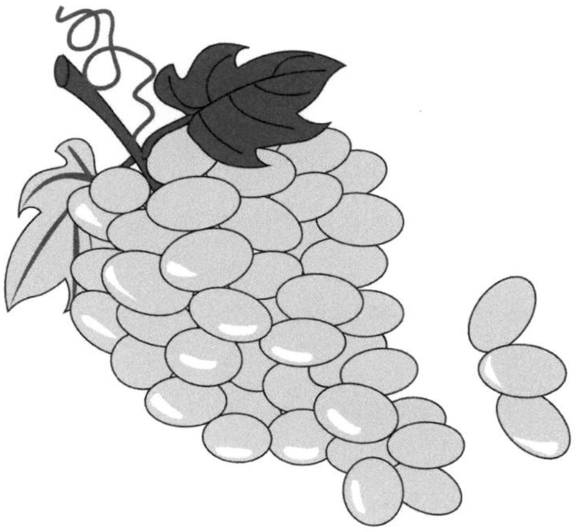

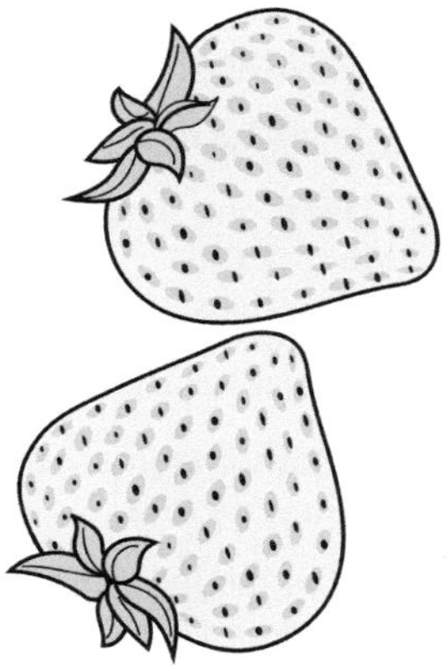

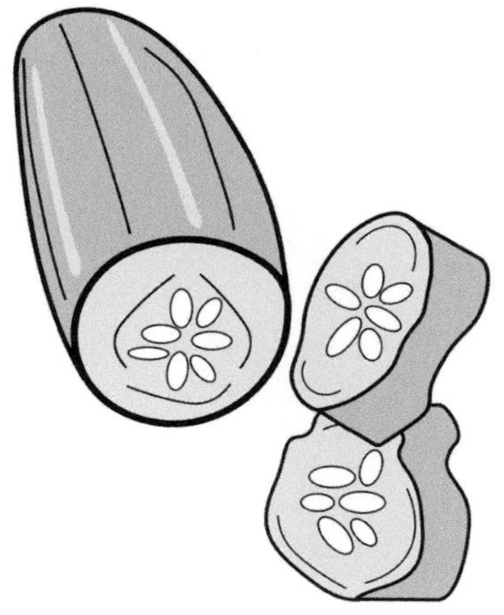

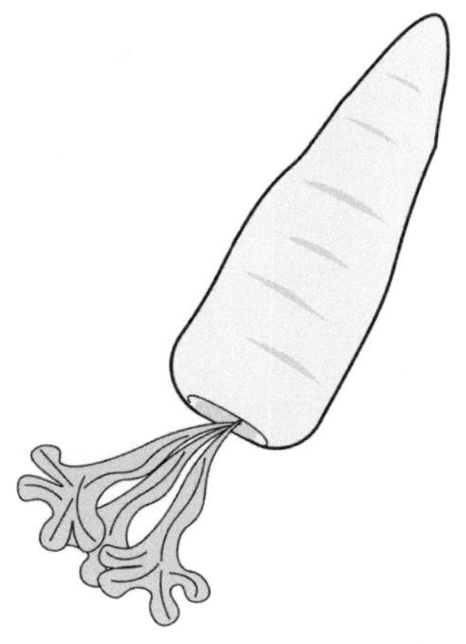

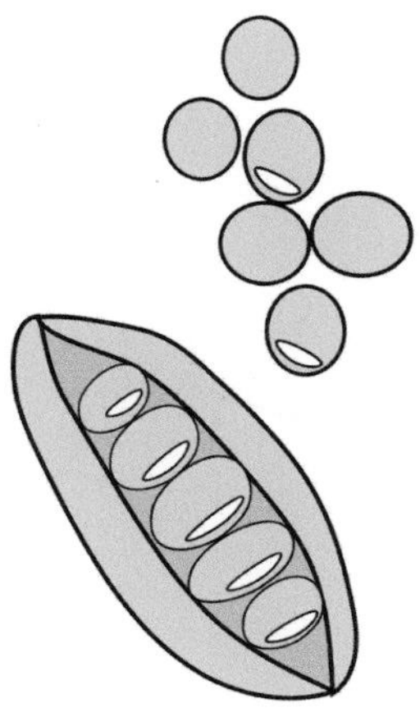

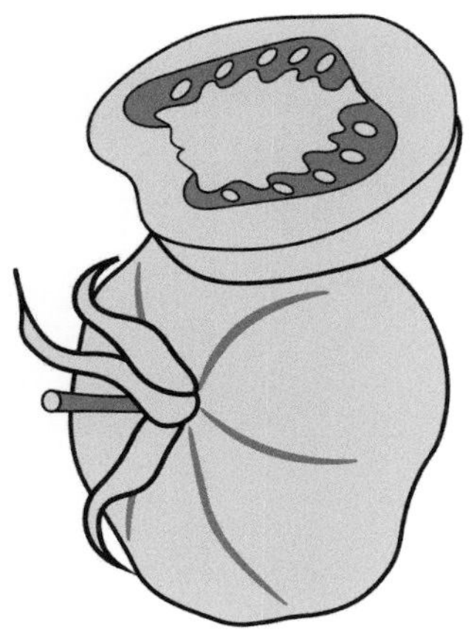

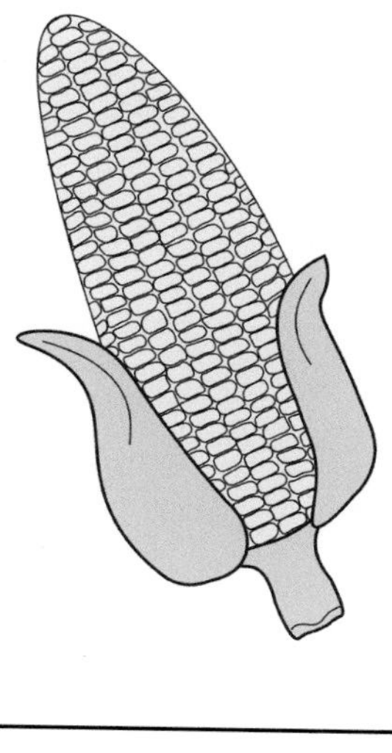

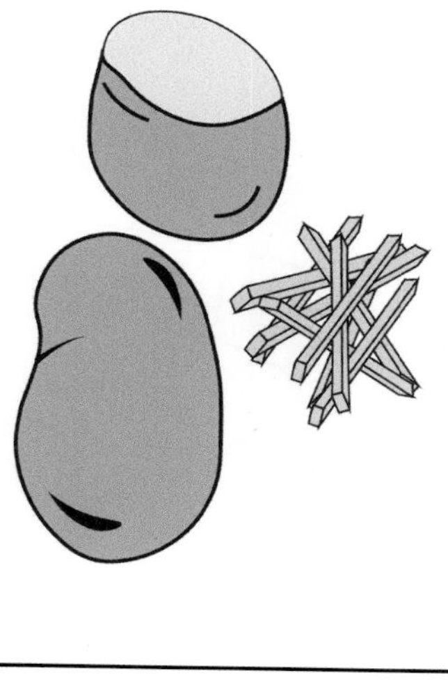

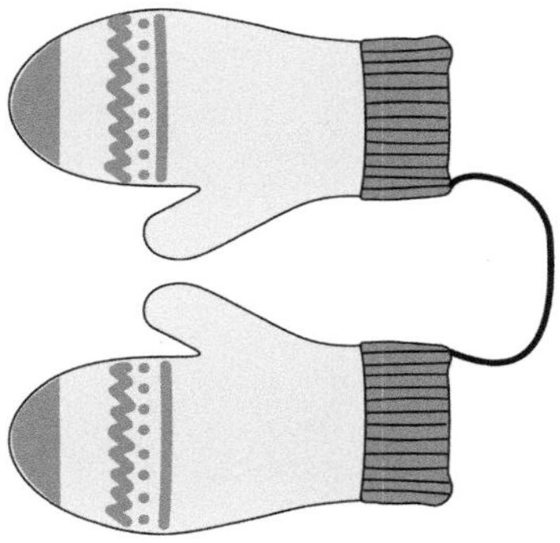

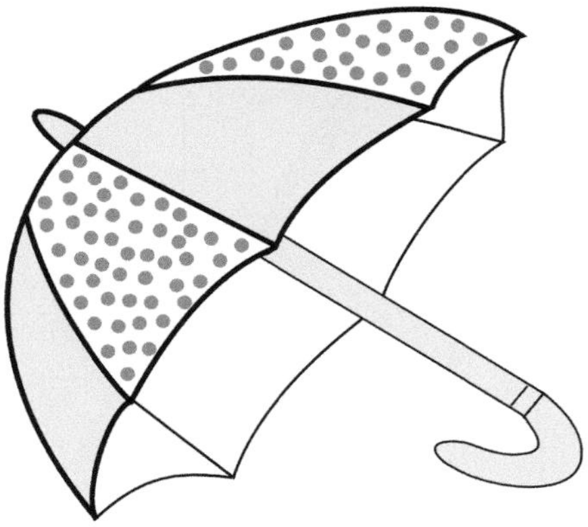

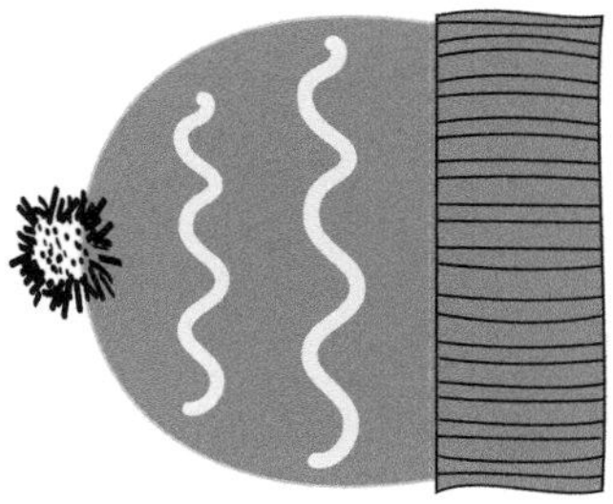

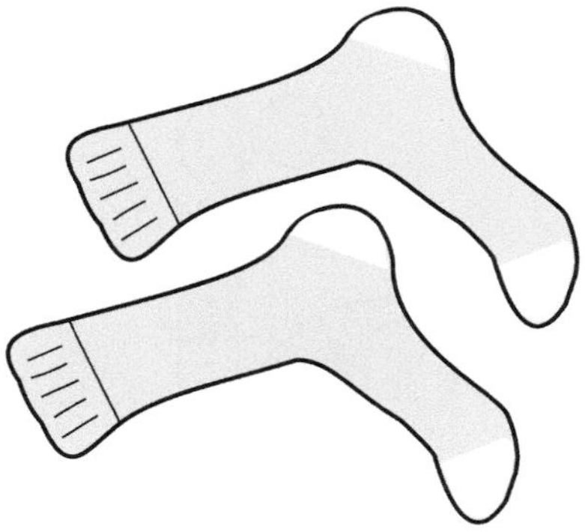

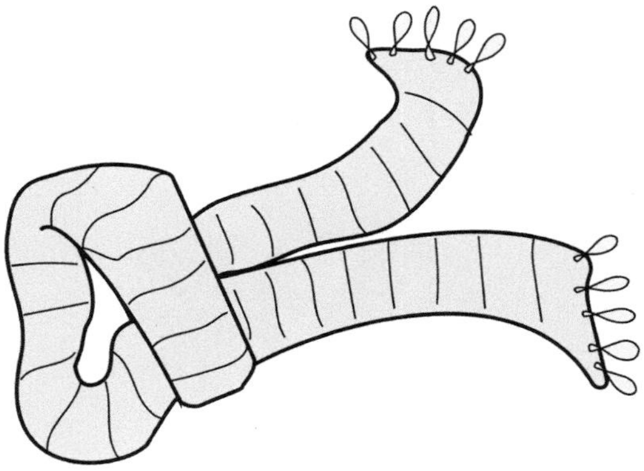

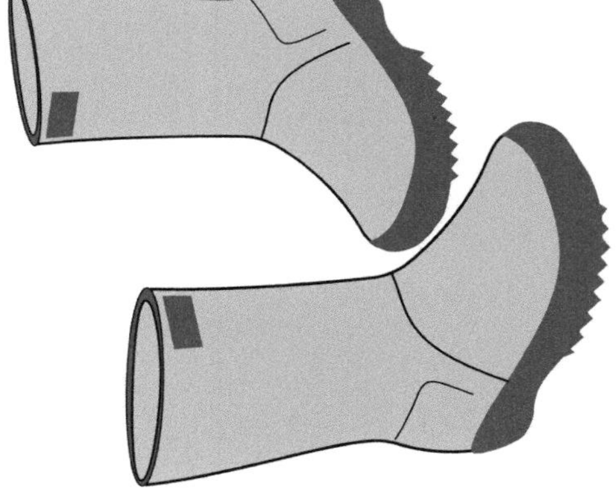

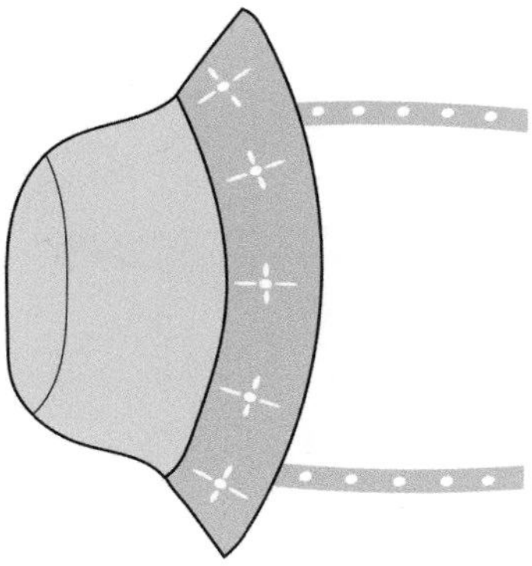

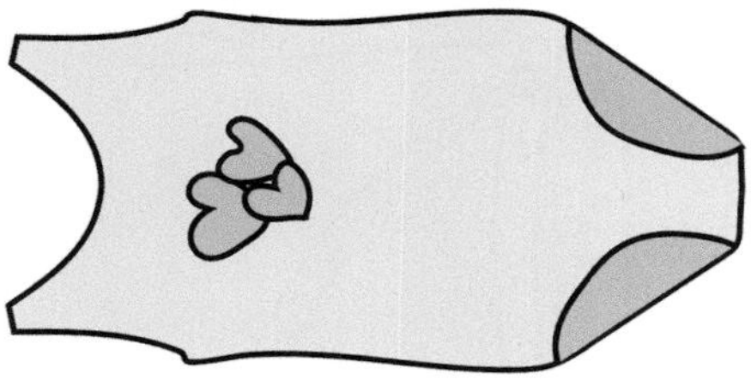

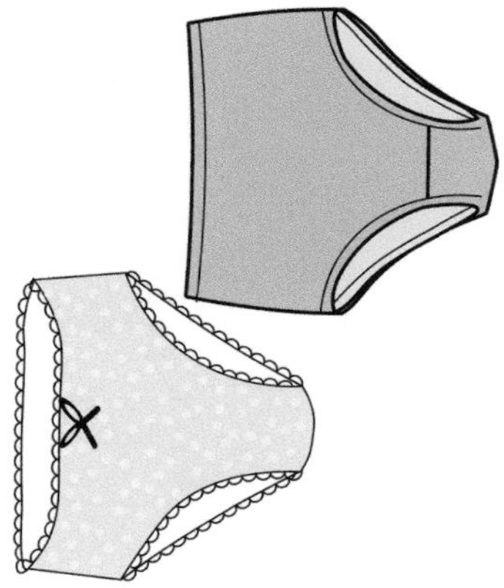

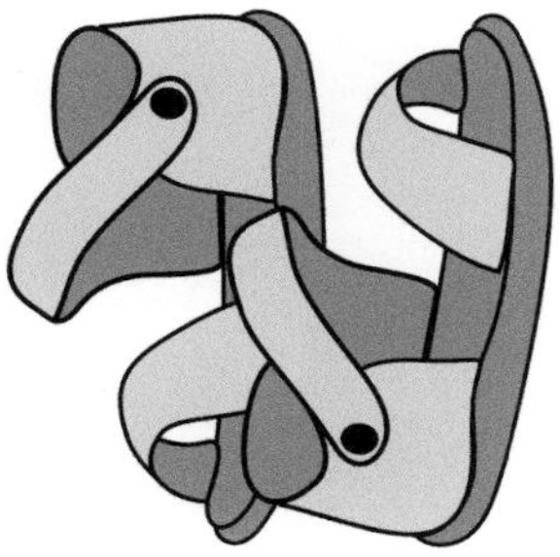

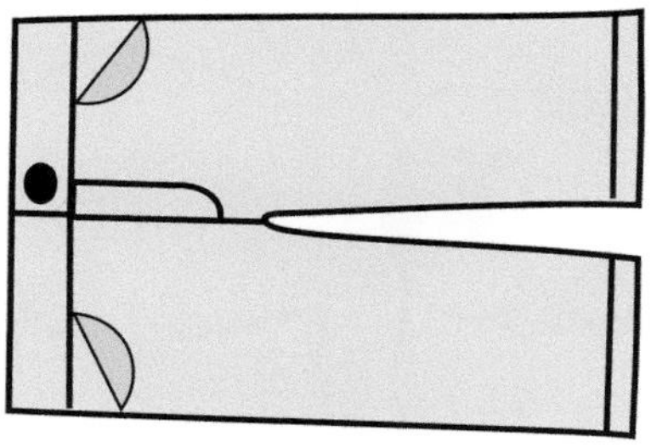

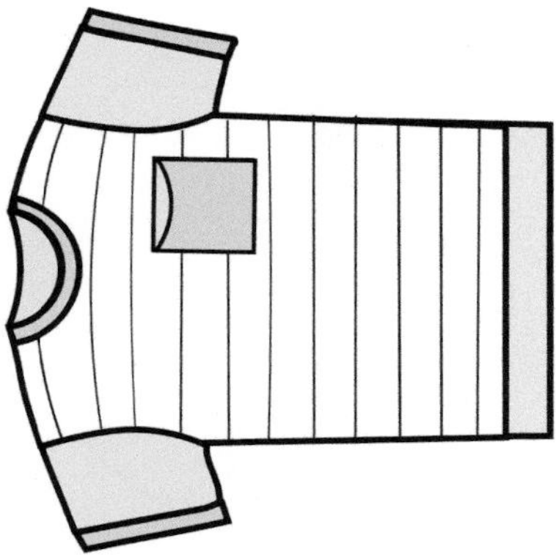

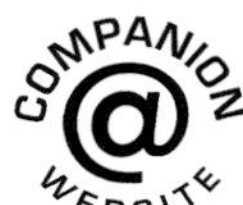
COMPANION
@
WEBSITE

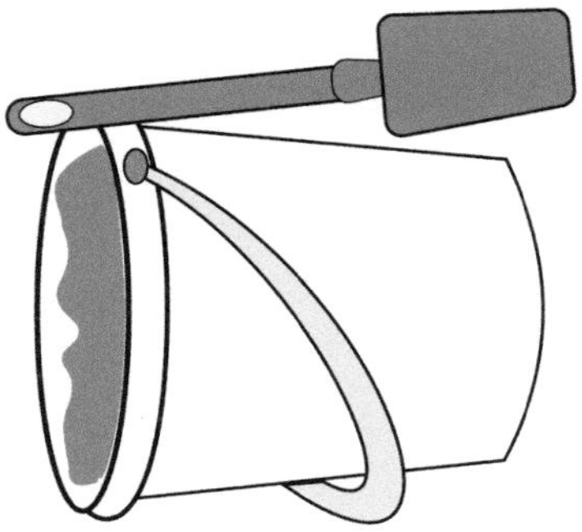

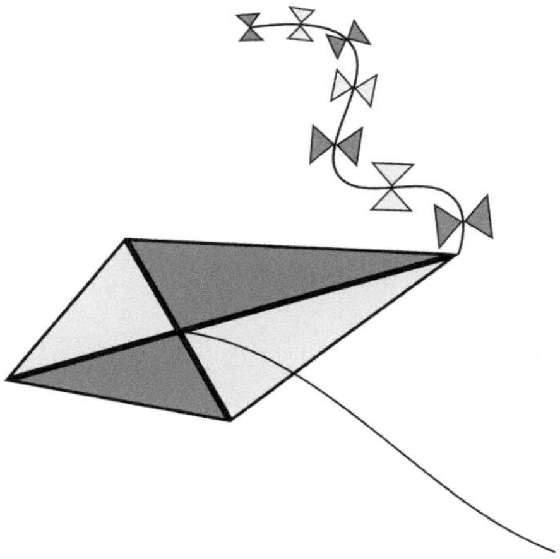

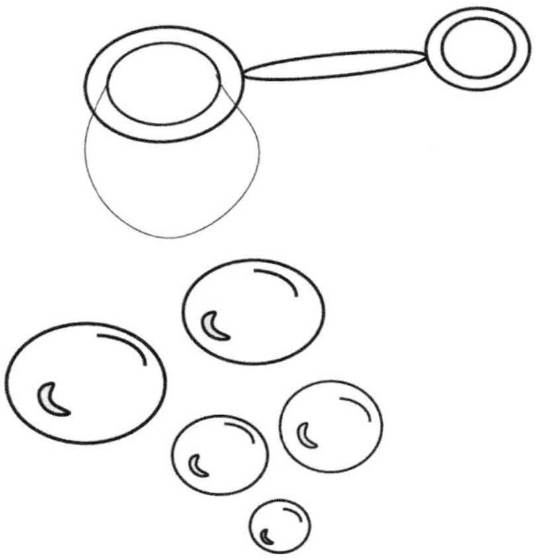

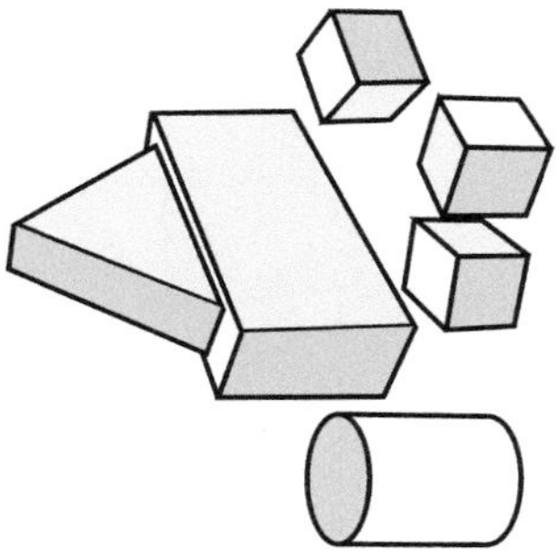

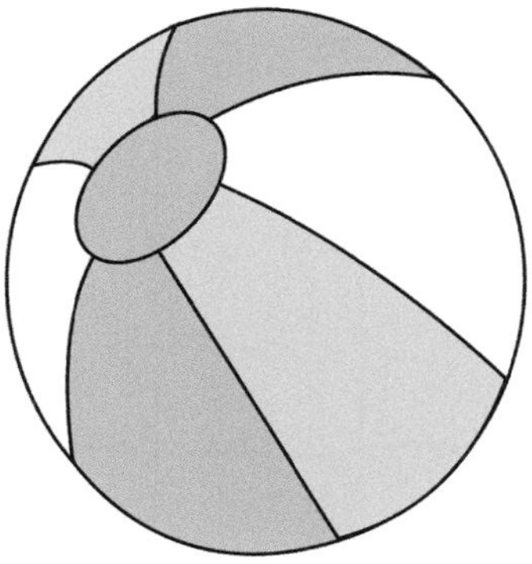

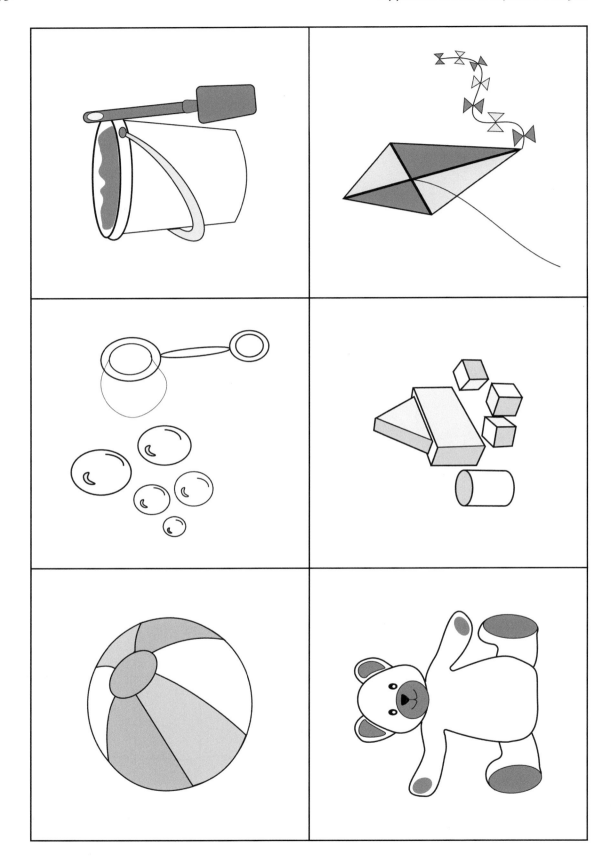

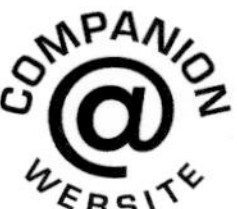
COMPANION
@
WEBSITE

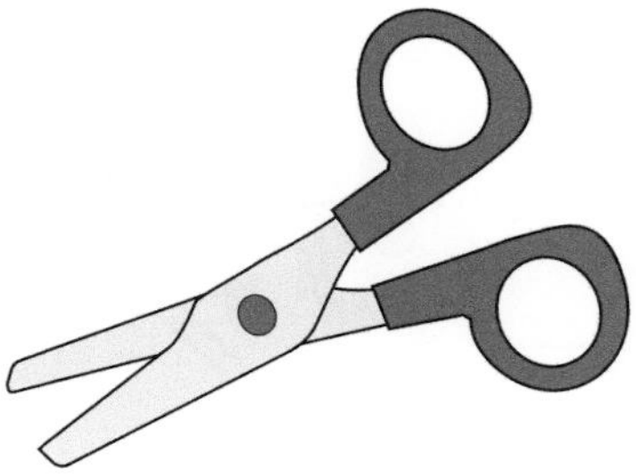

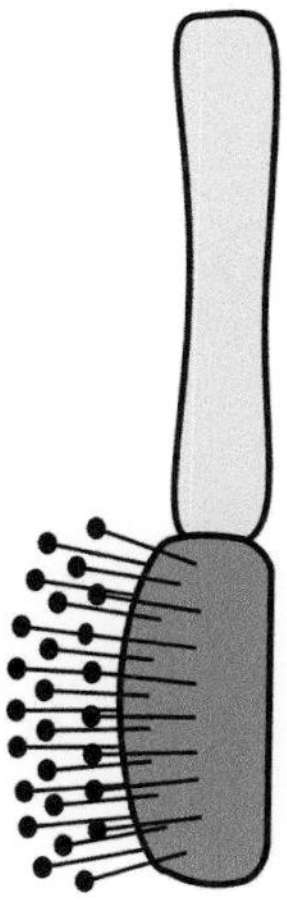

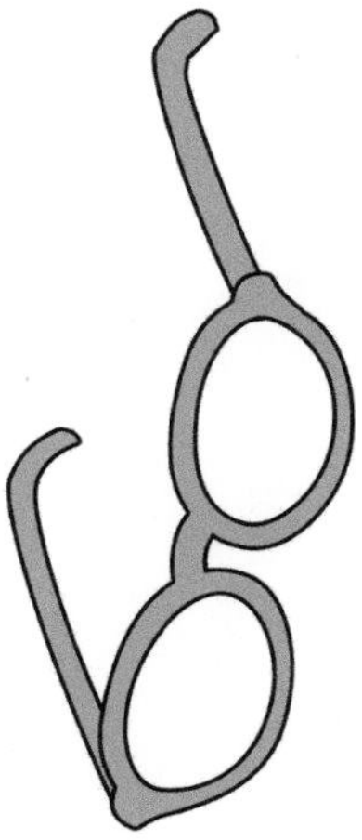

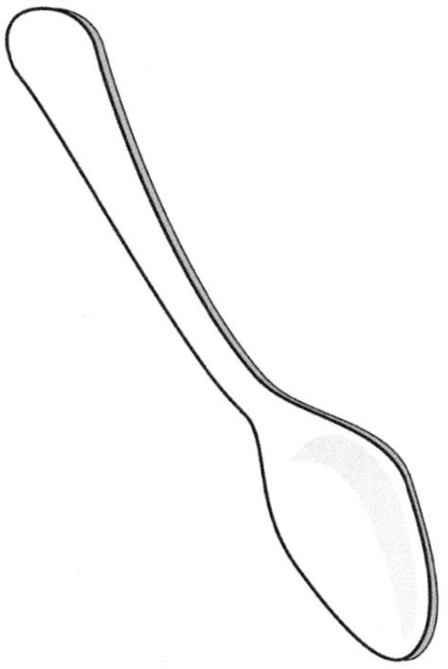

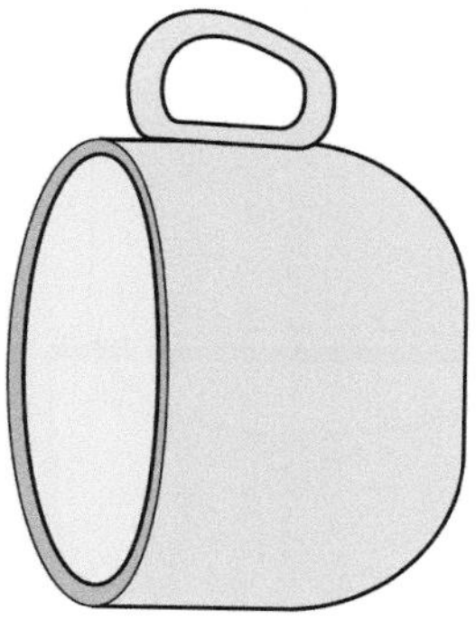

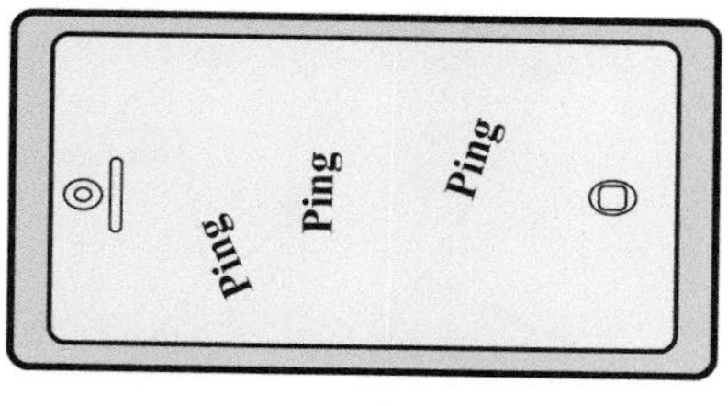

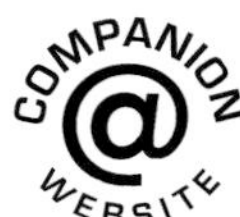
COMPANION
@
WEBSITE

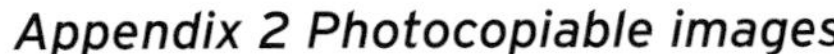

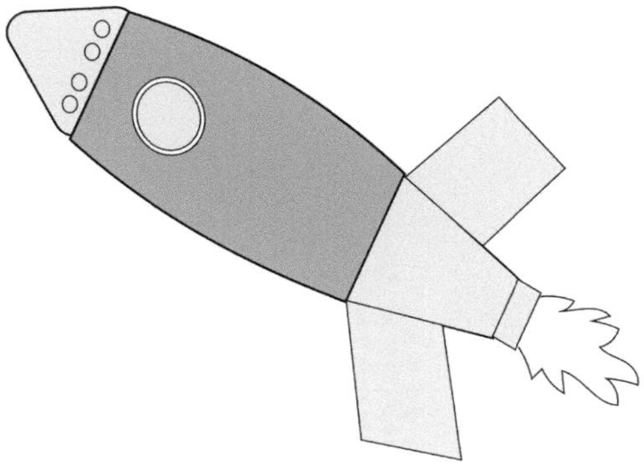

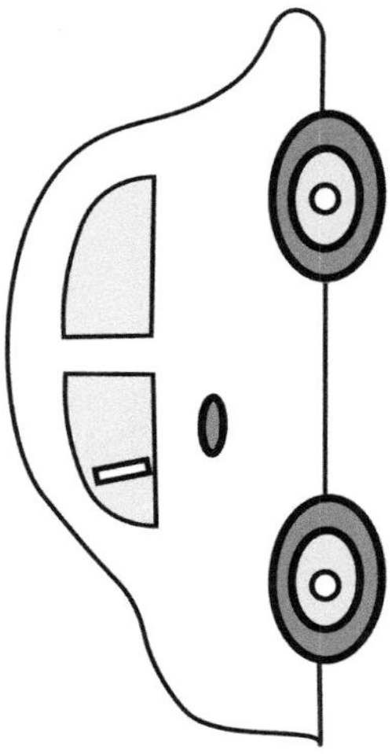

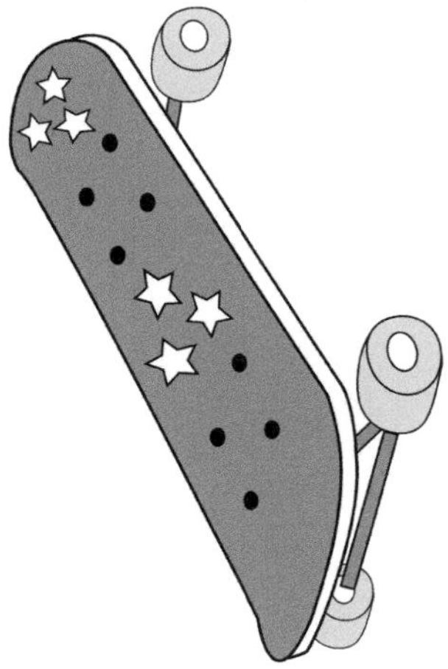

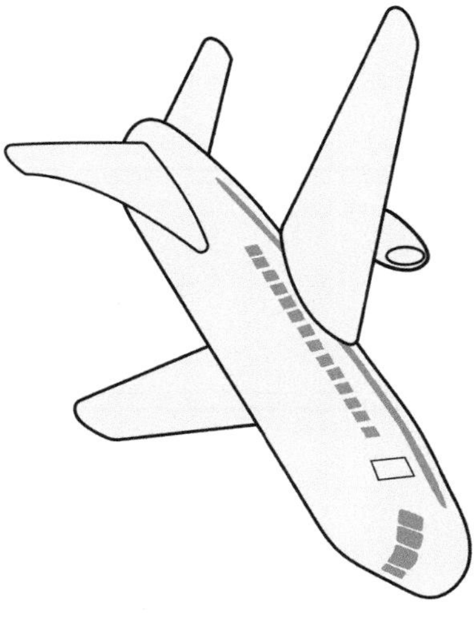

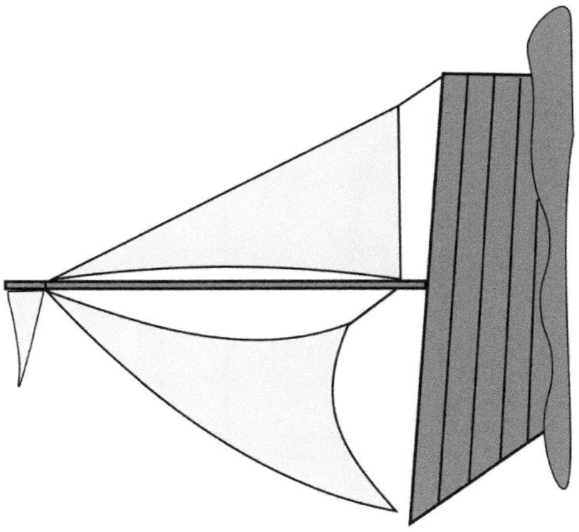

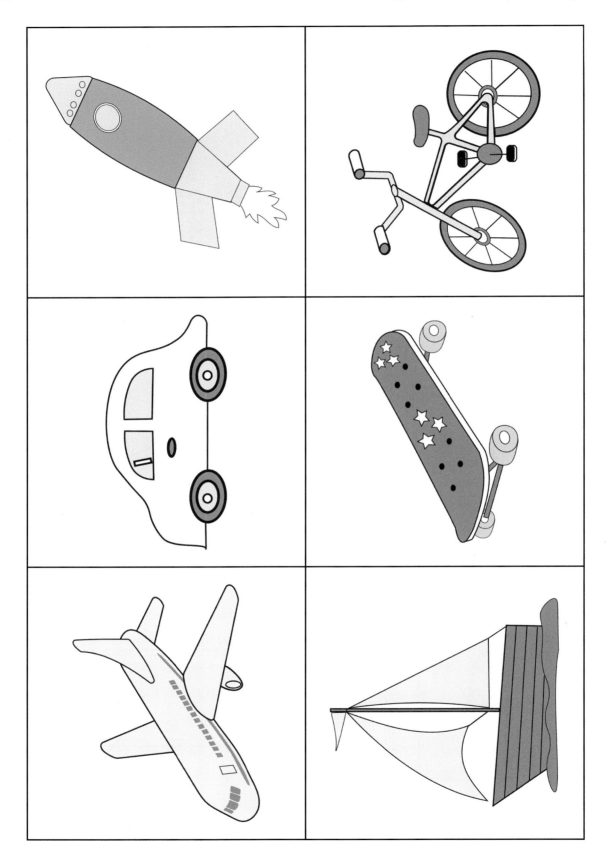

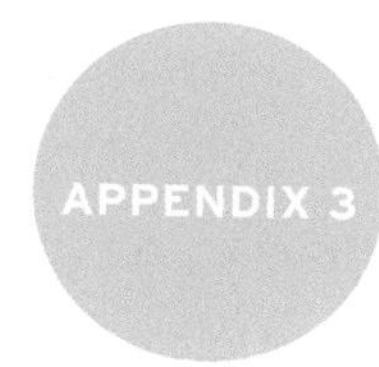

RESOURCES

Toys, materials and equipment are available from the following companies:

Consortium

142B Park Drive
Milton Park
Milton
Abingdon
Oxon OX14 4S
www.consortiumeducation.com

Early Learning Centre

Boughton Business Park
Bell Lane
Little Chalfont
Amersham
Buckinghamshire HP6 6GL
www.elc.co.uk

Hope Education

2 Gregory Street
Hyde
Cheshire SK14 4TH
www.hope-education.co.uk

LDA

2 Gregory Street
Hyde

Cheshire SK14 4TH
www.ldalearning.com

Sensory Education Limited
Unit W1
Westpoint Business Park
Middlemore Lane West
Aldridge WS9 8DT
www.cheapdisabilityaids.co.uk

Speechmark
Routledge| Taylor & Francis Group
2-4 Park Square
Milton Park
Abingdon
Oxon OX14 4RN
www.routledge.com/go/speechmark

TFH
Special Needs Toys
Unit 5-7 Severnside Business Park
Severn Road
Stourport-on-Severn
Worcestershire DY13 9HT
www.specialneedstoys.com

Winslow Resources
Goyt Side Road
Chesterfield
Derbyshire S40 2PH
www.winslowresources.com

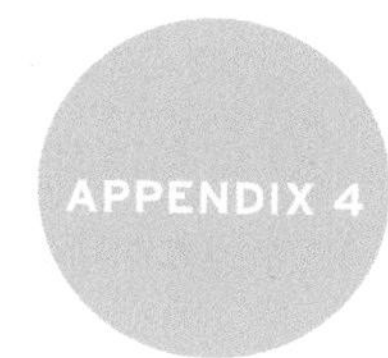

USEFUL ADDRESSES

AFASIC

St Margaret's House
15 Old Ford Road
London E2 9PJ
www.afasic.org.uk

A parent-led organisation providing information and support services for children and young people with speech, language and communication disabilities and their families.

I CAN

31 Angel Gate (Gate 5)
Goswell Road
London EC1V 2PT
ican.org.uk

A communication charity supporting children and young people's speech, language and communication needs (SLCN), providing information and resources for families and professionals at ican.org.uk/i-cans-talking-point/

MENCAP

123 Golden Lane
London EC1Y 0RT
www.mencap.org.uk

The Royal Mencap Society is a charity supporting people with a learning disability, and their families and caregivers.

National Autistic Society

393 City Road
London EC1V 1NG
www.autism.org.uk

A charity providing support, guidance and advice for people on the autism spectrum and their families, as well as campaigning to protect the rights and interests of autistic people.

National Deaf Children's Society

Ground Floor South
Castle House
37–45 Paul Street
London EC2A 4LS
www.ndcs.org.uk

A charitable organisation of professionals and parents working together to support deaf children and young people in overcoming the social and educational barriers that hold deaf children back.

RADLD

RADLD provides information and resources to raise awareness of developmental language disorder.
www.radld.org

The Royal College of Speech & Language Therapists

2–3 White Hart Yard
London SE1 1NX,
www.rcslt.org

The professional body for speech and language therapists and support workers in the United Kingdom provides information for the public about speech and language therapy.

BIBLIOGRAPHY

Adamson, L.B. (2019) *Communication development during infancy*. Abingdon, Oxon: Routledge.

Aljahlan, Y., & Spaulding, T.J. (2019) 'The impact of manipulating attentional shifting demands on preschool children with specific language impairment', *Journal of Speech, Language, and Hearing Research*, 62(2), pp. 324–333.

Apicella, F., Chericoni, N., Costanzo, V., Baldini, S., Billeci, L., Cohen, D., & Muratori, F. (2013) 'Reciprocity in interaction: A window on the first year of life in autism', *Autism Research and Treatment*, 2013, pp. 1–12.

Baddeley, A. (2007) *Working memory, thought, and action*. Oxford: Oxford University Press. Oxford psychology series: Vol. 45.

Barkley, R.A. (2006) *Attention deficit hyperactivity disorder: A handbook for diagnosis and treatment*. (3rd ed.) New York: Guilford Press.

Bates, E. (1976) *Language in context: The acquisition of pragmatics*. New York: Academic Press.

Bates, E., Dale, P., & Thal, D. (1995) 'Individual differences and their implications for theories of language development', in Fletcher, P. & MacWhinney, B. (eds.) *Handbook of Child Language*. Oxford: Basil Blackwell, pp. 96–151.

Bates, E., & Dick, F. (2002) 'Language, gesture, and the developing brain', *Developmental Psychobiology*, 40(3), pp. 293–310.

Bates, E., Thal, D., Finlay, B., & Clancy, B. (2003) 'Early language development and its neural correlates', in Rapin, I. & Segalowitz, S. (eds.) *Handbook of Neuropsychology*. Vol. 8: Child Neurology (2nd ed.) Amsterdam: Elsevier, pp. 109–176.

Bee, H., & Boyd, D. (2019) *Lifespan development*. Harlow: Pearson Education Ltd.

Bergelson, E., & Swingley, D. (2015) 'Early word comprehension in infants: Replication and extension', *Language Learning and Development*, 11(4), pp. 69–380.

Bishop, D.V.M., Snowling, M.J., Thompson, P.A., Greenhalgh, T., & the CATALISE-2 consortium. (2017) 'Phase 2 of CATALISE: A multinational and multidisciplinary Delphi consensus study of problems with language development: Terminology', *Journal of Child Psychology & Psychiatry*, 58(10), pp. 1068–1080.

Black, M.M., & Rollins, H.A. (1982) 'The effects of instructional variables on young children's organization and free recall', *Journal of Experimental Child Psychology*, 33(1), pp. 1–19.

Bloom, K. (1988). 'Quality of adult vocalizations affects the quality of infant vocalizations', *Journal of Child Language*, 15(3), pp. 469–480.

Bloom, L. (1973) *One word at a time: The use of single-word utterances before syntax*. The Hague: Mouton.

Bloom, L., & Lahey, M. (1978) *Language development and language disorders*. New York: John Wiley & Sons.

Bloom, L., Lightbown, P., Hood, L., Bowerman, M., Maratsos, M., & Maratsos, M. (1975) 'Structure and variation in child language', *Monographs of the Society for Research in Child Development*, 40(2), pp. 1–97.

Booth, A.E. (2009) 'Causal supports for early word learning', *Child Development*, 80(4), pp.1243–1250.

Borg, E., Risberg, A., McAllister, B., Undemar, B.M., Edquist, G., Reinholdson, A.C., & Willstedt-Svensson, U. (2002) 'Language development in hearing-impaired children. Establishment of a reference material for a "language test for hearing-impaired children," LATHIC', *International Journal of Pediatric Otorhinolaryngology*, 65(1), pp. 15–26.

Brady, T.F., Störmer, V.S., Shafer-Skelton, A., Williams, J.R., Chapman, A.F., & Schill, H.M., (2019) 'Scaling up visual attention and visual working memory to the real world', *Psychology of Learning and Motivation, Academic Press*, 70, pp. 29–69.

Braine, M.D.S. (1963) 'On learning the grammatical order of words', *Psychology Review*, 70(4), pp. 323–348.

Brignell, A., Williams, K., Jachno, K., Prior, M., Reilly, S., & Morgan, A.T. (2018) 'Patterns and predictors of language development from 4 to 7 years in verbal children with and without autism spectrum disorder', *Journal of Autism & Developmental Disorders*, 48, pp. 3282–3295.

Broen, P. (1972) 'The verbal environment of the language-learning child', *Monographs of the American Speech & Hearing Association*, 17, pp. 1–96.

Brown, R. (1973) *A first language: The early stages*. London: Allen & Unwin.

Bruner, J. (1975) 'The ontogenesis of speech acts', *Journal of Child Language*, 2, pp. 1–19.

BSA. (2018) *Position statement & practice guidance – auditory processing disorder (APD)*. Available online at: www.thebsa.org.uk/wp-content/uploads/2018/02/Position-Statement-and-Practice-Guidance-APD-2018.pdf

Buckley, B. (2003) *Children's communication skills: From birth to five years*. London: Routledge.

Caballo, C., & Verdugo, M. (2007) 'Social skills assessment of children and adolescents with visual impairment: Identifying relevant skills to improve quality of social relationships', *Psychological Reports*, 100, pp. 1101–1106.

Cai, T., & McPherson, B. (2017) 'Hearing loss in children with otitis media with effusion: A systematic review', *International Journal of Audiology*, 56(2), pp. 65–76.

Carter, A.L. (1979) 'Pre-speech meaning relations: An outline of one infant's sensorimotor development', in Fletcher, P. & Garman, M. (eds.) *Language acquisition: studies in first language development*. Cambridge: Cambridge University Press, pp. 71–92.

Choudhury, N., & Gorman, K.S. (2000) 'The relationship between sustained attention and cognitive performance in 17–24-month-olds', *Infant and Child Development*, 9, pp. 127–146.

Clark, E.V. (1970) 'How young children describe events in time', in Flores D'arcais, G.B. & Levelt, W.J.M. (eds.) *Advances in psycholinguistics*. Amsterdam: North-Holland Publishing Co., pp. 275–284.

Clark, E.V. (2016) *First language acquisition*. (3rd ed.) Cambridge: Cambridge University Press.

Clark, E.V. (2017) *Language in children*. London: Routledge & Linguistic Society of America.

Clark, E.V. (2018) 'Conversation and language acquisition: A pragmatic approach', *Language Learning and Development*, 14(3), pp. 170–185.

Cleave, P.L., Becker, S.D., Curran, M.K., Van Horne, A.J., & Fey, M.E. (2015) 'The efficacy of recasts in language intervention: A systematic review and meta-analysis', *American Journal of Speech-Language Pathology*, 4(2), pp. 237–55.

Cole, P. (1982) *Language disorders in children*. Englewood Cliffs, NJ: Prentice-Hall.

Cooper, J., Moodley, M., & Reynell, J. (1974) 'Intervention programmes for preschool children with delayed language development. A preliminary report', *British Journal of Disorders of Communication*, 9(2), pp. 81–91.

Cromer, R. (1974) 'The Development of Language and Cognition: The cognition hypothesis', in Foss, B. (ed.) *New perspectives in child development*. New York: Penguin.

Crystal, D., Fletcher, P., & Garman, M. (1976) *The grammatical analysis of language disability: A procedure for assessment and remediation*. (2nd ed.) London: Edward Arnold.

de Villiers, J., & de Villiers, P. (1978) *Language acquisition*. Cambridge, MA: Harvard University Press.

Delack, J.B. (1976) 'Aspects of infant speech development in the first year of life', *Canadian Journal of Linguistics*, 21, pp. 17–37.

Deluzio, J., & Girolametto, L. (2011) 'Peer interactions of preschool children with and without hearing loss', *Journal of Speech, Language, & Hearing Research*, 54, pp. 1197–1210.

Department for Education. (2021) *Statutory framework for the early years foundation stage*. Available at: www.gov.uk/government/publications/early-years-foundation-stage-framework-2

Dickinson, D.K., Golinkoff, R.M., & Hirsh-Pasek, K. (2010) 'Speaking out for language: Why language is central to reading development', *Educational Researcher*, 39(4), pp. 305–310.

Dockrell, J. (2019) 'Language learning challenges in the early years', in Whitebread, D., Grau, V., & Kumpulainen, K. (eds.) *The SAGE handbook of developmental psychology and early childhood education*. London: Sage Publishing, pp. 435–452.

Dockrell, J.E., & Shield, B.M. (2006) 'Acoustical barriers in classrooms: The impact of noise on performance in the classroom', *British Educational Research Journal*, 32(3), pp. 509–525.

Dore, J. (1974) 'A pragmatic description of early language development', *Journal of Psycholinguistic Research*, pp. 343–350.

Ebert, K.D., & Kohnert, K. (2011) 'Sustained attention in children with primary language impairment: A meta-analysis', *Journal of Speech, Language, and Hearing Research*, 54(5), pp. 1372–1384.

Elmlinger, S.L., Schwade, J.A., & Goldstein, M.H. (2019) 'The ecology of prelinguistic vocal learning: Parents simplify the structure of their speech in response to babbling', *Journal of Child Language*, 16, pp. 1–14.

Erickson, L.C., & Newman, R.S. (2017) 'Influences of background noise on infants and children', *Current Directions in Psychological Science*, 26(5), pp. 451–457.

Esteve-Gilbert, N., & Prieto, P. (2014) 'Infants temporally coordinate gesture-speech combinations before they produce their first words', *Speech Communication*, 57, pp. 301–316.

Fagan, M.K. (2009) 'Mean length of utterance before words and grammar: Longitudinal trends and developmental implications of infant vocalizations', *Journal of Child Language*, 36(3), pp. 495–527.

Fagan, M.K. (2014) 'Frequency of vocalization before and after cochlear implantation: Dynamic effect of auditory feedback on infant behavior', *Journal of Experimental Child Psychology*, 126, pp. 328–338.

Feldman, R., & Eidelman, A.I. (2006) 'Neonatal state organization, neuromaturation, mother-infant interaction, and cognitive development in small-for-gestational-age premature infants', *Pediatrics* 118(3), pp. 869–878.

Fenson, L., Dale, P., Reznick, J., Bates, E., Thal, D., & Pethick, J. (1994) 'Variability in early communication development', *Monographs of the Society for Research in Child Development*, 59(5), pp. 1–185.

Fenson, L., Marchman, V.A., Thal, D.J., Dale, P.S., Reznick, J.S., & Bates, E. (2007) *Macarthur-bates communicative development inventories (cdi): Words and gestures*. Baltimore, MD: Brookes Publishing.

Franklin, B., Warlaumont, A.S., Messinger, D., Bene, E., Iyer, S.N., Lee, C.C., Lambert, B., & Oller, D.K. (2014) 'Effects of parental interaction on infant vocalization rate, variability and vocal type', *Language Learning & Development: The Official Journal of the Society for Language Development*, 10(3), pp. 279–296.

Frizelle, P., Harte, J., O'Sullivan, K., Fletcher, P., & Gibbon, F. (2017) 'The relationship between information carrying words, memory and language skills in school age children with specific language impairment', *PLOS one*, 12, p. e0180496.

Gill, C.B., Klecan-Aker, J., Roberts, T., & Fredenburg, K.A. (2003) 'Following directions: Rehearsal and visualisation strategies for children with specific language impairment', *Child Language Teaching and Therapy*, 19, pp. 85–104.

Gillham, B. (1979) *The first words language programme*. London: Croom Helm.

Gnanavel, S., Sharma, P., Kaushal, P., & Hussain, S. (2019) 'Attention deficit hyperactivity disorder and comorbidity: A review of literature', *World Journal of Clinical Cases*, 7(17), pp. 2420–2426.

Goldin-Meadow, S., Goodrich, W., Sauer, E., & Iverson, J. (2007) 'Young children use their hands to tell their mothers what to say', *Developmental Science*, 10(6), pp. 778–785.

Gomes, H., Molholm, S., Christodolou, C., Ritter, W., & Cowan, N. (2000) 'The development of auditory attention in children', *Frontiers in Bioscience*, 5, pp. 108–120.

Gratier, M., Devouche, E., Guellai, B., Infanti, R., Yilmaz, E., & Parlato-Oliveira, E. (2015) 'Early development of turn-taking in vocal interaction between mothers and infants', *Frontiers in Psychology*, 6, p. 1167.

Green, B.C., Johnson, K.A., & Bretherton, L. (2014) 'Pragmatic language difficulties in children with hyperactivity and attention problems: An integrated review', *International Journal of Language & Communication Disorders*, 49, pp. 15–29.

Hadley, E.B., Dickinson, D.K., Hirsh-Pasek, K., Golinkoff, R.M., & Nesbitt, K.T. (2016) 'Examining the acquisition of vocabulary knowledge depth among preschool students', *Reading Research Quarterly*, 51(2), pp. 181–198.

Halliday, M.A.K. (1975) *Learning how to mean: Explorations in the development of language*. London: Edward Arnold.

Halliday, M.A.K. (2004) *Language of early childhood (Vol.4)*. Edited by Jonathan J. Webster. London: Bloomsbury Publishing PLC.

Heft, H. (1979) 'Background and focal environmental conditions of the home and attention in young children', *Journal of Applied Social Psychology*, 9, pp. 47–69.

Hendry, A., Jones, E.J.H., & Charman, T. (2016) 'Executive function in the first three years of life: Precursors, predictors and patterns', *Developmental Review*, 42, pp. 1–33.

Hoff, E. (2006) 'How social contexts support and shape language development', *Developmental Review*, 26(1), pp. 55–88.

Hoff, E. (2013) 'Interpreting the early language trajectories of children from low-SES and language minority homes: Implications for closing achievement gaps', *Developmental Psychology*, 49(1), pp. 4–14.

Hood, L.H. (1977) 'A longitudinal study of the development of the expression of causal relations in complex sentences', *Dissertation Abstracts International*, 38(5-B), pp. 2341–2342.

Houston-Price, C., Plunkett, K., & Duy, H. (2006) 'The use of social and salience cues in early word learning', *Journal of Experimental Child Psychology*, 95, pp. 27–55.

Howard, J. (2019) 'Securing the future of play in early childhood education: Journeying with children toward the essence of play to evidence its function and value', in Whitebread, D., Grau, V. & Kumpulainen, K. (eds.) *The SAGE handbook of developmental psychology and early childhood education*. London: Sage publishing, pp. 201–222.

Hudry, K., Leadbitter, K., Temple, K., Slonims, V., McConachie, H., Aldred, C., Howlin, P., & Charman, T., Pact Consortium, (2010) 'Preschoolers with autism show greater impairment in receptive compared with expressive language abilities', *International Journal of Language & Communication Disorders*, 45(6), pp. 81–90.

Humphreys, K.L., Machlin, L.S., Guyon-Harris, K.L., Nelson, C.A., Fox, N.A., & Zeanah, C.H. (2020) 'Psychosocial deprivation and receptive language ability: A two-sample study', *Journal of Neurodevelopmental Disorders*, 12(1), p. 36.

Iverson, J.M., & Fagan, M.K. (2004) 'Infant vocal-motor coordination: Precursor to the gesture-speech system?' *Child Development*, 75(4), pp. 1053–1066.

Iyer, S.N., & Oller, D.K. (2008) 'Prelinguistic vocal development in infants with typical hearing and infants with severe-to-profound hearing loss', *The Volta Review*, 108(2), pp. 115–138.

Jackson, E., Leitão, S., Claessen, M., & Boyes, M. (2019) 'The evaluation of word-learning abilities in people with developmental language disorder: A scoping review', *International Journal of Language and Communication Disorders*, 54(5), pp. 742–755.

Jeffree, D., McConkey, R., & Hewson, S. (1977) *Let Me Play*. London: Human Horizons Series, Souvenir Press.

Jones, G., & Rowland, C.F. (2017) 'Diversity not quantity in caregiver speech: Using computational modeling to isolate the effects of the quantity and the diversity of the input on vocabulary growth', *Cognitive Psychology*, 98, pp. 1–21.

Kannass, K.N., Colombo, J., & Wyss, N. (2010) 'Now, pay attention! The effects of instruction on children's attention', *Journal of Cognition and Development: Official Journal of the Cognitive Development Society*, 11(4), pp. 509–532.

Kim, S.H., Paul, R., Tager-Flushberg, H., & Lord, C. (2014) 'Language and communication in autism', in Volkmar, F.R., Rogers, S.J., Paul, R., & Pelphry, K.A. (eds.) *Handbook of autism and pervasive developmental disorders*. (4th ed.) Hoboken, NJ: Wiley, pp. 230–262.

Knowles, W., & Masidlover, M. (1982) *The Derbyshire Language Scheme*. Derby: Derbyshire County Council.

Koehlinger, K.M., Van Horne, A.J., & Moeller, M.P. (2013) 'Grammatical outcomes of 3- and 6- year-old children who are hard of hearing', *Journal of Speech, Language, and Hearing Research*, 56(5), pp. 1701–1714.

Kröger, T., & Nupponen, A-M. (2019) 'Puppet as a pedagogical tool: A literature review', *International Electronic Journal of Elementary Education*, 11(4), pp. 393–401.

Lahey, M. (1988) *Language disorders and language development*. (Rev. ed.) New York: Macmillan.

Lang, S., Bartl-Pokorny, K.D., Pokorny, F.B., Garrido, D., Mani, N., Fox-Boyer, A.V., Zhang, D., & Marschik, P.B. (2019) 'Canonical babbling: A marker for earlier identification of late detected developmental disorders?', *Current Developmental Disorders Report*, 6, pp. 111–118.

Leonard, L. (2014) 'Specific language impairment across languages', *Child Development Perspectives*, 8(1), pp. 1–5.

Leslie, A.M. (1987) 'Pretence and representation: The origins of 'theory of mind'', *Psychological Review*, 94, pp. 412–426.

Lüke, C., Ritterfeld, U., Grimminger, A., Liszkowski, U., & Rohlfing, K.J. (2017) 'Development of pointing gestures in children with typical and delayed language acquisition', *Journal of Speech, Language, and Hearing Research*, 60(11), pp. 3185–3197.

Manlove, E.E., Frank, T., & Vernon-Feagans, L. (2001) 'Why should we care about noise in classrooms and child care settings?', *Child & Youth Care Forum*, 30, pp. 55–64.

Massey-Abernathy, A.R., & Haseltine, E. (2019) 'Power talk: Communication styles, vocalization rates and dominance', *Journal of Psycholinguist Research*, 48, pp. 107–116.

McCune, L., & Vihman, M.M. (2001) 'Early phonetic and lexical development: A productivity approach', *Journal of Speech, Language, & Hearing Research*, 44(3), pp. 670–684.

McDade, H.L, (1981) 'A parent-child interactional model for assessing and remediating language disabilities', *British Journal for Disorders of Communication*, 16(3), pp. 175–183.

McNeil, N., Alibali, M., & Evans, J. (2000) 'The role of gesture in children's comprehension of spoken language: Now they need it, now they don't', *Journal of Nonverbal Behavior*, 24, pp. 131–150.

Mirsky, A., Anthony, B., Duncan, C., Ahearn, M., & Kellam, S. (1991) 'Analysis of the elements of attention: A neuropsychological approach', *Neuropsychology Review*, 2, pp. 109–145.

Moore, D.R. (2018) 'Editorial: Auditory processing disorder', *Ear & Hearing*, 39(4), pp. 617–620.

Morgan, L., & Wren, Y.E. (2018) 'A systematic review of the literature on early vocalizations and babbling patterns in young children', *Communication Disorders Quarterly*, 40(1), pp. 3–14.

Morgan, P.L., Farkas, G., Hillemeier, M.M., Hammer, C.S., & Maczuga, S. (2015) '24-Month-old children with larger oral vocabularies display greater academic and behavioral functioning at kindergarten entry', *Child Development*, 86(5), pp. 1351–1370.

Naber, F.B.A., Swinkels, S.H.N., Buitelaar, J.K., Dietz, C., van Daalen, E., & Bakermans-Kramerburg, M.J. (2007) 'Joint attention and attachment in toddlers with autism', *European Child & Adolescent Psychiatry*, 17, pp. 143–152.

Nakazima, S. (1975) 'Phonemicisation and symbolisation in language Development', in Lenneberg, E.H. & Lenneberg, E. (eds.) *Foundations of language: A multidisciplinary approach: Vol 1*. New York: Academic Press, pp. 181–187.

Nassrallah, F., Fitzpatrick, E.M., Whittingham, J.A., Sun, H., Na, E., & Grandpierre, V. (2020) 'A descriptive study of language and literacy skills of early school-aged children with unilateral and mild to moderate bilateral hearing loss', *Deafness & Education International*, 22(1), pp. 74–92.

Nathani, S., Ertmer, D.J., & Stark, R.E. (2006) 'Assessing vocal development in infants and toddlers', *Clinical Linguistics & Phonetics*, 20(5), pp. 351–369.

National Autistic Society. (2021) 'What is autism?'. Available at: www.autism.org.uk/advice-and-guidance/what-is-autism

National Deaf Children's Society. (2017) 'Glue ear'. Available at: www.ndcs.org.uk/information-and-support/childhood-deafness/causes-of-deafness/glue-ear/

Neijenhuis, K., Campbell, N.G., Cromb, M., Luinge, M.R., Moore, D.R., Rosen, S., & de Wit, E. (2019) 'An evidence-based perspective on "misconceptions" regarding pediatric auditory processing disorder', *Frontiers in Neurology*, 10(287).

Nomikou, I., Rohlfing, K.J., & Szufnarowska, J. (2013) 'Educating attention: Recruiting, maintaining and framing eye contact in early natural mother-infant interactions', *Interaction Studies*, 14, pp. 240–267.

Norbury, C.F., Gooch, D., Wray, C., Baird, G., Charman, T., Simonoff, E., Vamvakas, G., & Pickles, A. (2016) 'The impact of nonverbal ability on prevalence and clinical presentation of language disorder: Evidence from a population study', *Journal of Child Psychology and Psychiatry*, 57(11), pp. 1247–1257.

Ogundele, M.O. (2018) 'Behavioural and emotional disorders in childhood: A brief overview for paediatricians', *World Journal of Clinical Pediatrics*, 7(1), pp. 9–26.

Oller, D.K., Caskey, M., Yoo, H., Bene, E.R., Jhang, Y., Lee, C.C., Bowman, D.D., Long, H.L., Buder, E.H., & Vohr, B. (2019) 'Preterm and full term infant vocalization and the origin of language', *Scientific Reports*, 9(1), p. 14734.

Oller, K.D. (2000) *The emergence of the speech capacity*. Mahwah, NJ: Lawrence Erlbaum.

Operto, F.F., Pastorino, G., Marciano, J., de Simone, V., Volini, A.P., Olivieri, M., Buonaiuto, R., Vetri, L., Viggiano, A., & Coppola, G. (2020) 'Digital devices use and language skills in children between 8 and 36 months', *Brain Sciences*, 10(9), p. 656.

Orr, E. (2020) 'Object play as a mediator of the role of exploration in communication skills development', *Infant Behaviour and Development*, 60, p. 101467.

Ouellette, G.P. (2006) 'What's meaning got to do with it: The role of vocabulary in word reading and reading comprehension', *Journal of Educational Psychology*, 98(3), pp. 554–566.

Paul, R. (1981) 'Analyzing complex sentences development', in Miller, J.F. (ed.) *Assessing language production in children*. Baltimore: University Park Press, pp. 36–40.

Paul, R., Norbury, C., & Gosse, C. (2018) *Language disorders from infancy through adolescence: listening, speaking, reading, writing, and communicating*. (5th ed.) Missouri, USA: Mosby.

Petersen, S.E., & Posner, M.I. (2012) 'The attention system of the human brain: 20 years after', *Annual Review of Neuroscience*, 35, pp. 73–89.

Piaget, J. (1929) *The child's conception of the world*. London: Kegan Paul, Trench & Trubner & Co.

Piaget, J. (1962) 'The stages of the intellectual development of the child', *Bulletin of the Menninger Clinic*, 26(3), pp. 120–128.

Posner, M.I. (2016) 'Orienting of attention: Then and now', *Quarterly Journal of Experimental Psychology*, 69(10), pp. 1864–1875.

Quinn, S., Donnelly, S., & Kidd, E. (2018) 'The relationship between symbolic play and language acquisition: A meta-analytic review', *Developmental Review*, 49, pp. 121–135.

Rączaszek-Leonardi, J., Nomikou, I., & Rohlfing, K. (2013) 'Young children's dialogical actions: The beginnings of purposeful intersubjectivity', *IEEE Transactions on Autonomous Mental Development*, 5(3), pp. 210–221.

Rahn, N., Coogle, C., & Ottley, J. (2019) 'Early childhood special education teachers' use of embedded learning opportunities within classroom routines and activities', *Infants & Young Children*, 32, pp. 3–19.

RCSLT, (2020) RCSLT briefing paper on 'Language disorder with a specific focus on developmental language disorder'. Available at: www.rcslt.org/wp-content/uploads/media/docs/Covid/language-disorder-briefing-paper-with-edit.pdf?la=en&hash=98B6A1E60824DEE9D52CCDFFACCE5EE6D67749D9

Rettig, M. (1998) 'Environmental influences on the play of young children with disabilities', *Education and Training in Mental Retardation and Developmental Disabilities*, 33(2), pp. 189–194.

Reyna, B.A., & Pickler, R.H. (2009) 'Mother – infant synchrony during infant feeding', *Infant Behavior and Development*, 38(4), pp. 470–477.

Reynell, J. (1977) *Reynell Developmental Language Scales*. (Rev. ed.). Windsor: NFER Publishing Company Ltd.

Reynell, J. (1980) *Language Development and Assessment*. London: Edward Arnold.

Rice, M.L., & Hoffman, L. (2015) 'Predicting vocabulary growth in children with and without specific language impairment: A longitudinal study from 2; 6 to 21 years of age', *Journal of Speech, Language, Hearing Research*, 58(2), pp. 345–359.

RNIB, (2021) 'Education and children, young people and families research'. Available at: www.rnib.org.uk/professionals/knowledge-and-research-hub/research-reports/education-research

Roseberry, S., Hirsh-Pasek, K., Parish-Morris, J., & Golinkoff, R.M. (2009) 'Live action: Can young children learn verbs from video?', *Child Development*, 80(5), pp. 1360–1375.

Ross, M.C. (2017) *Promoting joint attention in children with visual impairment: Proposing an intervention using modified strategies from joint attention symbolic play engagement regulation (JASPER)*. PhD thesis. The Ohio State University. Available at: https://etd.ohiolink.edu/apexprod/rws_olink/r/1501/10?clear=10&p10_accession_num=osu1500289755492111 (Accessed 31/12/2020).

Rowe, M.L. (2008) 'Child-directed speech: Relation to socioeconomic status, knowledge of child development and child vocabulary skill', *Journal of Child Language*, 35(1), pp. 185–205.

Rowe, M.L., Ozçalişkan. S., & Goldin-Meadow. S. (2008) 'Learning words by hand: Gesture's role in predicting vocabulary development', *First Language*, 28(2), pp. 182–199.

Rutter, M., & Martin, J. (eds) (1972) *The child with delayed speech*. London: William Heinemann Medical Books.

Schneider, R., Yurovsky, D., & Frank, M.C. (2015) 'Large-scale investigations of variability in children's first words', *Proceedings of the 37th Annual Meeting of the Cognitive Science Society*, Pasadena, California, 22–25 July. Austin, TX: Cognitive Science Society, pp. 2110–2115.

Schulz, L.E., Gopnik, A., & Glymour, C. (2007) 'Preschool children learn about causal structure from conditional interventions', *Developmental Science*, 10, pp. 322–332.

Sharma, A., & Cockerill, H. (2014) *Mary Sheridan's from birth to five years: Children's developmental progress*. (4th ed.) Abingdon, Oxon: Routledge.

Shield, B.M., & Dockrell, J.E. (2003) 'The effects of noise on children at school: A review', *Journal of Building Acoustics*, 10(2), pp. 97–106.

Singer Harris, N.G.S., Bellugi, U., Bates, E., Jones, W., & Rossen, M. (1997) 'Contrasting profiles of language development in children with Williams and Down syndromes', *Developmental Neuropsychology*, 13(3), pp. 345–370.

Sleigh, G. (1972) 'A study of some symbolic processes in young children', *British Journal of Disorders of Communication*, 7, pp. 163–175.

Slocum, S.K., & Tiger, J.H. (2011) 'An assessment of the efficiency of and child preference for forward and backward chaining', *Journal of Applied Behavior Analysis*, 44(4), pp. 793–805.

Smith, B., Brown-Sweeney, S., & Stoel-Gammon, C. (1989) 'A quantitative analysis of reduplicated and variegated babbling', *First Language*, 9, pp. 175–189.

Snow, C. (1972) 'Mother's speech to children learning language', *Child Development*, 43, pp. 549–565.

Snow, C. (1977) 'The development of conversation between mothers and babies', *Journal of Child Language*, 4(1), pp. 1–22.

Soderburgh, R. (1974) 'The fruitful dialogue: The child's acquisition of his first language: Implications for education at all stages', *Project Child Language Syntax*, reprint No 2, Stockholm: Stockholm University.

St. Clair-Thompson, H.L., & Holmes, J. (2008) 'Improving short-term and working memory: Methods of memory training', in Johansen, N.B. (ed.) *New research on short-term memory*. New York: Nova Science, pp. 125–154.

Stark, R.E. (1980) 'Stages of speech development in the first year of life', in Yeni-Komshian, G., Kavanagh, J., & Ferguson, CA. (eds.) *Child phonology: Vol.1, Production*. New York: Academic Press, pp. 73–90.

Steffani, S.A., & Dachtyl, L.A. (2007) 'Identifying embedded and conjoined complex sentences: Making it simple', *Contemporary Issues in Communication Science and Disorders*, 34, pp. 44–54.

Stern, D. (1974) 'Mother and infant at play: The dyadic interaction involving facial, vocal and gaze behaviors', in Lewis, M. & Rosenblum, L.A. (eds.) *The effect of the infant on its caregiver*. New York: John Wiley & Sons, pp. 187–213.

Stern, D. (1977) *The First Relationship: Infant and mother*. Cambridge, MA: Harvard University press.

Taylor, C.L., Christensen, D., Lawrence, D., Mitrou, F., & Zubrick, S.R. (2013) 'Risk factors for children's receptive vocabulary development from four to eight years in the longitudinal study of Australian children', *PLoS One*, 8(9), p. e73046.

Thiemann-Bourque, K., Johnson, L.K., & Brady, N.C. (2019) 'Similarities in functional play and differences in symbolic play of children with autism spectrum disorder', *American Journal on Intellectual and Developmental Disabilities*, 124(1), pp. 77–91.

Tomblin, J.B., Harrison, M., Ambrose, S.E., Walker, E.A., Oleson, J.J., & Moeller, M.P. (2015) 'Language outcomes in young children with mild to severe hearing loss', *Ear and Hearing*, 36, pp. 76S-91S.

Umiker-Sebeok, D.J. (1979) 'Preschool children's intraconversational narratives', *Journal of Child Language*, 6(1), pp. 91–109.

van den Broek, E.G.C., van Eijden, A.J.P.M., Overbeek, M.M., Kef, S., Sterkenburg, P.S., & Schuengel, C. (2017) 'A systematic review of the literature on parenting of young children with visual impairments and the adaptions for video-feedback intervention to promote positive parenting (VIPP)', *Journal of Developmental & Physical Disabilities*, 29(3), pp. 503–545.

van den Heuvel, M., Ma, J., Borkhoff, C.M., Koroshegyi, C., Dai, D.W.H., Parkin, P.C., Maguire, J.L., Birken, C.S., & TARGet Kids! Collaboration. (2019) 'Mobile media device use is associated with expressive language delay in 18-month-old children', *Journal of Developmental Behavioral Pediatrics*, 40(2), pp. 99–104.

Venuti, P., de Falco, S., Esposito, G., & Bornstein, M.H. (2009) 'Mother-child play: Children with Down syndrome and typical development', *American Journal on Intellectual and Developmental Disabilities*, 114(4), pp. 274–288.

Vygotsky, L.S. (1977) 'Play and its role in the mental development of the child', in Cole, M. (ed.) *Soviet Developmental Psychology*. White Plains, NY: M.E. Sharpe, pp. 76–99.

Weisberg, D., Zosh, J., Hirsh-Pasek, K., & Golinkoff, R. (2013) 'Talking it up: Play, language, and the role of adult support', *American Journal of Play*, 6, pp. 39–54.

Weisburg, P. (1963) 'Social and non-social conditioning of infant vocalisations', *Child Development*, 34, pp. 377–388.

Weiss, C.E., & Lillywhite, H.S. (1981) *Communicative Disorders: Prevention and early intervention*. (2nd ed.) Missouri, USA: C.V. Mosby Company.

Whitebread, D., Neale, D., Jensen, H., Liu, C., Solis, S.L., Hopkins, E., Hirsh-Pasek, K., & Zosh, J.M. (2017) *The role of play in children's development: A review of the evidence*. Billund, Denmark: The LEGO Foundation.

Wie, O.B., Torkildsen, J.V.K., Schauber, S., Busch, T., & Litovsky, R. (2020) 'Long-term language development in children with early simultaneous bilateral cochlear implants', *Ear and Hearing*, 41(5), pp. 1294–1305.

Winsler, A., Carlton, M.P., & Barry, M.J. (2000) 'Age-related changes in preschool children's systematic use of private speech in a natural setting', *Journal of Child Language*, 27, pp. 665–687.

Xiaoxue He, A., Maxwell, K., & Arunachalam, S. (2020). 'Linguistic context in verb learning: Less is sometimes more', *Language Learning and Development*, 16(1), pp. 22–42.

Zauche, L.H., Thul, T.A., Mahoney, D.A.E., & Stapel-Wax, J.L. (2016) 'Influence of language nutrition on children's language and cognitive development: An integrated review', *Early Childhood Research Quarterly*, 36, pp. 318–333.

Index